Lecture Notes in Computer Science 11046

Commenced Publication in 1973
Founding and Former Series Editors:
Gerhard Goos, Juris Hartmanis, and Jan van Leeuwen

More information about this series at http://www.springer.com/series/7412

Yinghuan Shi · Heung-Il Suk
Mingxia Liu (Eds.)

Machine Learning in Medical Imaging

9th International Workshop, MLMI 2018
Held in Conjunction with MICCAI 2018
Granada, Spain, September 16, 2018
Proceedings

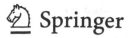 Springer

Editors
Yinghuan Shi
Nanjing University
Nanjing
China

Mingxia Liu
University of North Carolina at Chapel Hill
Chapel Hill, NC
USA

Heung-Il Suk
Korea University
Seoul
Korea (Republic of)

ISSN 0302-9743   ISSN 1611-3349 (electronic)
Lecture Notes in Computer Science
ISBN 978-3-030-00918-2   ISBN 978-3-030-00919-9 (eBook)
https://doi.org/10.1007/978-3-030-00919-9

Library of Congress Control Number: 2018954931

LNCS Sublibrary: SL6 – Image Processing, Computer Vision, Pattern Recognition, and Graphics

This Springer imprint is published by the registered company Springer Nature Switzerland AG
The registered company address is: Gewerbestrasse 11, 6330 Cham, Switzerland

Preface

The 9th International Workshop on Machine Learning in Medical Imaging (MLMI 2018) was held in Granada, Spain, on September 16, 2018, in conjunction with the 21st International Conference on Medical Image Computing and Computer-Assisted Intervention (MICCAI).

In recent years, machine learning is playing an essential role in the medical imaging field, including computer-assisted diagnosis, image segmentation, image registration, image fusion, image-guided therapy, image annotation, and image database retrieval. With advances in medical imaging, new imaging modalities and methodologies, as well as new machine learning algorithms/applications, are taking center stage in medical imaging. Owing to large inter-subject variations and complexities, it is generally difficult to derive analytic formulations or simple equations to represent objects such as lesions and anatomy in medical images. Therefore, tasks in medical imaging require learning from patient data for heuristics and prior knowledge, in order to facilitate the detection/diagnosis of abnormalities in medical images.

The main aim of the MLMI 2018 workshop was to help advance scientific research within the broad field of machine learning in medical imaging. The workshop focused on major trends and challenges in this area, and presented works aimed to identify new cutting-edge techniques and their use in medical imaging. We hope that the MLMI workshop becomes an important platform for translating research from the bench to the bedside.

The range and level of submissions for this year's meeting were of very high quality. Authors were asked to submit full-length papers for review. A total of 82 papers were submitted to the workshop in response to the call for papers. Each of the 82 papers underwent a rigorous double-blinded peer-review process, with each paper being reviewed by at least two reviewers from the Program Committee, composed of 50 well-known experts in the field. Based on the reviewing scores and critiques, the 46 best papers (56%) were accepted for presentation at the workshop and chosen to be included in this Springer LNCS volume. The large variety of machine-learning techniques applied to medical imaging were well represented at the workshop.

We are grateful to the Program Committee for reviewing the submitted papers and giving constructive comments and critiques, to the authors for submitting high-quality papers, to the presenters for excellent presentations, and to all the MLMI 2018 attendees coming to Granada from all around the world.

August 2018

Yinghuan Shi
Heung-Il Suk
Mingxia Liu

Organization

Workshop Organizers

Yinghuan Shi   Nanjing University, China
Heung-Il Suk   Korea University, Republic of Korea
Mingxia Liu   University of North Carolina at Chapel Hill, USA

Steering Committee

Dinggang Shen   University of North Carolina at Chapel Hill, USA
Pingkun Yan   Philips Research North America, USA
Kenji Suzuki   Illinois Institute of Technology, USA and World
         Research Hub Initiative, Tokyo Institute of
         Technology, Japan
Fei Wang   AliveCor Inc., USA

Program Committee

Amin Zarshenas   Illinois Institute of Technology, USA
Antonios Makropoulos   Imperial College London, UK
Chunfeng Lian   University of North Carolina at Chapel Hill, USA
Francesco Ciompi   Radboud University Medical Center, The Netherlands
Gang Li   University of North Carolina at Chapel Hill, USA
Gerard Sanrom   Pompeu Fabra University, Spain
Ghassan Hamarneh   Simon Fraser University, Canada
Guoyan Zheng   University of Bern, Switzerland
Hanbo Chen   University of Georgia, USA
Heang-Ping Chan   University of Michigan Medical Center, USA
Holger Roth   NVIDIA
Hoo-Chang Shin   National Institutes of Health, USA
Jaeil Kim   Kyungpook National University, Republic of Korea
Janne Nappi   Massachusetts General Hospital, USA
Jong-Hwan Lee   Korea University, Republic of Korea
Jun Zhang   University of North Carolina at Chapel Hill, USA
Junchi Liu   Illinois Institute of Technology, USA
Jurgen Fripp   Australian e-Health Research Centre
Kelei He   Nanjing University, China
Ken'ichi Morooka   Kyushu University, Japan
Kilian Pohl   SRI International, USA
Kim-Han Thung   University of North Carolina at Chapel Hill, USA
Li Shen   University of Pennsylvania, USA
Li Wang   University of North Carolina at Chapel Hill, USA

Contents

Developing Novel Weighted Correlation Kernels for Convolutional Neural Networks to Extract Hierarchical Functional Connectivities from fMRI for Disease Diagnosis

Biao Jie[1,2], Mingxia Liu[1], Chunfeng Lian[1], Feng Shi[3], and Dinggang Shen[1(✉)]

[1] Department of Radiology and BRIC, University of North Carolina at Chapel Hill, Chapel Hill, NC 27599, USA
dgshen@med.unc.edu
[2] Department of Computer Science and Technology, Anhui Normal University, Anhui 241003, China
[3] Shanghai United Imaging Intelligence Co., Ltd., Shanghai 201807, China

Abstract. Functional magnetic resonance imaging (fMRI) has been widely applied to analysis and diagnosis of brain diseases, including Alzheimer's disease (AD) and its prodrome, *i.e.*, mild cognitive impairment (MCI). Traditional methods usually construct connectivity networks (CNs) by simply calculating Pearson correlation coefficients (PCCs) between time series of brain regions, and then extract low-level network measures as features to train the learning model. However, the valuable observation information in network construction (*e.g.*, specific contributions of different time points) and high-level (*i.e.*, high-order) network properties are neglected in these methods. In this paper, we first define a novel weighted correlation kernel (called wc-kernel) to measure the correlation of brain regions, by which weighting factors are determined in a data-driven manner to characterize the contribution of each time point, thus conveying the richer interaction information of brain regions compared with the PCC method. Furthermore, we propose a wc-kernel based convolutional neural network (CNN) (called wck-CNN) framework for extracting the hierarchical (*i.e.*, from low-order to high-order) functional connectivities for disease diagnosis, by using fMRI data. Specifically, we first define a layer to build dynamic CNs (DCNs) using the defined wc-kernels. Then, we define three layers to extract local (region specific), global (network specific) and temporal high-order properties from the constructed low-order functional connectivities as features for classification. Results on 174 subjects (a total of 563 scans) with rs-fMRI data from ADNI suggest that the our method can *not only* improve the performance compared with state-of-the-art methods, *but also* provide novel insights into the interaction patterns of brain activities and their changes in diseases.

© Springer Nature Switzerland AG 2018
Y. Shi et al. (Eds.): MLMI 2018, LNCS 11046, pp. 1–9, 2018.
https://doi.org/10.1007/978-3-030-00919-9_1

1   Introduction

As a challenging and interesting task, accurate diagnosis of Alzheimer's disease (AD) and its prodromal stage, *i.e.*, mild cognitive impairment (MCI), is very important for early treatment and possible delay of disease progression. A large number of pattern analysis methods have been proposed and applied to identifying disease-related imaging markers from advanced medical imaging techniques, *e.g.*, functional magnetic resonance imaging (fMRI). Compared with other imaging techniques, fMRI provides a non-invasive way to quantify the functional interaction of the cerebrum, thus providing an insight into the basic mechanism and cognitive processes of the human brain [1]. These interaction patterns among brain regions are usually characterized as connectivity networks (CNs), and used for brain disease analysis and diagnosis by using graph/network based methods, thus helping us better understand the pathological underpinnings of neurological disorder. Hence, functional CNs using resting-state fMRI (rs-fMRI) have been widely applied to automated diagnosis of AD/MCI [2].

Studies on functional CNs currently focus on two aspects: (1) *traditional CNs* and (2) *dynamic CNs (DCN)*. The former usually implicitly assumes that functional connectivity is a constant (*i.e.*, temporal stationary) throughout recording period in rs-fMRI. However, the dynamics of CNs are neglected in these studies. The latter focuses on the temporal changes of functional connectivities between specific brain regions. Numerous studies have indicated that the changes of functional connectivity over time may be related to cognitive and vigilance state [3], and is critical for better understanding the underpinnings of pathology of brain diseases [4]. And, studies have found that AD is associated with changes of functional connectivity over time [5]. All these studies usually construct the CNs by simply calculating the Pearson correlation coefficients (PCCs) between time series from brain regions, and then extract the low-level measures (*e.g.*, clustering coefficients) from constructed CNs as features to train the learning model (*e.g.*, support vector machine, SVM). However, *first*, in network construction, the valuable observation information (*e.g.*, specific contributions of different time points) is neglected in these studies. Intuitively, different time points should have different contributions for characterizing interaction between brain regions. *Second*, the high-level (*i.e.*, high-order) network properties that could further improve the performance are also neglected in feature learning step. In addition, since network construction, feature learning and classification are separately performed, it could yield sub-optimal learning model, thus decreasing the classification performance.

To address these problems and motivated by recent successful applications of convolutional neural network (CNN) in the natural image analysis field, in this paper we first define a weighted correlation kernel (called wc-kernel) for calculating the correlation between brain regions by using learned weights to characterize the contributions of different time points. Compared with the PCC method, the proposed wc-kernel can capture the specific contributions of different time points, thus conveying the richer interaction information among brain regions. Furthermore, we propose a wc-kernel based CNN (called wck-CNN) framework

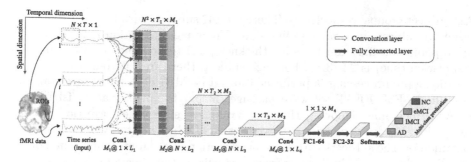

Fig. 1. Architecture of the proposed wck-CNN framework for DCN construction and analysis using fMRI data. There are four convolutional layers, *i.e.*, con1: connectivity construction layer, con2: regional feature layer, con3: brain-network feature layer and con4: temporal feature layer, and two fully connected layers (*i.e.*, FC1 and FC2) including 64 and 32 units, respectively. Here, the kernel sizes in four layers are $1 \times L_1$, $N \times L_2$, $N \times L_3$ and $1 \times L_4$ (with the corresponding kernel numbers of M_1, M_2, M_3, M_4), respectively. T_1, T_2 and T_3 denote the total operations of using kernel along temporal dimension for con1, con2 and con3 layers, respectively. T is the length of time series of each ROI, and N is the number of ROIs.

for defining/extracting the hierarchical (*i.e.*, from low-order to high-order) functional connectivities for disease diagnosis, by using fMRI data. To the best of our knowledge, our proposed method is among the first attempt to define the correlation kernel in CNN for characterizing the interactions among brain regions, and explore a unified CNN framework for DCN construction and analysis using fMRI data. Figure 1 shows the architecture of the proposed wck-CNN framework. Specifically, we first define a layer to build DCNs using the defined wc-kernels. Here, multiple DCNs can be constructed using multiple wc-kernels, with each DCN reflecting changes of CNs over time, thus conveying richer dynamic information of brain network. Then, we build other three layers to extract local (brain-region specific), global (network specific) and temporal high-order properties from the constructed low-order functional connectivities as features for classification. Results on 174 subjects (a total of 563 scans) with rs-fMRI data from the Alzheimer's Disease Neuroimaging Initiative (ADNI) database demonstrate the efficacy of our method.

2 Method

2.1 Subjects and Image Preprocessing

We use a total of 174 subjects, including 48 NCs (28female (F)/20male (M), aged 76.0 ± 6.8 years), 50 early MCI (eMCI) (30F/20M, aged 72.4 ± 7.1 years), 45 late MCI (lMCI) (18F/27M, aged 72.3 ± 8.1 years) and 31 AD (15F/16M, aged 73.2 ± 7.3 years), with rs-fMRI data from ADNI database. Totally, there are 563 scans covering nine possible stages (*i.e.*, baseline, 6, 12, 24, 36, 48, 60, 72 and 84 months), including 154, 165, 145, 99 scans for NC, eMCI, lMCI and

AD subject groups, respectively. There are 147 subjects with baseline scans, and other 27 subjects without baseline scan. The image resolution is 2.29–3.31 mm for inplane and 3.31 mm for slice thickness, TE (echo time) is 30 ms and TR (repetition time) is 2.2–3.1 s. For each subject, there are 140 volumes.

Image pre-processing is performed for all rs-fMRI data by using a standard pipeline in FSL FEAT software package (http://fsl.fmrib.ox.ac.uk/fsl/fslwiki/FEAT), including removing the first 3 volumes, slice time correction, motion correction, bandpass filtering, and regression of white matter, CSF, and motion parameters. The subjects with large head motion (i.e., larger than 2.0 mm or 2°) are discarded, since the head motion has substantial effects on functional CN measures [6]. Structural skull stripping is performed using FSL, which is used to register the fMRI to the Montreal Neurological Institute (MNI) space. The fMRI data are then spatially smoothed using a 6 mm Gaussian kernel. The subjects with more than 2.5 min of large frame-wise displacement (>0.5) are excluded in this study. The BOLD signals are band-pass filtered ($0.015 \leq f \leq 0.15$ Hz). The mean time series are extracted from each of the 116 regions of interest (ROIs) by the automated anatomical labeling (AAL) template [7]. The time point signal from each ROI i is normalized using the following scheme:

$$g(z) = (z - \mu_i)/\sigma_i \tag{1}$$

where z corresponds to the time point signal from the ROI i, μ_i and σ_i are the mean and standard deviation of time series from the ROI i, respectively.

2.2   Proposed Weighted Correlation Kernel

To capture the specific contributions of different time points, we defined a weighted correlation kernel for calculating the correlation between brain regions, i.e.,

$$k(\mathbf{x}_i, \mathbf{x}_j) = \sum_{l=1}^{L_1} \mathbf{w}^l \mathbf{x}_i^l \mathbf{x}_j^l \tag{2}$$

where $\mathbf{x}_i$ is the normalized (using Eq. 1) time series of the ROI i, $\mathbf{x}_i^l$ is the lth time point, $\mathbf{w} = [\mathbf{w}^1, \mathbf{w}^2, \ldots, \mathbf{w}^{L_1}]$ is a weight vector, and the kernel size is $1 \times L_1$.

According to the definition in Eq. 2, the wc-kernel calculates the correlation between time series of a pair of ROIs by using a weight $\mathbf{w}^l$ to characterize the specific contribution of each time point, thus conveying richer interaction information of brain regions compared with the PCC method, since the latter computes the correlation of brain regions using the same contribution for all time points (i.e., with all weights in $\mathbf{w}$ equaling to 1). Therefore, the defined wc-kernel is actually an extension of the PCC.

2.3   Architecture of the Proposed Wc-Kernel Based CNN

As shown in Fig. 1, the proposed wck-CNN framework includes four convolutional layers (i.e., Con1, Con2, Con3 and Con4) and two fully connected layers (*i.e.*, FC1 and FC2). Each layer uses a rectified linear unit (ReLU) as the activation function, and each fully connected layer is followed by dropout with a rate of 0.50. The input of this model is time series of all ROIs, and the output (via soft-max) is the probability of the subject belonging to four categories (*i.e.*, NC, eMCI, lMCI and AD). Here, M_1, M_2, M_3 and M_4 denote the numbers of kernels in four convolutional layers, respectively. Next, we will present the details of the four convolutional layers.

Con1: Connectivity Construction Layer We define a connectivity construction layer for CN construction using the defined wc-kernels, with time series of ROIs as the input. The output of this layer with a given wc-kernel is a matrix $\mathbf{C} \in R^{N^2 \times T_1}$ as

$$\mathbf{C}_{i+j-1,t} = k(\mathbf{S}_i^t, \mathbf{S}_j^t) \tag{3}$$

where k is the wc-kernel defined in Eq. 2, $\mathbf{S}_i \in R^T$ denotes the whole time series from the ith ROI, $\mathbf{S}_i^t$ denotes the corresponding segment of time series when performing the tth operation of sliding kernel along the temporal dimension (corresponding to time series of ROIs), T is the length of time series, T_1 is the total operations of sliding kernel along the temporal dimension, and N is the number of ROIs.

In connectivity construction layer, the convolution along the spatial dimension (corresponding to any pair of ROIs) computes the functional connectivity between ROIs, reflecting their interactions. Thus, each column in $\mathbf{C}$ denotes a CN. The convolution along the temporal dimension computes different functional connectivities of the same pair of ROIs within different segments of time series (similar to the sliding window method in conventional DCN construction), reflecting the changes of functional connectivity over time. Thus, the matrix $\mathbf{C}$ denotes a DCN, reflecting dynamics of CNs. Finally, the output of this layer with M_1 wc-kernels is a $3D$ tensor, which includes M_1 DCNs, conveying richer dynamic information of brain networks.

Con2: Regional Feature Layer Following the connectivity construction layer, we build a regional feature layer to learn local (*i.e.*, brain-region specific) high-order features by using the DCNs in connectivity construction layer. Specifically, we use the kernels with the size of $N \times L_2$, and set the size of stride along both dimensions (*i.e.*, temporal and spatial dimensions) to $(N, 1)$. Thus, the convolution along the spatial dimension is a feature mapping for each ROI by computing the weighted combination of functional connectivities connected to that ROI across $L_2(>1)$ neighboring time points (*i.e.*, CNs). The convolution along the temporal dimension corresponds to the different feature mappings for the same ROI over time, reflecting temporal variability of ROI. Note that features learned in this layer are high-order since they are calculated based on series of functional connectivities of specific ROI across multiple CNs, thus characterizing temporal properties of functional connectivity series of specific ROI.

Con3: Brain-Network Feature Layer Following the regional feature layer, we build a brain-network feature layer to learn the global (*i.e.*, brain-network specific) high-order features of whole CN using brain-region specific features. Specifically, we use the kernels with the size of $N \times L_3$, and set the size of stride along both dimensions to $(1, 1)$. Therefore, the convolution along the spatial dimension is a feature mapping for the whole CN by computing the weighted combination of all brain-region specific features across L_3 (>1) neighboring time points. The convolution along the temporal dimension corresponds to different mappings of the whole CN over time, reflecting the temporal variability of the whole brain network. Similar to the regional feature layer, the features learned in this layer are also high-order.

Con4: Temporal Feature layer To reduce the feature dimensionality, we further build a temporal feature layer to learn high-level temporal feature. Specifically, we use a kernel with the size of $1 \times L_4$, set the size of stride along both dimensions to $(1, 1)$, and perform an average-pooling (AP) operation after convolution for mapping all features into a feature. Thus, the output of this layer with a learned kernel can be used as a measure for the temporal variability of the whole CN.

3 Experiments

Experimental Settings: We perform a multi-class task, *i.e.*, NC *vs.* eMCI *vs.* lMCI *vs.* AD classification, by using a 5-fold cross-validation. Specifically, the set of 147 subjects with baseline scan is (roughly) equivalently partition into five subsets. One subset is selected as the testing data. The remaining four subsets and the set of 27 subjects without baseline scan are combined as the training subjects. Note, to enhance the generalization of model, all scans of each training subject are used as training data, with each scan as an independent sample but with the same class label. We evaluate the performance by computing the overall accuracy of four categories, and the accuracy for each category. In the experiment, we set the parameters $M_1 = 16$, $M_2 = 32$, $M_3 = 64$, $M_4 = 64$, $L_1 = 70$, $L_2 = 2$, $L_3 = 2$, $L_4 = 8$. In connectivity construction layer, we set the size of stride along temporal dimension to 2. Note that other scans (excepting for the baseline) of the testing subjects are not used for training or testing.

We first compare the proposed method with two traditional learning methods, including (1) baseline method (donted as **BL**) and (2) SVM method with local clustering coefficients (denoted as **SVM**). In both methods, the CN of each subject is first built by computing the PCC between the whole time series of a pair of ROIs, and the connectivity strengths and the local clustering coefficients are then extracted from constructed CNs as features, respectively. A t-test method with the threshold (*i.e.*, $p-$value < 0.05) is used for feature selection, followed by a linear SVM with default parameters for classification. Here, a one-to-all strategy is used for multi-class task.

To further evaluate the contributions of the proposed method, we compare wck-CNN with its three variants. These variants include (1) CNN method using traditional CNs (denoted as **CNN**), (2) CNN method using DCNs (denoted as **DCN-CNN**), and (3) wck-CNN framework without using high-order feature information (denoted as **wck-CNN-1**). In the CN-CNN and DCN-CNN methods, there don't include the proposed wc-kernel based network construction layer, while use the traditional CNs and DCNs as input of CNN, respectively. Here, the DCNs are constructed using overlapping sliding window method with the window length equal to 70, and the translation step equal to 2. In wck-CNN-1 method, no high-order features are extracted in regional feature layer and brain-network feature layer, *i.e.*, setting L_1 and L_2 to 1.

Table 1. Performance of all methods in NC vs. eMCI vs. lMCI vs. AD classification.

	Method	Accuracy	Accuracy$_{NC}$	Accuracy$_{eMCI}$	Accuracy$_{lMCI}$	Accuracy$_{AD}$
CN-based methods	BL	30.6	20.0	38.9	30.0	33.3
	SVM	35.0	22.0	69.5	21.0	6.7
	CNN	44.2	32.2	**74.6**	28.3	22.2
DCN-based methods	DCN-CNN	50.0	38.3	53.0	53.8	**58.3**
	wck-CNN-1	54.5	52.2	62.7	45.0	55.6
	wck-CNN	**57.0**	**68.9**	52.4	**56.7**	44.4

Results: Experimental results of all methods are summarized in Table 1. As can be seen from Table 1, our proposed method achieves the overall accuracy of 57.0% for four classes, while the best overall accuracy of competing methods is 50.0% (by regarding wck-CNN-1 still our method), suggesting the effectiveness of our proposed wck-CNN method. In addition, from Table 1, we can make four interesting observations. *First*, compared with traditional learning methods (*i.e.*, BL and SVM), CNN-based methods (*i.e.*, CNN, DCN-CNN wck-CNN-1 and wck-CNN) can achieve much higher performance, indicating that CNN can capture the underlying properties of brain networks, and thus can be better applied for brain network analysis. *Second*, compared with traditional CN-based methods (*i.e.*, BL, SVM and CNN), DCN-based methods (*i.e.*, DCN-CNN, wck-CNN-1 and wck-CNN) can achieve higher accuracies, suggesting that the dynamics of CNs can provide useful clues for better understanding the underpinnings of brain disease pathology, which is consistent with existing studies [4]. *Third*, the wc-kernel based methods (*i.e.*, wck-CNN-1 and wck-CNN) perform better than conventional DCN based method (*i.e.*, DCN-CNN), further indicating the effectiveness of our defined wc-kernel in conveying the interaction information between brain regions. *Finally*, the wck-CNN method can achieve higher performance in comparison with wck-CNN-1 method, demonstrating the advantage of exploring high-order information from brain networks.

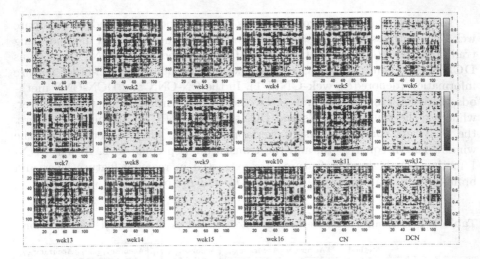

Fig. 2. The group difference of functional connectivity in the (dynamic) CNs constructed using different methods between AD and NC group. Here, p-values more than 0.05 are set to 1 (denoted as yellow points), wck1,..., wck16 correspond to the DCNs constructed by using the proposed method with 16 different wc-kernels, respectively. CN and DCN correspond to traditional CNs and DCNs constructed by using the overlapping sliding windows method, respectively.

Connectivity Analysis: Furthermore, we investigate the DCNs constructed by using the proposed wc-kernel based method. Specifically, we construct the DCNs (*i.e.*, the output of connectivity construction layer) for all subjects using the model learned in the first cross-validation. We obtained 16 DCNs for each subject with 16 wc-kernels. For simplicity, we compute the average network for each DCN of each subject. Then, for each wc-kernel, we compute the group difference of functional connectivity in average network using the standard t-test. Figure 2 gives the results (denoted as wck1 to wck16) between AD and NC groups. For comparison, in Fig. 2 we also report the group difference of functional connectivity in the traditional CNs and DCNs constructed by the overlapping sliding windows method, respectively. Here, we threshold the obtained p-values (*i.e.*, setting p-values more than 0.05 to 1) for clarity.

From Fig. 2, we can make three interesting observations for most of the proposed wc-kernel based DCNs, compared with traditional CNs and DCNs. *First*, there are more discriminative functional connectivities (with the corresponding p-value less than 0.05), indicating these DCNs are more discriminative. *Second*, there are more obvious patterns. For example, the discriminative functional connectivities focus on connection with specific regions, including lateral surface, parietal lobe, limbic lobe and sub-cortical gray nuclei, which have been widely reported in existing studies [8]. *Finally*, there are few discriminative functional connectivity among brain regions from the cerebellum, but have a few discriminative functional connectivities between brain regions from the cerebellum and the cerebrum, indicating that the cerebellum might be associated with AD and it may provide useful information for AD prognosis [9].

4 Conclusion

In this paper, we define a novel wc-kernel for characterizing the rich interaction information among brain regions, and propose a unified wck-CNN framework for DCN construction and analysis using fMRI data. Results on 174 subjects with a total of 563 scans from ADNI database demonstrate that our proposed method can *not only* improve the classification performance compared with state-of-the-art methods, *but also* provide insights into the interactions of brain activity and their changes in AD.

Acknowledgments. This study was supported by NSFC (61573023, 61703301), NIH grants (EB006733, EB008374, EB009634, MH100217, AG041721, AG042599, AG010129, AG030514).

References

1. Greicius, M.D., Krasnow, B., Reiss, A.L., Menon, V.: Functional connectivity in the resting brain: a network analysis of the default mode hypothesis. Proc. Natl. Acad. Sci. **100**(1), 253–258 (2003)
2. Jie, B., Liu, M., Zhang, D., Shen, D.: Sub-network kernels for measuring similarity of brain connectivity networks in disease diagnosis. IEEE Trans. Image Process. **27**(5), 2340–2353 (2018)
3. Thompson, G.J., et al.: Short-time windows of correlation between large-scale functional brain networks predict vigilance intraindividually and interindividually. Hum. Brain Mapp. **34**(12), 3280–3298 (2013)
4. Hutchison, R.M., et al.: Dynamic functional connectivity: promise, issues, and interpretations. NeuroImage **80**, 360–378 (2013)
5. Jie, B., Liu, M., Shen, D.: Integration of temporal and spatial properties of dynamic connectivity networks for automatic diagnosis of brain disease. Med. Image Anal. **47**, 81–94 (2018)
6. Van Dijk, K.R., Sabuncu, M.R., Buckner, R.L.: The influence of head motion on intrinsic functional connectivity MRI. NeuroImage **59**(1), 431–438 (2012)
7. Tzourio-Mazoyer, N., et al.: Automated anatomical labeling of activations in SPM using a macroscopic anatomical parcellation of the MNI MRI single-subject brain. NeuroImage **15**(1), 273–289 (2002)
8. Yao, H., et al.: Decreased functional connectivity of the amygdala in Alzheimer's disease revealed by resting-state fMRI. Eur. J. Radiol. **82**(9), 1531–1538 (2013)
9. Jie, B., Wee, C.Y., Shen, D., Zhang, D.: Hyper-connectivity of functional networks for brain disease diagnosis. Med. Image Anal. **32**, 84–100 (2016)

Robust Contextual Bandit via the Capped-ℓ_2 Norm for Mobile Health Intervention

Feiyun Zhu[1,3], Xinliang Zhu[1], Sheng Wang[1], Jiawen Yao[1], Zhichun Xiao[3],
and Junzhou Huang[1,2(✉)]

[1] Department of CSE, University of Texas at Arlington, Arlington, TX 76013, USA
[2] Tencent AI Lab, Shenzhen 518057, China
jzhuang@uta.edu
[3] Walmart (Sam's Club) Technology, Dallas, TX 75202, USA

Abstract. This paper considers the actor-critic contextual bandit for the mobile health (mHealth) intervention. The state-of-the-art decision-making methods in the mHealth generally assume that the noise in the dynamic system follows the Gaussian distribution. Those methods use the least-square-based algorithm to estimate the expected reward, which is prone to the existence of outliers. To deal with the issue of outliers, we are the first to propose a novel robust actor-critic contextual bandit method for the mHealth intervention. In the critic updating, the capped-ℓ_2 norm is used to measure the approximation error, which prevents outliers from dominating our objective. A set of weights could be achieved from the critic updating. Considering them gives a weighted objective for the actor updating. It provides the ineffective sample in the critic updating with zero weights for the actor updating. As a result, the robustness of both actor-critic updating is enhanced. There is a key parameter in the capped-ℓ_2 norm. We provide a reliable method to properly set it by making use of one of the most fundamental definitions of outliers in statistics. Extensive experiment results demonstrate that our method can achieve almost identical results compared with the state-of-the-art methods on the dataset without outliers and dramatically outperform them on the datasets noised by outliers.

1 Introduction

Nowadays, billions of people frequently use various kinds of smart devices, such as smart-phones and wearable activity sensors [7,8]. It is increasingly popular among the scientist community to make use of the mobile health (mHealth) technologies to collect and analyze real-time data from users. Based on that, the goal of mHealth is to decide when, where, and how to deliver the in-time intervention to best serve users, helping them to lead healthier lives. For example,

This work was partially supported by NSF IIS-1423056, CMMI-1434401, CNS-1405985, IIS-1718853 and the NSF CAREER grant IIS-1553687.

Y. Shi et al. (Eds.): MLMI 2018, LNCS 11046, pp. 10–18, 2018.
https://doi.org/10.1007/978-3-030-00919-9_2

mHealth guides people how to reduce alcohol abuses, increase physical activities and regain the control of eating disorders, obesity/weight management [4, 7, 8].

The tailoring of mHealth interventions is generally modeled as a sequential decision-making (SDM) problem. The contextual bandit provides a paradigm for the SDM [11, 12]. In mHealth, the first contextual bandit [5] was proposed in 2014. It is in an actor-critic setting and has an explicit parameterized stochastic policy. Such setting has two advantages: (1) the actor-critic algorithm has good properties of quick convergence with low variance [3]; (2) we could understand the key features that contribute most to the policy by analyzing the estimated parameters. This is important for the behavior scientists to design the state (feature). After then, Lei [4] improved the method by emphasizing the explorations and introducing the stochasticity constraint on the policy coefficients.

Those two methods serve a good start for the mHealth. However, they assume that there is no outlier in the data. They use the least-square-based algorithm to learn the expected reward, which, however, is prone to the presence of outliers. In practice, there are various kinds of complex noise in the mHealth system. For example, the wearable devices are unable to accurately record the states and rewards from users under various conditions. The mHealth requires self-report to deliver effective interventions to device users. However, some users are unwilling to accomplish the self-reports. They sometimes randomly fill out the report to save time. We treat the various of complex noises in the system as outliers. We want to get rid of the extreme observations. However, there is no such actor-critic contextual bandit method focusing on the robust learning.

In this paper, a novel robust actor-critic contextual bandit is proposed to deal with the outlier issue in the mHealth system. The capped-ℓ_2 norm is used in the estimation of the expected reward in the critic updating. As a result, we obtain a set of weights. With them, we propose a weighted objective for the actor updating, which gives the samples that are ineffective for the critic updating zero weights. As a result, the robustness of both actor-critic updating is greatly enhanced. There is a key parameter in the capped-ℓ_2 norm. We propose a solid method to set it properly, which is based on a solid method to detect outliers in statistics. With it, we can achieve the conflicting goal of enhancing the robustness of our algorithm and obtaining almost same results compared with the state-of-the-art method on the datasets without outliers. Extensive experiment results show that in a variety of parameter settings our method obtains clear gains compared with the state-of-the-art methods.

2   Preliminaries

The expected reward $\mathbb{E}(r \mid s, a)$ is a core concept in the contextual bandit to evaluate the policy for the dynamic system. In case of large state or action spaces, the parameterized approximation is widely accepted: $\mathbb{E}(r \mid s, a; \mathbf{w}) = \mathbf{x}(s, a)^T \mathbf{w}$ is assumed to be in a low dimensional space, where $\mathbf{w} \in \mathbb{R}^u$ is the unknown coefficients and $\mathbf{x}(s, a)$ is the contextual feature for the state-action $\{s, a\}$ pair.

The aim of the actor-critic algorithm is to learn an optimal policy to maximize the reward for all the state-action pairs. The objective is $\pi_{\theta^*} = \arg\max_{\theta} \widehat{J}(\theta)$, where $\widehat{J}(\theta) = \sum_{s\in\mathcal{S}} d(s) \sum_{a\in\mathcal{A}} \pi_\theta(a \mid s) \mathbb{E}(r \mid s,a;\mathbf{w})$ is the average reward over all the possible states & actions; $d(s)$ is a reference distribution over states. To make the actor updating a well-posed objective, various constraints on θ are considered [5]. Specifically, the stochasticity constraint is introduced to reduce the habituation and facilitate learning [4]. The stochasticity constraint specifies the probability of selecting both actions is at least p_0 for more than $100(1-\alpha)\%$ contexts: $P[p_0 \le \pi_\theta(a=1 \mid s_t) \le 1-p_0] \ge 1-\alpha$. Via the Markov inequality, a relaxed and smoother stochasticity constraint is as follows $\theta^\mathsf{T}\mathbb{E}[g(s)^\mathsf{T} g(s)]\theta \le \alpha\{\log[p_0/(1-p_0)]\}^2$ [4], leading to the objective $\widehat{J}(\theta)$ as

$$\widehat{J}(\theta) = \sum_{s\in\mathcal{S}} d(s) \sum_{a\in\mathcal{A}} \pi_\theta(a \mid s)\mathbb{E}(r \mid s,a;\mathbf{w}) - \lambda\theta^\mathsf{T}\mathbb{E}[g(s)g(s)^\mathsf{T}]\theta, \qquad (1)$$

where $g(s_i) = g(s_i, 1) - g(s_i, 0)$; $g(s,a)$ is the feature for the policy [4].

According to (1), we need the estimation of the expected reward to form the objective. This process is called the critic updating [3]. Current methods generally use the ridge regression to learn it. The objective is defined as follows

$$\min_{\mathbf{w}} \sum_{i=1}^{T} \|\mathbf{x}(s_i, a_i)^\mathsf{T}\mathbf{w} - r_i\|_2^2 + \zeta\|\mathbf{w}\|_2^2. \qquad (2)$$

It has a closed-form solution: $\widehat{\mathbf{w}} = (\mathbf{X}\mathbf{X}^\mathsf{T} + \zeta\mathbf{I}_u)^{-1}\mathbf{X}\mathbf{r}$, where $\mathbf{X} \in \mathbb{R}^{u\times T}$ is a designed matrix with the i-th column as $\mathbf{x}_i = \mathbf{x}(s_i, a_i)$; $\mathbf{r} = [r_1, \cdots, r_T]^\mathsf{T} \in \mathbb{R}^T$ consists of all the immediate rewards. However similar to the existing least square based algorithms, the objective is sensitive to the existence of outliers [9,13,14].

3   Robust Contextual Bandit with Capped-ℓ_2 Norm

To boost the robustness of the actor-critic learning, the capped-ℓ_2 norm is used to measure the approximation error:

$$\min_{\mathbf{w}} O(\mathbf{w}) = \sum_{i=1}^{M} \min\left\{\|r_i - \mathbf{x}_i^T\mathbf{w}\|_2^2, \epsilon\right\} + \zeta\|\mathbf{w}\|_2^2. \qquad (3)$$

By properly setting the value of ϵ, we can get rid of the outliers that distribute far away from the majority of samples while keep the effective samples. Otherwise when ϵ is too large, there are outliers left in the data; while ϵ is too small, lots of effective samples will be removed, leading to unstable estimations.

It is important to properly set the value of ϵ. We propose an effective method to set ϵ. It is derived from one of the most widely accepted outlier definitions in the statistics community. When we use the boxplot to give a descriptive illustration of the distribution of a dataset, the samples that are $1.5 \times IQR$ more above the third quartile are treated as outliers. Thus, we set ϵ as:

$$\epsilon = q_3 + 1.5 \times IQR \qquad (4)$$

where $IQR = q_3 - q_1$ is the interquartile range.

3.1 Algorithm for the Critic Updating

Proposition 1. *The critic objective* (3) *is equivalent to the following objective*

$$\min_{\mathbf{w}} \sum_i u_i \left\| r_i - \mathbf{x}_i^T \mathbf{w} \right\|_2^2 + \zeta \left\| \mathbf{w} \right\|_2^2, \tag{5}$$

where ζ is the balancing parameter for the ℓ_2-norm based smooth constraint; $u_i = 1_{\left\{ \left\| r_i - \mathbf{x}_i^T \mathbf{w} \right\|_2^2 < \epsilon \right\}}$ is dependent on the unknown variable $\mathbf{w}$.

According to Proposition 1, we obtain a simplified objective for the critic updating. However, it is still complex to minimize (5) since the weight term depends on the unknown variable $\mathbf{w}$. In this section, an iteratively re-weighted algorithm is proposed for the optimization of (5). It assumes the weight $\mathbf{u}$ is fixed when optimizing for the optimal $\mathbf{w}$ and vice versa. When $\mathbf{u}$ is fixed, the objective (5) is convex over $\mathbf{w}$. We may get the solver by differentiating (5) and setting the derivative to zero, leading to the following linear system

$$\mathbf{w}^{(t)} = \left(\mathbf{X} \mathbf{U}^{(t-1)} \mathbf{X}^T + \zeta \mathbf{I} \right)^{-1} \mathbf{X} \mathbf{U}^{(t-1)} \mathbf{r}, \tag{6}$$

where $\mathbf{U}^{(t-1)} = \text{diag}\left(\mathbf{u}^{(t-1)} \right)$ is the weight at the $(t-1)$-th iteration. Then we update the weight term as $u_i^{(t)} = 1_{\left\{ \left\| r_i - \mathbf{x}_i^T \mathbf{w}^{(t)} \right\|_2^2 < \epsilon \right\}}$ for $i = 1, \cdots, T$.

3.2 Algorithm for the Actor Updating

Since the distribution of $d(s)$ in the objective (1) is generally unavailable, we consider the T-trial based objective as follows

$$\hat{J}(\theta) = \frac{1}{T} \sum_{i=1}^{T} \sum_{a \in \mathcal{A}} u_i \pi_\theta (a \mid s_i) \mathbb{E}(r \mid s_i, a; \mathbf{w}) - \lambda \theta^T \left[\frac{1}{T} \sum_{i=1}^{T} u_i g(s_i) g(s_i)^T \right] \theta, \tag{7}$$

where $\{u_i\}_{i=1}^{T}$ is the weighted term learned from the critic updating, cf. Section 3.1. With the weight $\{u_i\}_{i=1}^{T}$, the outlier tuples that have large approximation errors are removed for the actor updating. As a result, the robustness is boosted. The actor updating aims to maximize the objective (7) over θ. We use the Sequential Quadratic Programming (SQP) algorithm for the optimization. Specially, the implementation of SQP with finite-difference approximation to the gradient in FMINCON is utilized in our algorithm.

4 Experiments

4.1 Datasets

To evaluate the performance, we utilize a dataset from the mHealth study (called HeartSteps) to approximate the generative model. The HeartSteps is a 42-day mHealth study, resulting in 210 decision points per user [5,7]. It aims to increase the users' daily activities (i.e. steps) by sending them positive interventions, for example, suggesting them to go for a hike on the sunny weekend etc.

For each user, a trajectory of $T = 210$ tuples of observations $\mathcal{D} = \{(s_i, a_i, r_i)\}_{i=1}^T$ are generated via the micro-randomized trials [7,8]. The initial state is drawn from the Gaussian distribution $S_0 \sim \mathcal{N}_p\{0, \Sigma\}$, with the pre-defined covariance matrix $\Sigma \in \mathbb{R}^{p \times p}$. The random policy provides a method to select actions. $\forall t \geq 0$, $a_t = 1$ is chosen with a probability of 0.5, i.e. $\mu(1 \mid s_t) = 0.5$ for all states s_t. When $t \geq 1$, the state and immediate reward are generated as

$$
\begin{aligned}
S_{t,1} &= \beta_1 S_{t-1,1} + \xi_{t,1}, \\
S_{t,2} &= \beta_2 S_{t-1,2} + \beta_3 A_{t-1} + \xi_{t,2}, \\
S_{t,3} &= \beta_4 S_{t-1,3} + \beta_5 S_{t-1,3} A_{t-1} + \beta_6 A_{t-1} + \xi_{t,3}, \\
S_{t,j} &= \beta_7 S_{t-1,j} + \xi_{t,j}, \qquad \text{for } j = 4, \ldots, p
\end{aligned}
\tag{8}
$$

$$
R_t = \beta_{14} \times [\beta_8 + A_t \times (\beta_9 + \beta_{10} S_{t,1} + \beta_{11} S_{t,2}) + \beta_{12} S_{t,1} - \beta_{13} S_{t,3} + \varrho_t], \tag{9}
$$

where $\beta = \{\beta_i \mid i = 1, \cdots, 14\}$ is the main coefficient for the dynamic system. It is set as $\beta = [0.4, 0.3, 0.4, 0.7, 0.05, 0.6, 0.25, 3, 0.25, 0.25, 0.4, 0.1, 0.5, 500]$. $\{\xi_{t,i}\}_{i=1}^p \sim \mathcal{N}(0, \sigma_s^2)$ is the Gaussian noise in the state (8) and $\varrho_t \sim \mathcal{N}(0, \sigma_r^2)$ is the Gaussian noise in the reward model (9).

To mimic the outliers in the trajectory, there are two processing steps: (a) a fixed ratio (i.e. $\psi = 4\%$) of tuples is randomly selected in each user's trajectory; (b) we add a large noise (ν times the average value in the trajectory) to the states and rewards in the selected tuples. Additionally, the actions in the selected tuples are randomly set to simulate the random failure of sending interventions due to the weak mobile network.

4.2 Experiments Settings

In the experiment, there are three contextual bandit methods for comparison: (1) Lin-UCB (linear upper confidence bound) is a famous contextual bandit method that achieves great successes in the Internet advertising [1,6,11]; (2) S-ACCB is the stochasticity constrained actor-critic contextual bandit for the mHealth [4]; (3) RS-ACCB is the proposed Robust ACCB with the stochasticity constraint.

We use the the expected long-run average reward (ElrAR) [8] to evaluate the estimated policies $\pi_{\hat{\theta}_n}$ for $n \in \{1, \cdots, N\}$. There are two processing steps to obtain the ElrAR: (a) get the average reward $\eta^{\pi_{\hat{\theta}_n}}$ for the n-th user by averaging the rewards over the last 4,000 elements in a trajectory of 5,000 tuples under the policy $\pi_{\hat{\theta}_n}$; (b) the ElrAR $\mathbb{E}[\eta^{\pi_{\hat{\theta}}}]$ is achieved by averaging the 50 $\eta^{\pi_{\hat{\theta}}}$'s.

There are $N = 50$ users' MDPs used in the experiment. Each user has a trajectory of $T = 210$ tuples. There are $p = 3$ variables in the state. The noises in the MDP are set as $\sigma_r = 3$ and $\sigma_s = 1$ respectively. The parameterized policy is assumed to be the Boltzmann distribution $\pi_\theta(a \mid s) = \frac{\exp[-\theta^\mathsf{T} g(s,a)]}{\sum_{a'} \exp[-\theta^\mathsf{T} g(s,a')]}$ [8], where $\theta \in \mathbb{R}^m$ is the unknown coefficients, $g(s,a) = [as^\mathsf{T}, a]^\mathsf{T}$ is the policy feature and $m = p + 1$. The feature vector for the estimation of expected rewards is set as $\mathbf{x}(s, a) = [1, s^\mathsf{T}, a, s^\mathsf{T}a]^\mathsf{T} \in \mathbb{R}^u$, where $u = 2p + 2$. The tuning parameters for the actor-critic learning are set as $\zeta = \lambda = 0.001$. The outlier ratio and strength are set $\psi = 4\%$ and $\nu = 5$ respectively.

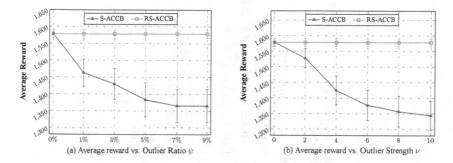

(a) Average reward vs. Outlier Ratio ψ (b) Average reward vs. Outlier Strength ν

Fig. 1. Average reward of two contextual bandit methods. The left sub-table shows the results when the trajectory is short, i.e. $T = 42$; the right one shows the results when $T = 100$. RS-ACCB is our method. A larger value is better.

4.3 Results and Discussion

In this section, the experiments are carried out to verify the performance of three contextual bandit methods from the following two aspects:

(**S1**) We change the ratio ψ of tuples that contain outliers from 0% to 9%. The experiment results are displayed in the left sub-table in Table 1 and Fig. 1(a). As we can see, when $\psi = 0$, there is zero percentage of outliers in the dataset. Under such condition, our method achieves almost identical results compared with the S-ACCB [4]. This results verify that though our method aims at the robust learning, it is well adapted to the dataset without outliers. As ψ rises, the performance of both Lin-UCB and S-ACCB drops obviously. While their standard deviations increases dramatically. Compared with those two methods, both the performance and the standard deviation of our method keep stable. As a result, our method averagely improves the performance by 146.8 steps, i.e. 10.26%, compared with the best of state-of-the-art methods.

(**S2**) The strength of outliers ν ranges from 0 to 10 times of the average value in the trajectory. The right sub-table in Table 1 and Fig. 1(b) summarize the experiment results. As we shall see, when ν rises, the strength of outliers increases gradually. We have the following observations from the experiment results: (1) when there is no outlier in the trajectory, our method achieves similar results compared with S-ACCB; (2) as ν rises, the performances of S-ACCB and Lin-UCB decrease obviously and their standard deviations increase dramatically; (3) as ν rises, both the performance of our method and the standard deviation keep stable. Compared with the state-of-the-art methods, our method get clear gains

Table 1. Average reward vs. outlier ratio ψ (setting **S1**) and outlier strength ν (setting **S2**) on the two sub-tables. The three methods are (a) Lin-UCB [6], (b) S-ACCB [4] and (c) RS-ACCB (is our method). A larger value is better.

ψ	Average reward vs. outlier ratio ψ			ν	Average reward vs. outlier strength ν		
	Lin-UCB	S-ACCB	RS-ACCB		Lin-UCB	S-ACCB	RS-ACCB
0%	1578.7 ± 13.75	1578.3 ± 12.70	1578.3 ± 12.55	0	1578.7 ± 13.75	1578.3 ± 12.70	1578.3 ± 12.55
1%	1462.5 ± 40.24	1462.9 ± 39.88	1578.4 ± 12.61	2	1535.6 ± 21.94	1527.7 ± 30.71	1578.3 ± 12.68
3%	1428.1 ± 49.69	1429.5 ± 45.79	1578.2 ± 12.57	4	1431.7 ± 44.13	1424.7 ± 46.53	1578.2 ± 12.65
5%	1391.0 ± 49.42	1383.2 ± 50.40	1578.6 ± 12.66	6	1380.8 ± 49.03	1377.2 ± 48.83	1578.2 ± 12.62
7%	1370.6 ± 50.20	1365.0 ± 49.02	1578.7 ± 12.62	8	1359.8 ± 49.76	1357.1 ± 48.51	1578.2 ± 12.63
9%	1358.9 ± 48.43	1365.0 ± 49.02	1578.7 ± 12.62	10	1346.8 ± 48.83	1344.9 ± 46.94	1578.2 ± 12.64
Avg	1431.6	1430.7	1578.5	Avg	1438.9	1435.0	1578.2

in a variety of parameter settings. Averagely, it improves the performance by 139.3 steps and 143.3 steps compared with Lin-UCB and S-ACCB respectively.

5   Conclusions and Future Directions

To alleviate the influence of outliers in the mHealth study, a robust actor-critic contextual bandit method is proposed to form robust interventions. We use the capped-ℓ_2 norm to boost the robustness for the critic updating, which results in a set of weights. With them, we propose a weighted objective for the actor updating. It gives the tuples that have large approximate errors zero weights, enhancing the robustness against those tuples. Additionally, a solid method is provided to properly set the thresholding parameter in the capped-ℓ_2 norm. With it, we can achieve the conflicting goal of enhancing the robustness of the actor-critic algorithm as well as obtaining almost identical results compared with the state-of-the-art method on the datasets without outliers. Extensive experiment results show that in a variety of parameter settings the proposed method obtains significant improvements compared with the state-of-the-art contextual bandit methods. In the future, we may explore the robust learning on the reinforcement learning method. It could be on both the discount reward setting and the average reward setting [3,8]. Those two directions are much more challenging since it is not a general regression task to estimate the value function.

Appendix: The Proof of Proposition 1

Proof. The objective of (3) is non-convex and non-differentiable [2,10]. We could obtain its sub-gradient: $\partial O\left(\mathbf{w}\right) = \sum_i \partial \min\left\{\left\|r_i - \mathbf{x}_i^T \mathbf{w}\right\|_2^2, \epsilon\right\} + 2\zeta\mathbf{w}$, where

$$
\partial \min\left\{\left\|r_i - \mathbf{x}_i^T \mathbf{w}\right\|_2^2, \epsilon\right\} = \begin{cases} 0, & \text{if } \left\|r_i - \mathbf{x}_i^T \mathbf{w}\right\|_2^2 > \epsilon \\ [-1,0]\,\partial\left(\left\|r_i - \mathbf{x}_i^T \mathbf{w}\right\|_2^2\right) & \text{if } r_i - \mathbf{x}_i^T \mathbf{w} = -\sqrt{\epsilon} \\ [0,1]\,\partial\left(\left\|r_i - \mathbf{x}_i^T \mathbf{w}\right\|_2^2\right) & \text{if } r_i - \mathbf{x}_i^T \mathbf{w} = \sqrt{\epsilon} \\ \partial\left(\left\|r_i - \mathbf{x}_i^T \mathbf{w}\right\|_2^2\right) & \text{if } \left\|r_i - \mathbf{x}_i^T \mathbf{w}\right\|_2^2 < \epsilon \end{cases}
\tag{10}
$$

Letting $u_i = 1_{\left\{\left\|r_i - \mathbf{x}_i^T \mathbf{w}\right\|_2^2 < \epsilon\right\}}$ for $i \in \{1, \cdots, T\}$ gives a simplified partial derivative of (3) that satisfies the sub-gradient (10). It is defined as

$$
\partial O\left(\mathbf{w}\right) = \sum_i u_i \partial\left(\left\|r_i - \mathbf{x}_i^T \mathbf{w}\right\|_2^2\right) + 2\zeta\mathbf{w},
$$

which is equivalent to the partial derivative of the following objective

$$
\max_{\mathbf{w}} \sum_i u_i \left\|r_i - \mathbf{x}_i^T \mathbf{w}\right\|_2^2 + \zeta \left\|\mathbf{w}\right\|_2^2.
\tag{11}
$$

From the perspective of optimization, the objective (11) is equivalent to (3). $\square$

References

1. Dudík, M., Langford, J., Li, L.: Doubly robust policy evaluation and learning. In: ICML, pp. 1097–1104 (2011)
2. Gao, H., Nie, F., Cai, T.W., Huang, H.: Robust capped norm nonnegative matrix factorization: capped norm NMF. In: ACM International Conference on Information and Knowledge, pp. 871–880 (2015)
3. Grondman, I., Busoniu, L., Lopes, G.A.D., Babuska, R.: A survey of actor-critic reinforcement learning: standard and natural policy gradients. IEEE Trans. Syst. Man Cybern. **42**(6), 1291–1307 (2012)
4. Lei, H.: An online actor critic algorithm and a statistical decision procedure for personalizing intervention. Ph.D. thesis, University of Michigan (2016)
5. Lei, H., Tewari, A., Murphy, S.: An actor-critic contextual bandit algorithm for personalized interventions using mobile devices. In: NIPS 2014 Workshop: Personalization: Methods and Applications, pp. 1–9 (2014)
6. Li, L., Chu, W., Langford, J., Schapire, R.E.: A contextual-bandit approach to personalized news article recommendation. In: International Conference on World Wide Web (WWW), pp. 661–670 (2010)
7. Liao, P., Tewari, A., Murphy, S.: Constructing just-in-time adaptive interventions. Ph.D. Section Proposal, pp. 1–49 (2015)
8. Murphy, S.A., Deng, Y., Laber, E.B., Maei, H.R., Sutton, R.S., Witkiewitz, K., et al.: A batch, off-policy, actor-critic algorithm for optimizing the average reward. CoRR abs/ arXiv:1607.05047 (2016)
9. Nie, F., Wang, H., Cai, X., Huang, H., Ding, C.: Robust matrix completion via joint schatten p-norm and lp-norm minimization. In: IEEE International Conference on Data Mining (ICDM), pp. 566–574. Washington, DC, USA (2012)
10. Sun, Q., Xiang, S., Ye, Y.: Robust principal component analysis via capped norms. In: ACM SIGKDD International Conference on Knowledge Discovery and Data Mining, pp. 311–319 (2013)
11. Tewari, A., Murphy, S.A.: From ads to interventions: contextual bandits in mobile health. In: Rehg, J., Murphy, S.A., Kumar, S. (eds.) Mobile Health: Sensors, Analytic Methods, and Applications. Springer, Berlin (2017)
12. Zhou, L., Brunskill, E.: Latent contextual bandits and their application to personalized recommendations for new users. In: International Joint Conference on Artificial Intelligence, pp. 3646–3653 (2016)
13. Zhu, F., Fan, B., Zhu, X., Wang, Y., Xiang, S., Pan, C., et al.: 10,000+ times accelerated robust subset selection (ARSS). Proc. Assoc. Adv. Artif. Intell. (AAAI). 3217–3224 (2015). http://arxiv.org/abs/1409.3660
14. Zhu, F., Wang, Y., Fan, B., Meng, G., Pan, C.: Effective spectral unmixing via robust representation and learning-based sparsity. CoRR abs/1409.0685 (2014). http://arxiv.org/abs/1409.0685

Dynamic Multi-scale CNN Forest Learning for Automatic Cervical Cancer Segmentation

Nesrine Bnouni[1,2(✉)], Islem Rekik[2], Mohamed Salah Rhim[3], and Najoua Essoukri Ben Amara[1]

[1] LATIS- Laboratory of Advanced Technology and Intelligent Systems, ENISo, Sousse University, Sousse, Tunisia
nesrine.bnouni@gmail.com
https://www.latis-eniso.org
[2] BASIRA Lab, CVIP, School of Science and Engineering, Computing, University of Dundee, Dundee, UK
https://www.basira-lab.com
[3] Department of Gynecology Obstetrics, Faculty of Medicine of Monastir, Monastir, Tunisia

Abstract. Deep-learning based labeling methods have gained unprecedented popularity in different computer vision and medical image segmentation tasks. However, to the best of our knowledge, these have not been used for cervical tumor segmentation. More importantly, while the majority of innovative deep-learning works using convolutional neural networks (CNNs) focus on developing more sophisticated and robust architectures (e.g., ResNet, U-Net, GANs), there is very limited work on how to *aggregate* different CNN architectures to improve their *relational learning* at multiple levels of CNN-to-CNN interactions. To address this gap, we introduce a Dynamic Multi-Scale CNN Forest (C^{K+1}DMF), which aims to address three major issues in medical image labeling and ensemble CNN learning: (1) *heterogeneous* distribution of MRI training patches, (2) a *bi-directional* flow of information between two consecutive CNNs as opposed to cascading CNNs—where information passes in a directional way from current to the next CNN in the cascade, and (3) *multiscale* anatomical variability across patients. To solve the first issue, we group training samples into K clusters, then design a forest with $(K + 1)$ trees: a *principal tree* of CNNs trained using all data samples and *subordinate trees*, each trained using a cluster of samples. As for the second and third issues, we design each dynamic multiscale tree (DMT) in the forest such that each node in the tree nests a CNN architecture. Two successive CNN nodes in the tree pass bidirectional contextual maps to progressively improve the learning of their relational non-linear mapping. Besides, as we traverse a path from the root node to a leaf node in the tree, the architecture of each CNN node becomes shallower to take in smaller training patches. Our C^{K+1}DMF significantly ($p < 0.05$) outperformed several conventional and ensemble CNN architectures, including conventional CNN (improvement by 10.3%) and CNN-based DMT (improvement by 5%).

Electronic supplementary material The online version of this chapter (https://doi.org/10.1007/978-3-030-00919-9_3) contains supplementary material, which is available to authorized users.

© Springer Nature Switzerland AG 2018
Y. Shi et al. (Eds.): MLMI 2018, LNCS 11046, pp. 19–27, 2018.
https://doi.org/10.1007/978-3-030-00919-9_3

1 Introduction

Nearly more than a quarter of a million patients, diagnosed with cervical cancer, die every year [1]. Magnetic Resonance Imaging (MRI) of the pelvis is the most reliable imaging modality for staging, treatment planning, and following-up the cervical cancer. In particular, clinical staging of cervical cancer is based on the nodal status [2] and the tumor volume. However, this heavily relies on developing accurate segmentation techniques of cervical cancer on MR images that can effectively capture the large variability in the shape, location, and size of the tumor. To the best of our knowledge, a few fully automatic segmentation methods have been applied to diagnose cervical cancer. In this work [3], a Fisher's linear discriminant analysis approach was used for cervical cancer segmentation. Related works on pelvic organ segmentation leveraged machine learning techniques for automated tissue labeling using Computed Tomography (CT) and MRI data. For instance, advanced organ segmentation methods such as male pelvic organs using non-linear classifiers were proposed in [4, 5]. In [4], a new deformable MR method was devised to segment prostate by integrating deep feature learning with sparse patch matching. In [5], displacement regressors were estimated by multi-task Random Forest (RF) for guiding a deformable segmentation model. On the other hand, several studies showed that the aggregation of multiple classifiers improved the performance of a single classifier. In [6], Choi *et al.* combined different classifier approaches such as RF and Gentle AdaBoost learning techniques for improved classification of mammographic lesion. The approach achieved better results compared to each individual classifier model. However, these methods [3–6] are somewhat limited as they require hand-crafted features and may not be robust against varying image appearances. This motivates us to use Deep Learning (DL) method based on Convolutional Neural Networks (CNNs), where features are extracted and learned automatically for robust segmentation.

Recently, CNNs [7] and Fully Convolutional Network (FCN) [8] have gained more popularity in medical image high-resolution synthesis and organ segmentation as they automatically learn features and have defined the state-of-the-art performance in several tasks. For instance, Bahrami *et al.* [7] devised and trained a deep CNN architecture using appearance (intensity) and anatomical (brain-tissue labels) patches to non-linearly map 3T MRI to 7T MRI. In a different work, Alansary *et al.* [8] used CNN to segment the placenta from the structural T2-w MR scans of the whole uterus. To further boost up the performance of a single CNN, other approaches [9–11] chained a set of CNNs for image labeling and reconstruction. Bahrami *et al.* [9] cascaded deep CNN architectures proposed in [7]. In [10], a combination of three ConvNets was used to detect the heart in a different orthogonal plane. In [11], a cascaded architecture that simultaneously exploits local and global contextual features was utilized to segment brain tumor. However, deep learning methods developed in [7–11] mostly leverage a single CNN architecture. To address this limitation, CNN ensemble learning strategies were developed to leverage the strength of multiple CNN architectures. For example, Kamnitsas *et al.* [12] used ensemble of multiple CNN architectures for brain tumor segmentation. In [13], three paralleled CNNs with the same architecture trained following different image preprocessing methods were used for cervical cancer segmentation. Dolz *et al.* [14] also utilized an ensemble of deep CNNs to segment infant brains in MRI images, where 10 CNNs were combined using majority voting to refine the quality of segmentation. Ju and *et al.* [15] investigated a wide spectrum of ensemble learning methods, including the super learner, the Bayes optimal classifier, unweighted averaging and majority voting, with deep neural networks for image recognition tasks. Guan *et al.* [16] demonstrated that their ensemble of deep long short-term memory (LSTM) networks improved the performance of individual LSTM networks for activity recognition.

All previous ensemble DL methods [7–16] developed for image segmentation and other tasks overlooked three major aspects, which if leveraged would further improve the target results: (1) the *heterogeneity* of MRI training patches distribution, (2) *relational learning* at multiple levels of CNN-to-CNN interactions in the ensemble model (absence of *dynamic* learning), and (3) *multiscale* anatomical variability across patients.

On the other hand, recently, Amiri *et al.* [17] designed a Dynamic Multiscale Tree (DMT) structure for brain tumor segmentation, where each node embeds a structured RF classifier or a Bayesian Network (BN) classifier. The DMT cascades classifiers along different traversal paths in a binary tree for multi-label brain image segmentation. Ascending and descending feedbacks between each parent node and its children nodes are dynamically communicated and gradually refined to boost the overall performance of the tree. To address the limitations of aforementioned methods [3–17] while leveraging their appealing aspects, we unprecedentedly propose a *Cluster-based Dynamic Multi-scale Forest* ($C^{K+1}DMF$) for automatic cervical cancer segmentation. The proposed $C^{K+1}DMF$ comprises $(K+1)$ dynamic multiscale trees (DMTs): a *principal tree* trained using all data samples, and K *subordinate trees*, each trained with a more homogeneous cluster of data samples. In particular, each node, in our proposed DMT, nests a CNN architecture. As we go deeper along the tree edges nearing its CNN leaf nodes, the training patch size decreases and the architecture of each visited CNN node becomes shallower. Ultimately, in the testing stage, a testing intensity patch passes through each of these paralleled DMTs, then majority voting is used to fuse labels from all trees in our dynamic forest.

2 Proposed Cluster-Based Dynamic Multi-scale Dynamic Forest

Figure 1 shows the proposed $C^{K+1}DMF$ architecture. Our method comprises several steps. *First*, we cluster the training intensity patches into K clusters using k-means clustering using squared Euclidean distance. *Second*, we design a dynamic forest, where each tree is defined as a DMT [17], and each node in the DMT nests a CNN architecture. We define a principal tree which will be trained using all patches, and K subordinate trees, each trained using patches belonging to each of the clusters. *Next*, the directional flow $F(n_i \rightarrow n_j)$ from node n_i to node n_j in the tree is defined as: $F(n_i \rightarrow n_j) = L(n_i)$, where $L(n_i)$ is the label map outputted by node n_i. This auto-contextual flow enforces spatial consistency between neighboring patches during

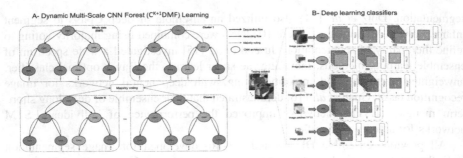

Fig. 1. (**A**) Proposed clustering-based paralleled C^{K+1}DMF for cervical cancer segmentation. We first define a DMT where the training of each tree is dynamic comprising an ascending (red arrow) and descending (black arrow) contextual flow, i.e., probability segmentation map between each parent node and its children nodes. Thus, the two children nodes of the same parent communicate together (via red arrows). Then, we cluster training patches into K clusters. Next, we define C^{K+1}DMF, where the principal DMT is trained using the whole training samples, while the subordinate K paralleled DMTs are trained using samples in each cluster. Final segmentation map is obtained by applying majority voting to segmentation maps of all C^{k+1}DMF. (**B**) Proposed multiscale CNN architectures to define nodes in each tree in our dynamic forest.

training. Finally, to generate the target tumor label map, we apply majority voting to the segmentation maps outputted by each DMT in our forest.

2.1   Root Node CNN Architecture

Figure 1-B displays the designed multiscale CNN architectures, including the tree root CNN node in green (i.e., CNN1). To train and test our model, we first automatically define a region of interest (ROI) around the tumor in the cervix, and then we extract 2D intensity patches of size 15×15 from each sagittal slice for each training subject.

Convolutional layers of root node CNN. Our architecture is composed of four layers. The first CNN layer aims to learn a feature representation of the input intensity patch of size 15×15. The activation function of the first layer is defined as $a_1 = max(0, M(f_1, x) + b_1)$, where 1 corresponds to 64 filters with size 7×7, denotes the biases, and (.) is the mapping convolution function, followed by ReLU function $(0,.)$. The activation function in the second layer is formulated as $a_2 = max(0, (f_2, a_1) + b_2)$, where denotes the learned 128 filters of size of 5×5 and the corresponding biases. Similarly, the activation function of the third layer is defined as $a_3 = max(0, (f_3, a_2) + b_3)$. We basically convolve the 128 feature maps of the second layer with 256 filters of size 3×3, followed by ReLU. Finally, we estimate the 256 feature maps of the fourth layer with one filter of size of 3×3, followed by ReLU, using $a_4 = max(0, (f_4, a_3) + b_4)$.

Fully connected layer and regression function. The final layer in our architecture is a fully connected layer followed by a regression function to produce the target label value at the center pixel of the input intensity patch x. In fact, during training, each intensity patch is mapped to the center voxel value in its corresponding label patch. The final label map is obtained through probability map thresholding. However, a single CNN has a poor invariance scaling, hence the value of cascaded CNNs [9–11].

2.2 Cascaded CNNs

To further boost the performance of a single CNN, we nest it into a cascade of CNNs while leveraging the performance of the previous CNN using an auto-context model. This is achieved through feed-forwarding the outputted segmentation map of each CNN in the cascade as a context information along with the original intensity map to the next CNN as in [9]. By generating the whole image segmentation map after each CNN, we can enforce spatial consistency as neighboring patches coordinate with each other for joint improvement of tumor segmentation using the next CNN (Supplementary Fig. 1). However, a CNN nested in such a cascaded architecture, will only benefit from the learning of the previous CNN in the chain. To address this limitation, we leverage the binary dynamic multiscale tree architecture proposed in [17] to define a CNN-based DMT, where each node embeds a specific single-scale CNN architecture.

2.3 Proposed CNN-Based Dynamic Multi-scale Tree (DMT)

Specifically, our CNN-based DMT is a binary tree $T(V, E)$, where $V = \{n_1, \ldots, n_N\}$ denotes the set of N nodes in T and E is a finite set of directed edges connecting two nodes in T. Each parent node nests a CNN architecture, and has two children CNN nodes (one left and one right). At the mth iteration of our DMT learning, a parent node n_i receives the ascending flows $F^m(n_j \rightarrow n_i)$ and $F^m(n_{j'} \rightarrow n_i)$ from its left and right children nodes n_j and $n_{j'}$, which are first fused then passed on, in a second round $(m + 1)$, as contextual information $F^{m+1}(n_i \rightarrow n_j) = L^{m+1}(n_i)$ and $F^{m+1}(n_i \rightarrow n_{j'}) = L^{m+1}(n_i)$ to the children nodes (Fig. 2). We note that each parent CNN node is trained using the fusion of the segmentation maps passed on by its children nodes along with the original input intensity images to produce a new probability map, then communicate it to its two children nodes. Hence, the children CNN nodes of the same parent CNN node cooperate to enhance their parent learning as well as their own learning. This progressively improves the training of each

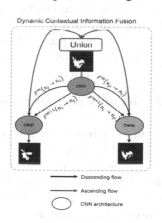

Fig. 2. Binary tree architecture. Ascending and descending flows in our dynamic CNN-DMT.

CNN classifier node at each scale level of the tree. Our CNN-DMT is generated automatically as described in Supplementary Fig. 3 and Algorithm 1.

In addition, to learn how to label anatomical details of the tumor at different scales, we propose a *coarse-to-fine tree learning strategy*, where the root node of the tree embeds the first CNN architecture with a largest patch of size s_1. Next, the architecture of parent node along with its associated training patch size will be copied into its left node (only once as it is not propagated to its grand-child node). The right node, on the other hand, nests a shallower CNN trained with a smaller patch size $s_{l+1} < s_l$ at the next level $l + 1$. We note that after copying one CNN architecture once to the left, the left node of the copied CNN will nest a shallower CNN trained at a finer scale. Our proposed CNN-based DMT has two strengths: (1) it captures fine-to-coarse variability in tumor shape and intensity, and (2) both the scale and the patch size influence the performance of parent and children nodes. In fact, to further boost the performance of a single CNN node of the same architecture and to handle unbalanced distribution of negative and positive patches, the left node is copied once to the left. The dynamic tree models the relationships between maps generated from different CNN architecture and at different scales, which helps further reduce the segmentation errors.

2.4 Proposed C^{K+1}DMF Learning Framework

Although promising, our CNN-based DMT overlooks the heterogeneity of the training patches. To better explore the heterogeneous intensity patch distribution, we divide all training intensity patches including both positive (inside tumor) and negative (outside tumor) samples into K clusters to define homogeneous patch clusters using k-means algorithm. Next, we introduce our C^{K+1} Dynamic Multi-scale Forest (DMF), aggregating $(K + 1)$ paralleled DMT learners in a unified dynamic architecture. Specifically, our C^{K+1}DMF includes a principal DMT, which is trained using all training patches, and K subordinate DMTs, each trained using patches within a specific cluster. In the testing stage, each testing patch passes through each DMT to eventually estimate the label of its center pixel. Ultimately, we apply majority voting to the segmentation maps outputted by the $(K + 1)$ DMTs (**Fig.** 1).

3 Results and Discussion

Dataset, parameters and evaluation. We evaluated our method on 12 clinical T2-weighted MR images of patients with cervical cancer using leave-one-out cross-validation. We use affine registration to align all training MR images to a common space. Each testing subject is then affinely aligned to the training samples. To speed up CNN training, we extract intensity patches within a bounding box of size 141×141 automatically drawn around the cervix and its neighboring regions on sagittal views. For each subject, we extracted 2D intensity patches of size of 15×15 from each sagittal slice for each training subject, thereby producing 363,000 patches for each subject. We used about 4 million patches for training our CNN models. For evaluation, we used the Dice ratio defined as: $Dice = 2A \cap B / A + B$, where denotes the ground-truth (GT) label map, manually delineated by an expert radiologist, and the estimated label map.

Evaluation and comparison methods. We compared our C^{K+1}DMF with several segmentation methods (**Table** 1): (1) single CNN [7], (2) Contextual CNN Cascade-1 (CNN-C2), (3) CNN-C3 [9], (4) DMT($d = 1$), and (5) DMT($d = 2$) [17]. We note that CNN-C2 cascades two CNNs while CNN-C3 cascades three CNNs. We stop at depth

$d = 2$ as the improvement in the classification accuracy becomes negligible. Our $C^{k+1}DMF(d = 2)$ is a binary tree with 3 levels (root node + 2 levels). On the other hand, for cluster-based methods, we used the squared Euclidean distance for k-means algorithm. The optimal number of clusters is 3. We note that the number of clusters was empirically set. We also note that DMT($d = 1$) uses $n = 2^{d+1} - 1$ nodes (i.e., 3 nodes). DMT($d = 2$) uses 7 nodes. The proposed cluster-based methods include (6) $C^{K+1}DMF(d = 1)$, and (7) $C^{K+1}DMF(d = 2)$. We note that $C^{K+1}DMF(d = 1)$ uses (k + 1) × n nodes (i.e., 12 nodes). For instance, C^4DMF ($d = 2$) has 28 nodes.

The detailed experimental results are reported in Table 1. We visually inspect the results using our framework and comparison methods for 3 representative patients displayed in Fig. 3. Our proposed C^4DMF ($d = 2$) significantly outperformed all comparison methods (p < 0.05) and produced the best segmentation maps. We note that we report results after applying a post-process using Savitzky–Golay filter for smoothing the tumor boundary outputted by each method. We also note a significant increase in the average Dice ratio from 74.6% by the conventional CNN and 79.9% by the conventional DMT to 84.9% when using $C^4DMF(d = 2)$. Our C^4DMF multi-architecture boosted the segmentation accuracy up to 79.9%, in comparison to 76.2%

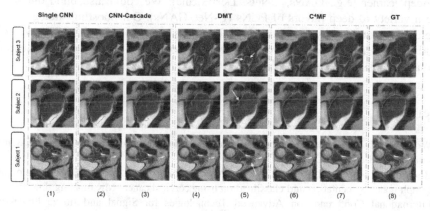

Fig. 3. *Cervical cancer results for 3 representative patients.* Comparison methods and our proposed methods: (1) CNN, (2) CNN-C2, (3) CNN-C3, (4) DMT(1), (5) DMT(2), (6) C^4DMF (1), (7) C^4DMF(2), and (8) GT.

Table 1. Average Dice ratio mixg comparison and proposed methods.

Methods	Average Dice (%)
CNN [7]	74.6 = 4.3
CNN-C2	75.7 = 6.0
CNN-C3 [9]	76.0 = 6.1
DMT($d = 1$)	78.1 ± 7.0
DMTM($d = 2$) [17]	79.9 = 6.5
C^4-DMF($d = 1$)	84.0 = 6.3
C^4-DMF($d = 2$)	**84.9 ± 6.7**

obtained when solely cascaded CNN. Since the subordinate trees in $C^4DMF(d = 2)$ are able to better capture the boundary of the tumor, they helped significantly (p = 0.002) boost up the performance of the principal. This shows that disentangling heterogeneous training samples can help improve CNN training and boost its performance. Both quantitatively and qualitatively, we observed that each cluster captures a unique anatomical detail of the tumor boundary that might be overlooked by other clusters (yellow arrows in Fig. 3 and Supplementary Fig. 2). A theoretical proof is out of the scope of the current paper.

4 Conclusion

In this paper, we proposed a novel fully automated ensemble deep learning architecture for cervical tumor segmentation on T2-w MR images, leveraging auto-context model to enforce spatial consistency between neighboring patches and introducing paralleled CNN-based dynamic multi-scale trees to handle training-sample heterogeneity. The focus of our paper is not on the choice of the deep learners (CNN or GANs) but on the *boosting* strategy itself by our *generic* clustered forest, which should be applicable to any deep learner (e.g., GANs, UNets, DeepMedic). We could also build our forest using a variety of deep flavors of FCNs (U-Net, GANs). Our boosting strategy is not complex compared to typical boosting algorithms such as ADABOOST. We will extend our $C^{K+1}DMF$ boosting architecture to further handle fine-to-coarse anatomical variability across subjects.

References

1. World Health Organization: Comprehensive Cervical Cancer Control: A Guide to Essential Practice, 2nd edn, p. 2014. WHO, Geneva (2017)
2. Bnouni, N., Mechi, O., Rekik, I., Rhim, M.S., Essoukri Ben Amara, N.: Semi-automatic lymph node segmentation and classification using cervical cancer MR imaging. In: 2018 4th International Conference on Advanced Technologies for Signal and Image Processing (ATSIP), pp. 1–6. IEEE (2018)
3. Torheim, T., Malinen, E., Hole, K.H., Lund, K.V., Indahl, U.G., Lyng, H., et al.: Autodelineation of cervical cancers using multiparametric magnetic resonance imaging and machine learning. Acta Oncol. **56**(6), 806–812 (2017)
4. Guo, Y., Gao, Y., Shen, D.: Deformable MR prostate segmentation via deep feature learning and sparse patch matching. In: Deep Learning for Medical Image Analysis, pp. 197–222 (2017)
5. Gao, Y., Shao, Y., Lian, J., Wang, A.Z., Chen, R.C., Shen, D.: Accurate segmentation of CT male pelvic organs via regression-based deformable models and multi-task random forests. IEEE Trans. Med. Imaging **35**(6), 1532–1543 (2016)
6. Choi, J.Y., Kim, D.H., Plataniotis, K.N., Ro, Y.M.: Classifier ensemble generation and selection with multiple feature representations for classification applications in computer-aided detection and diagnosis on mammography. Expert Syst. Appl. **46**, 106–121 (2016)
7. Bahrami, Khosro, Shi, Feng, Rekik, Islem, Shen, Dinggang: Convolutional neural network for reconstruction of 7T-like images from 3T MRI using appearance and anatomical features. In:

Carneiro, Gustavo, Mateus, Diana, Peter, Loïc, Bradley, Andrew, Tavares, João Manuel R.S., Belagiannis, Vasileios, Papa, João Paulo, Nascimento, Jacinto C., Loog, Marco, Lu, Zhi, Cardoso, Jaime S., Cornebise, Julien (eds.) LABELS/DLMIA -2016. LNCS, vol. 10008, pp. 39–47. Springer, Cham (2016). https://doi.org/10.1007/978-3-319-46976-8_5

8. Alansary, A., et al.: Fast fully automatic segmentation of the human placenta from motion corrupted MRI. In: International Conference on Medical Image Computing and Computer-Assisted Intervention, pp. 589–597. Springer, Cham (2016)

9. Bahrami, K., Rekik, I., Shi, F., Shen, D.: Joint reconstruction and segmentation of 7T-like MR images from 3T MRI based on cascaded convolutional neural networks. In: International Conference on Medical Image Computing and Computer-Assisted Intervention, pp. 764–772. Springer, Cham (2017)

10. Wolterink, J.M., Leiner, T., de Vos, B.D., van Hamersvelt, R.W., Viergever, M.A., Išgum, I.: Automatic coronary artery calcium scoring in cardiac CT angiography using paired convolutional neural networks. Med. Image Anal. **34**, 123–136 (2016)

11. Havaei, M., Davy, A., Warde-Farley, D., Biard, A., Courville, A., Bengio, Y., et al.: Brain tumor segmentation with deep neural networks. Med. Image Anal. **35**, 18–31 (2017)

12. Kamnitsas, K., et al. (2017). Ensembles of multiple models and architectures for robust brain tumour segmentation. arXiv preprint arXiv:1711.01468

13. Bnouni, N., Ben Amor, H., Rekik, I., Rhim, M. S., Solaiman, B., Essoukri Ben Amara, N.: Boosting CNN learning by ensemble image preprocessing methods for cervical cancer MR image segmentation. In: International Conference on Sensors, Systems Signals and Advanced Technologies (SSS) (2018)

14. Dolz, J., Desrosiers, C., Wang, L., Yuan, J., Shen, D., Ayed, I.B.: Deep CNN ensembles and suggestive annotations for infant brain MRI segmentation. arXiv preprint arXiv:1712.05319 (2017)

15. Ju, C., Bibaut, A., van der Laan, M.J.: The relative performance of ensemble methods with deep convolutional neural networks for image classification. arXiv preprint arXiv:1704.01664 (2017)

16. Guan, Y., Plötz, T.: Ensembles of deep lstm learners for activity recognition using wearables. Proc. ACM Interact. Mob. Wearable Ubiquitous Technol. **1**(2), 11 (2017)

17. Amiri, S., Mahjoub, M.A., Rekik, I.: Tree-based ensemble classifier learning for automatic brain glioma segmentation. Neurocomputing (2018). ISSN:0925-2312

Multi-task Fundus Image Quality Assessment via Transfer Learning and Landmarks Detection

Yaxin Shen[1], Ruogu Fang[2(✉)], Bin Sheng[1(✉)], Ling Dai[1], Huating Li[3], Jing Qin[4], Qiang Wu[3], and Weiping Jia[3]

[1] Department of Computer Science and Engineering, Shanghai Jiao Tong University, Shanghai, China
shengbin@sjtu.edu.cn
[2] Department of Biomedical Engineering, University of Florida, Gainesville, FL, USA
Ruogu.Fang@bme.ufl.edu
[3] Shanghai Jiao Tong University Affiliated Sixth People's Hospital, Shanghai, China
[4] School of Nursing, The Hong Kong Polytechnic University, Hong Kong, China

Abstract. The quality of fundus images is critical for diabetic retinopathy diagnosis. The evaluation of fundus image quality can be affected by several factors, including image artifact, clarity, and field definition. In this paper, we propose a multi-task deep learning framework for automated assessment of fundus image quality. The network can classify whether an image is gradable, together with interpretable information about quality factors. The proposed method uses images in both rectangular and polar coordinates, and fine-tunes the network from trained model grading of diabetic retinopathy. The detection of optic disk and fovea assists learning the field definition task through coarse-to-fine feature encoding. The experimental results demonstrate that our framework outperform single-task convolutional neural networks and reject ungradable images in automated diabetic retinopathy diagnostic systems.

Keywords: Fundus image quality assessment · Multi-task learning Optic disk detection · Fovea detection

1 Introduction

Fundus images are widely used in diagnosis of Diabetic Retinopathy (DR), age-related macular degeneration, and other retinal diseases [3]. Diagnosis requires high quality images, because blurred images may cause misdiagonsis. Recently, automatic DR diagnosis has gained significant research and clinical interests,

---

Y. Shen and R. Fang—These authors contribute equally to this work

Electronic supplementary material The online version of this chapter (https://doi.org/10.1007/978-3-030-00919-9_4) contains supplementary material, which is available to authorized users.

© Springer Nature Switzerland AG 2018
Y. Shi et al. (Eds.): MLMI 2018, LNCS 11046, pp. 28–36, 2018.
https://doi.org/10.1007/978-3-030-00919-9_4

while the image quality plays a key role in the diagnosis accuracy. Even though the technology used in digital fundus imaging has improved, non-biological factors resulting from improper operation can still reduce image quality. Therefore, image quality assessment (IQA) is essential for identifying ungradable images.

The IQA of fundus image belongs to No-Reference approaches without additional reference images. Lalonde et al. [6] used global edge histogram. Kohler et al. [5] used vessel segmentation. However, these methods only consider specific quality factor using hand-crafted features, neglecting the holistic picture of image quality. Deep convolutional neural networks (CNNs) have shown promising results in computer vision tasks. [9] proposed shallow CNNs to classify fundus image quality. [10] combined the CNN feature with salience map. These approaches lack analysis of quality factor. Hence, automatic retinal image quality assessment remains an open and important research direction.

In this paper, we propose a deep learning framework to extract fundus image features in both rectangular and polar coordinates to classify if input images are "gradable" as shown in Fig. 1. We analyze image quality in terms of artifact, clarity and field definition. To address a lack of data, we preinitialize weights by DR grading network. The field definition task is not reliable when the optic disk (OD) are invisible. The framework can filter clear and artifact-free images for fovea and OD localization and provide accurate field definition analysis. Our experimental results indicate that auxiliary tasks contribute to the image quality task while avoiding overfitting, and learning with both coordinate systems outperforms any single coordinate system. From these observations, our framework can provide reliable image quality assessment with quality factor analysis.

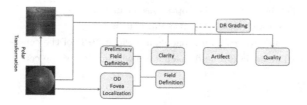

Fig. 1. The framework of the automatic fundus image quality assessment system.

2   Dataset

The dataset was collected from Shanghai Diabetic Retinopathy Screening Program (SDRSP). We used 11,653 retinal images for quality assessment and 275,146 for DR grading. The image quality is graded according to standards in terms of artifact, clarity, and field definition, as shown in Table 1. Figure 2 shows sample images with quality issues. Meanwhile graders also evaluate whether fundus images are adequate for grading. OD and fovea localization tasks use Indian Diabetic Retinopathy Image Dataset including 516 images without quality detects.

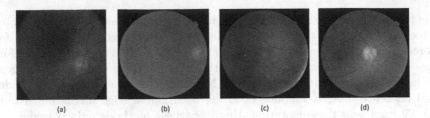

(a)   (b)   (c)   (d)

Fig. 2. From left to right, the images have problem on artifact, clarity and field definition respectively. Image (d) is a gradable image.

Table 1. Image quality scoring criteria

Type	Image quality specification	Score
Artifact	Do not contain artifacts	0
	Outside the aortic arch with range less than 1/4 of the image	1
	Do not affect the macular area with scope less than 1/4	4
	Cover more than 1/4, less than 1/2 of the image	6
	Cover more than 1/2 without fully cover the posterior pole	8
	Cover the entire posterior pole	10
Clarity	Only Level 1 vascular arch can be identified	1
	Can identify Level 2 vascular arch and a small number of lesions	4
	Can identify Level 3 vascular arch and some lesions	6
	Can identify Level 3 vascular arch and most lesions	8
	Can identify Level 3 vascular arch and all lesions	10
Field definition	Do not include the optic disc and macular	1
	Only contain either optic disc or macula	4
	Contain both optic disc and macula	6
	The optic disc and macula are within 2PD of the center	8
	The optic disc and macula are within 1PD of the center	10

3   Method

3.1   Multi-task Convolutional Neural Networks

Multi-task Learning. We propose an architecture with two input branches in rectangular and polar coordinates respectively and four output task branches as shown in Fig. 3. CNNs exploit spatially-local correlation, and through polar transformation, can better remove the black background of the original fundus image while extracting features of ringing artifacts. We preprocess images by cropping the circular region, and rescaled to 224 × 224 pixels. The proposed architecture uses hard parameter sharing [7] to optimize four tasks simultaneously: image artifact, clarity, field definition and overall quality. For the first three tasks, the network makes multiple predictions. The clarity task is a multilabel binary classification including whether the clarity score is greater than 1,

4, 6 and 8 respectively, while the artifact task and field definition task are similar based on Table 1. The overall image quality task makes a binary prediction on whether the image is gradable, where label 0 indicates gradable, and label 1 ungradable.

Transfer Learning. These tasks share same CNN encoders to extract structural features of retinal images. The network architecture of CNN encoder for each single coordinate branch includes the first 11 convolutional layers of ResNet-18 [1] as shown in Fig. 3. To speed up the training and to address the limited training data issue, we use two stage transfer learning method. (1) We perform DR grading using ResNet-18 network pretrained on ImageNet dataset. (2) We perform the second transfer learning using the model parameters from the trained DR grading network to initialize CNN encoders for image quality assessment.

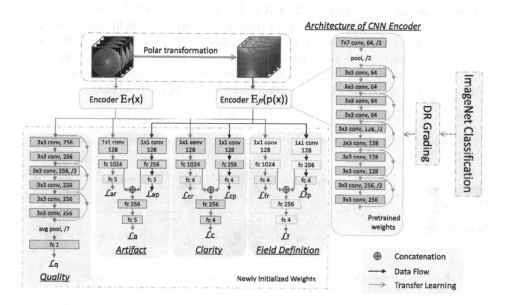

Fig. 3. Multi-task deep learning architecture of our proposed fundus image quality assessment network.

Architecture. Figure 3 shows the overall network architecture of our proposed multi-task retinal image quality assessment framework. Let $X = \{(x_i, y_i)\}_{i=0}^{N}$ represent labeled dataset of N samples. Let $p(x)$ represents a polar transformation function. Subscripts r, p represent rectangular and polar coordinate branches respectively, a, c, f and q represent artifact, clarity, field definition, and image quality tasks. Let $E(x, \theta_e)$ be a function parameterized by θ_e maps image x to a hidden representation shared by tasks. Batch normalization is used after each convolution layer. The polar coordinate branch encodes feature into 256-D embedding and the rectangular coordinate branch encodes feature into 1024-D embedding. The concatenation of these two embeddings is used for task-specific prediction. To ensure the representation of each single branch is useful and to improve generalizability, we optimize the losses after each branch and the concatenate representation at training stage, whereas at test stage, only the concatenate representations make the final prediction for quality factors. As depicted in Fig. 3, layers marked in yellow are only passed during training. The overall image quality task is optimized by the rectangular branch because polar image will lose some local structure features of vessels, OD and fovea.

3.2 Optic Disc and Fovea Detection

The field definition task relies on clear images, which is not reliable only depending on the network mentioned in Sect. 3.1. According to the clinical requirements, we choose score 8 to separate whether images are correct on field definition. We filter out images with adequate clarity and free of artifact through multi-task quality assessment network, and localize the OD center and fovea center to improve the performance of field definition by deciding whether they are within 2PD of the center of the image. The architecture is depicted in Fig. 4.

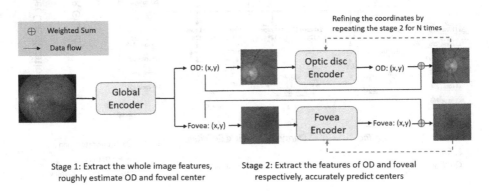

Fig. 4. The architecture for the detection of optic disc and fovea. This framework shows the data flow in inference stage. The global CNN encoder, the local optic disc encoder and the local fovea encoder are trained separately.

Global Encoder. The global CNN encoder is defined as a neural network component locating both the optic disc and fovea centers simultaneously. We extract the entire image feature and detect both the centers of OD and fovea through a global encoder with a backbone network of ResNet-50.

Local Encoder. The local encoders are designed as components that only focus on single object localization which refine the prediction of optic disc and fovea centers respectively. The retinal images in IDRiD dataset are only labeled with target center coordinates. The shapes and sizes of OD or fovea are basically invariant, but the sizes of target objects may vary due to the photographer's operation. Thus the bounding box can be located with the center coordinates and the approximate shape and scale. Square RoIs are directly cropped from the original image and will not be deformed after reducing the image size. The backbone network architecture of local encoder is VGG-16[8]. See Fig. 1 in the supplement for detail about RoIs selection.

For all encoders, we replace all the max pooling layers with average pooling layers compared with the original network architecture, due to the fact that the max pooling may lose some useful pixel-level information for our regression to predict the coordinates. The described algorithm won the first place on ISBI-2018 challenge for fovea and optic disc detection.

3.3   Learning

The goal of training the multi-task quality assessment network is to minimize the total loss:

$$L = \alpha \sum_{t=a,c,f} L_{tp} + \beta \sum_{t=a,c,f} L_{tr} + \gamma \sum_{t=a,c,f} L_t + \delta L_q \tag{1}$$

where α, β, γ and δ are the weights of loss terms, subscripts r, p represent rectangular and polar coordinate branches respectively, a, c, f and q represent artifact, clarity, field definition and image quality tasks. The classification loss L_{tp} and L_{tr} make task-specific prediction from polar and rectangular branch respectively, L_t makes prediction from the concatenate representation. The quality task loss L_q is the negative log-likelihood of the label for whether it is gradable:

$$L_q = -\sum_{i=0}^{N}(y_i^q \cdot log\hat{y}_i^q + (1 - y_i^q) \cdot log(1 - \hat{y}_i^q)) \tag{2}$$

where $y_i^q \in \{0,1\}$ is the class label and $\hat{y}_i^q = \frac{1}{1+e^{h_i}}$ represents the sigmoid prediction. The artifact, clarity and field definition tasks are learned by multi-label classification, and the losses of these tasks use sigmoid cross-entropy loss function as well.

For the OD and fovea localization task, the regression loss for the center location is Euclidean loss:

$$L = \frac{1}{2N} \sum_{i=1}^{N} \|y_i - \hat{y}_i\|_2^2 \tag{3}$$

where N is 2, y_0 and y_1 are the ground truth coordinates, $\hat{y}_0$ and $\hat{y}_1$ are the predicted coordinates. The loss functions are:

$$L_{global} = 0.0045 \cdot (L_{OD} + L_{fovea}) \tag{4}$$

$$L_{local} = 0.0045 \cdot L_{landmark} \tag{5}$$

We scale the loss since the original Euclidean distance is too large in practice to converge.

4   Experiments and Results

The quality labeled dataset contain 11,653 images including 3,373 un-gradable images and 8,280 gradable images. The training set contains 10,000 images selected by stratified sampling. We compare our proposed multi-task framework with baselines: (a) image quality task using the rectangular coordinate, (b) all tasks using the rectangular coordinate, (c) all tasks using both coordinates and (d) image quality task using the rectangular coordinate and quality factor tasks using both coordinates without transfer learning. Experiment (a) uses single-task learning, and (b) to (d) use multi-task learning with different architectures. For the OD and fovea localization, we randomly select 350 images from the IDRiD dataset as training set.

All the models are implemented in Caffe framework [4] and are trained using Stochastic Gradient with momentum. The multi-task quality networks are trained for 15 epochs and fine-tuned from DR grading network. The new initialized weights are initialized as in [2]. We use a mini-batch size of 128 and a weight decay of 0.0001. For the OD and fovea localization task, we train the global encoder for 200 epochs, local encoders for 30 epochs. The batch size for the global encoder is 16, and 64 for the other two local encoders. The learning rate is set as 0.01 and is divided by 10 when the error plateaus.

Table 2. Experimental results of overall image quality task we evaluated on all the methods. We replicated the experiments from [9] and [10] at the first two rows. The proposed methods in this paper is reported in the last row.

Method	Sensitivity	Specificity	AUC
Tennakoon et al. [9]	0.7235	0.8127	0.89073
Yu et al. [10]	0.8487	0.6418	0.92508
Quality task only(rectangular) single task learning	0.84194	0.83743	0.92287
All tasks(rectangular)	0.86774	0.80351	0.92363
All tasks(rectangular + polar)	0.83871	**0.83977**	0.92564
Quality task(rectangular)sub-tasks(rectangular + polar) without transfer learning	0.88387	0.78363	0.91829
Quality task(rectangular) sub-tasks(rectangular + polar)	**0.89677**	0.8	**0.93168**

Receiver operating characteristic (ROC) curves for the comparison methods of our proposed architecture are shown in Fig. 5. The weights of loss terms for Eq. 1 are set to: $\alpha = 0.2$, $\beta = 0.5$, $\gamma = 1.0$ and $\delta = 4.0$. Figure 5(a) shows the ROC for image quality task, the Area Under Curve (AUC) of the proposed method was 0.93168 which is the highest among the experiments. Table 2 reports sensitivity, specificity, and AUC for quality task of all comparing methods. We plot ROC curves of artifact, clarity and field definition as shown in Fig. 5. Image with field definition score larger than 6 can be consider to be image valid on field definition. The ROC curve of score 6 for field definition is corrected by OD and fovea detection and the AUC value is improved by 0.4%. The experimental results of OD and fovea localization are in supplement.

The proposed model outperforms all comparing approaches in our experiments, as it is able to improve the performance by multi-task learning through a representation that captures all tasks and avoids overfitting the overall image quality task. Multi-task learning is also an implicit data augmentation, as the model can learn a more general representation for multiple tasks.

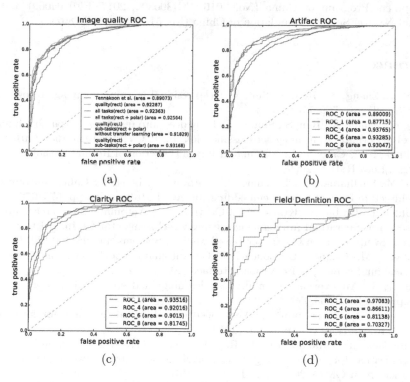

Fig. 5. ROC plots all tasks. (a) plots quality classification compared with different approaches. (b),(c),(d) plot sub-tasks of our proposed method according to different quality factor scores as described in Sect. 3.1. ROC_i plots ROC curve of binary classification on whether quality factor score is greater than score i.

5   Conclusion

In this paper, we have proposed an automated image quality assessment framework by deep multi-task learning, polar transformation and transfer learning which can predict image quality for DR diagnosis and provide interpretable quality factor scores in terms of artifact, clarity, and field definition. The experimental results demonstrate that the proposed multi-task architecture improves the performance on image quality classification. As image quality is an important pre-requisite of diabetic retinal image grading, the proposed technique can be incorporated with automated retinal image grading systems for DR screening programs.

Acknowledgement. This work is partially supported by National Key Research and Development Program of China (No: 2016YFC1300302, 2017YFE0104000) and by National Natural Science Foundation of China (No: 61525106, 61427807).

References

1. He, K., Zhang, X., Ren, S., Sun, J.: Deep residual learning for image recognition. In: CVPR, pp. 770–778 (2015)
2. He, K., Zhang, X., Ren, S., Sun, J.: Delving deep into rectifiers: Surpassing human-level performance on imagenet classification. In: ICCV, pp. 1026–1034 (2015)
3. Jelinek, H.F., Cree, M.J.: Automated Image Detection of Retinal Pathology. CRC Press, Boca Raton (2009)
4. Jia, Y., Shelhamer, E., Donahue, J., Karayev, S., Long, J.: Caffe: convolutional architecture for fast feature embedding. In: ACM Multimedia, pp. 675–678 (2014)
5. Kohler, T., Budai, A., Kraus, M.F., Odstrcilik, J.: Automatic no-reference quality assessment for retinal fundus images using vessel segmentation. In: IEEE International Symposium on Computer-Based Medical Systems, pp. 95–100 (2013)
6. Lalonde, M., Gagnon, L., Boucher, M.C.: Automatic visual quality assessment in optical fundus images. In: Vision Interface (2001)
7. Ruder, S.: An overview of multi-task learning in deep neural networks. arXiv preprint arXiv:1706.05098 (2017)
8. Simonyan, K., Zisserman, A.: Very deep convolutional networks for large-scale image recognition. Comput. Sci. (2014)
9. Tennakoon, R., Mahapatra, D., Roy, P., Sedai, S., Garnavi, R.: Image quality classification for DR screening using convolutional neural networks. In: MICCAI Workshop on OMIA 2016, pp. 113–120 (2016)
10. Yu, F.L., Sun, J., Li, A., Cheng, J., Cheng, W., Liu, J., et al.: Image quality classification for DR screening using deep learning. Eng. Med. Biol. Soc. 664–667 (2017)

End-to-End Lung Nodule Detection
in Computed Tomography

Dufan Wu[1], Kyungsang Kim[1], Bin Dong[2], Georges El Fakhri[1],
and Quanzheng Li[1]($\boxtimes$)

[1] Gordon Center for Medical Imaging, Massachusetts General Hospital
and Harvard Medical School, Boston, MA 02114, USA
{dwu6,li.quanzheng}@mgh.harvard.edu
[2] Beijing International Center for Mathematical Research, Peking University,
Beijing 100080, China

Abstract. Computer aided diagnostic (CAD) system is crucial for modern medical imaging. But almost all CAD systems operate on reconstructed images, which were optimized for radiologists. Computer vision can capture features that is subtle to human observers, so it is desirable to design a CAD system operating on the raw data. In this paper, we proposed a deep-neural-network-based detection system for lung nodule detection in computed tomography (CT). A primal-dual-type deep reconstruction network was applied first to convert the raw data to the image space, followed by a 3-dimensional convolutional neural network (3D-CNN) for the nodule detection. For efficient network training, the deep reconstruction network and the CNN detector was trained sequentially first, then followed by one epoch of end-to-end fine tuning. The method was evaluated on the Lung Image Database Consortium image collection (LIDC-IDRI) with simulated forward projections. With 144 multi-slice fanbeam projections, the proposed end-to-end detector could achieve comparable sensitivity with the reference detector, which was trained and applied on the fully-sampled image data. It also demonstrated superior detection performance compared to detectors trained on the reconstructed images. The proposed method is general and could be expanded to most detection tasks in medical imaging.

Keywords: Computer aided diagnosis · Artificial neural networks
Computed tomography

1 Introduction

Computer aided diagnostic (CAD) systems could effectively reduce the intensity of doctors' work by providing fast and high-quality candidates, therefore increase the efficiency of clinical process. Nearly all the current CAD systems operate on the reconstructed images, which are optimized for human observers rather than computers, which could potentially capture details that are subtle to human eyes. In some applications where low-dose or reduced sampling exist, it is often up to the radiologists to resolve the trade-off between accuracy and noise suppressing [1], but the solution may not be the best choice for CAD systems.

© Springer Nature Switzerland AG 2018
Y. Shi et al. (Eds.): MLMI 2018, LNCS 11046, pp. 37–45, 2018.
https://doi.org/10.1007/978-3-030-00919-9_5

In recent years, there were considerably number of works on using deep neural networks as CADs, for various applications including segmentation, detection, diagnosis, etc. [2]. They demonstrated superior performance compared against conventional handcrafted features when given enough training data. However, all these neural networks were still trained from the reconstructed images, thus they may suffer from the non-optimality of the image quality.

Reconstruction algorithms generate images from the original raw data by solving inverse problems. Recently proposed deep-neural-network-based reconstruction algorithms approximate iterative reconstruction process with neural networks, which was trained to minimize the errors between reconstructed images and the ground truth [3, 4]. When given enough training data, the deep-neural-network-based reconstruction algorithms could recover more details and maintain better signal-to-noise ratio (SNR) than conventional iterative or image-based methods.

There is an emerging trend on end-to-end signal processing with deep neural networks, and related works include voice recognition, self-driving cars, etc. [5, 6]. It was demonstrated that end-to-end deep neural networks had improved performance compared to multiple-step learning in these applications.

In this paper, we proposed an end-to-end deep neural network which predicts the location of lung nodules in the computed tomography (CT) images from raw data. The network first converted the raw data to image data with a reconstruction sub-network that approximate a 5-iteration-unrolled primal-dual algorithm; then a 3-dimensional convolutional neural network (3D-CNN) was incorporated as the detection sub-network to locate lung nodules in the images. For more efficient training, the reconstruction sub-network was trained first, followed by the training of the detection sub-network with the reconstructed images. Finally, an end-to-end fine tuning was done on the entire network to maximize the detection performance only. The method was implemented on The Lung Image Database Consortium image collection (LIDC-IDRI) [7], where undersampled CT was simulated from the images with 144 projections per rotation. The proposed method's detection performance and robustness to noises was evaluated and compared against the multiple-step method. The reconstructed images were also analyzed for better understanding of the neural networks.

2   Methodology

2.1   Overview

Although it is desirable to apply neural networks directly on the raw data, the low coherence between the acquisition and image made local signals in the image domain spreading out in the raw data domain, which lead to difficulty in utilizing the highly efficient CNNs. Furthermore, a detection CAD system should give the position of lesions in the image domain. Hence, our proposed end-to-end network was consisted of the reconstruction sub-network, which mapped the raw data to the image domain; and the detection sub-network, which gave the spatial position of the lesions.

Patch-based detector with fixed window size was used. Denote the raw data as $\mathbf{p}$, the reconstruction sub-network as $R(\mathbf{p}; \boldsymbol{\theta})$, the detection sub-network as $D(\mathbf{x}; \boldsymbol{\eta})$, the patch-wise cross entropy was minimized during training:

$$\boldsymbol{\theta}, \boldsymbol{\eta} = \arg \min \frac{1}{N} \sum_i \sum_j H\left(D\left(\mathbf{E}_{ij}R(\mathbf{p}_i; \boldsymbol{\theta}); \boldsymbol{\eta}\right), l_{ij}\right) \tag{1}$$

where N is the total number of patches; $\mathbf{p}_i$ is the raw data of the ith scan; E_{ij} is the patch extraction matrix for the jth patch from the ith scan; l_{ij} is the label of the patch ij, which was 1 for patches containing nodule centers and 0 for the rest. $H(\cdot, \cdot)$ is the cross entropy loss.

Directly solving (1) yields slow training due to the heavy computational loads of the reconstruction sub-network and the relatively slow convergence of the detection sub-network. To improve training speed, the training was split into 3 steps: training of the reconstruction sub-network, training of the detection sub-network, and end-to-end fine tuning.

2.2 Reconstruction Sub-network

The reconstruction sub-network R was firstly trained to minimize the L2 error between the reconstructed images and the ground truth:

$$\boldsymbol{\theta}_1 = \arg \min \frac{1}{N_1} \sum_i \|R(\mathbf{p}_i; \boldsymbol{\theta}) - \mathbf{x}_{Ti}\|_2^2 \tag{2}$$

where N_1 is the total number of training images and $\mathbf{x}_{Ti}$ is the ground truth image corresponding to the ith scan.

Many choices of R exist, most of which realize finite iteration of existing algorithms with neural network, by replacing the part related to the prior term with trainable CNNs [3, 4]. The entire neural network could then be trained through (2). Thorough studies are yet to be done for comparison between various network structures, and in this study the primal-dual framework was incorporated [3]. 5 unrolled iterations were used, and the model parameters were chosen so that the training could be accomplished in a reasonable time.

Furthermore, due to the relative large memory footprint of the reconstruction sub-network, it was infeasible to feed it with large number of slices. Instead, the primal-dual network took only a few adjacent slices (e.g. 3), and the final reconstructed images was the aggregation from different slices. Denote the primal-dual network as $R_{PD}(\mathbf{p}; \boldsymbol{\theta})$, then $R(\mathbf{p}; \boldsymbol{\theta})$ could be written as:

$$R(\mathbf{p}; \boldsymbol{\theta}) = \frac{\sum_k \mathbf{W}_k^T R_{PD}(\mathbf{W}_k \mathbf{p}; \boldsymbol{\theta})}{\sum_k \mathbf{W}_k^T \mathbf{W}_k \mathbf{1}} \tag{3}$$

where $\mathbf{W}_k$ is the matrix to extract the kth sub-slices from the raw data $\mathbf{p}$. $\mathbf{1}$ is an all-ones matrix with the same size of $\mathbf{p}$. The structure of the primal-dual network is demonstrated in Fig. 1.

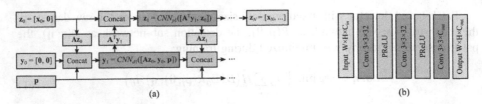

Fig. 1. The structure of the primal-dual network: (a) general structure; (b) structure of CNN_{pi} and CNN_{di}. z_i and y_i are primal and dual variables respectively, and we used $N_{primal} = N_{dual} = 2$ in the study. $\mathbf{x}_0$ had 3 slices (channels), so $\mathbf{z}_i$ and $\mathbf{y}_i$ both had 6 channels. $\mathbf{x}_N$ is the reconstructed image. C_{out} equals to the number of channels of $\mathbf{z}_i$ or $\mathbf{y}_i$.

2.3 Detection Sub-network

After training of $R(\mathbf{p}; \theta_1)$, patches were randomly extracted from the reconstructed images and the detection sub-network D was trained as:

$$\boldsymbol{\eta}_1 = \arg\min \frac{1}{N} \sum_i \sum_j H\big(D\big(\mathbf{E}_{ij} R(\mathbf{p}_i; \boldsymbol{\theta}_1); \boldsymbol{\eta}\big), l_{ij}\big) \qquad (4)$$

where the notations were the same with that of (1), except that only $\boldsymbol{\eta}$ was optimized.

The detector incorporated in this work was the 3D-CNN proposed in [8]. A patch was considered positive if the center of a non-small lung nodule is within the patch. Flips along the three axes were used for data augmentation because of its simplicity, but any augmentation that is expressible by matrix multiplication could fit into the proposed framework. The detection network is demonstrated in Fig. 2.

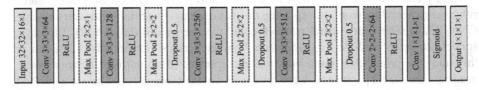

Fig. 2. The structure of the detection network. The modules with the dashed boxes did not use padding, and the rest used zero padding if applicable.

2.4 End-to-End Fine Tuning

After the two sub-networks were sequentially trained, one epoch of training of (1) was carried out with initial values set as θ_1 and $\boldsymbol{\eta}_1$. The gradient backpropagation from the detection sub-network to the reconstruction sub-network could be derived by chain rule of derivatives.

2.5   Inference

During inference from raw data $\mathbf{p}$, the detector D was applied on sliding windows on $R(\mathbf{p}; \boldsymbol{\theta})$, followed by a non-max suppressing (NMS) step to get the final detection.

3   Simulation Setup

3.1   Data Source

The LIDC-IDRI dataset was used for the simulation. It contains 1,018 chest CT scans from various scanners and each image was annotated by 4 radiologists. The detection task was set to detect the non-small nodules (nodules with ≥ 3 mm diameter), because imaging of small nodules is not stable for the used CT protocols.

All the images were resampled to $1 \times 1 \times 2$ mm^3, and forward projected in a multislice fanbeam geometry with equal angular detectors. 144 projections per rotation were used, and the detector had 736 units per layer with a pixel size of 1.2858×2 mm^2. The source-center and source-detector distances were 595 mm and 1086.5 mm.

The neural networks were trained on noiseless simulated data, but Poisson noise with equivalent initial photon number of 1×10^5 and 5×10^4 per ray were added at the test time to evaluate the robustness of the neural networks against inconsistency.

3.2   Training Parameters

The dataset was split into the training set and testing set with 916 and 102 scans respectively. The training parameters for the neural networks were as follows:

Reconstruction Sub-Network. The primal-dual network R_{PD} took 3 adjacent layers as input and realized 5 iterations of the primal-dual algorithm. The initial images were taken as the filtered backprojection (FBP) results. Adam optimizer with learning rate of 1×10^{-4} was used, with $\beta_1 = 0.9$ and $\beta_2 = 0.999$. 50 samples were randomly extracted from each scan, and 1 epoch was run for the training.

Detection Sub-Network. A patch size of $32 \times 32 \times 16$ was used for sampling. For each annotation on non-small nodules, the sampling was augmented by randomly translation between $[-8, 8]$ mm and flipping along 3 axes for 20 times, which generated 60–80 positive samples for each nodule (each nodule was annotated 3–4 times by different radiologists).

All the negative samplings kept a safe margin of 64 mm from any positive samplings. A 5-time augmented sampling was done for each non-nodule annotation. 400 patches were randomly extracted inside the lung whereas 100 patches were randomly extracted on the edge of the lung mask for each scan. The mask was derived from the FBP results.

The same Adam optimizer in the reconstruction sub-network was used here. 10 epochs of training were done with a minibatch size of 50.

End-to-End Fine Tuning. The same patch sampling coordinates were used with that for the detection sub-network. For each minibatch, 32 layers were extracted, and Adam optimizer was applied to the patches within the extracted layers. For each scan, multiple sub-layer extractions were done to cover all the patches once. 1 epoch of fine tuning was done with the same Adam optimizer in the previous steps.

3.3   Evaluation

For each testing scans, the detector was applied on sliding windows inside the lung masks with step size of 4 mm. NMS was then applied with intersection over union (IoU) threshold of 0.5. Free-response receiver operator curve (FROC) analysis was done with 1,000 bootstrapping to evaluate the detection performance [9], where a true positive was count if a nodule center was within the positive patch. Mean FROC scores were also calculated as the mean value of the sensitivities at 1/8, 1/4, 1/2, 1, 2, 4, 8 false positives per scan.

4   Results

4.1   FROC Analysis

Figure 3 gave the results of FROC for various detectors under 3 different noise levels. The end-to-end method was compared against the detector based on the FBP results and the two-step approach, where the primal-dual network was trained first and the detector was trained on its reconstruction results. Furthermore, the same detector was trained on the original resampled images to provide a reference FROC performance.

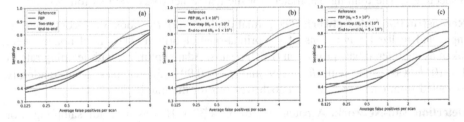

Fig. 3. FROC of different detectors: (a) noiseless performance; (b) performance with 1×10^5 photons per ray; (c) performance with 5×10^4 photons per ray. "Reference" refers to detection on original resampled images; "FBP" refers to detection on FBP results; "Two-step" refers to detection on primal-dual results; "End-to-end" refers to the proposed method. Only the mean value from the bootstrapping was shown for better visual effect.

The noiseless FROC results demonstrated significant improvement of the end-to-end approach over the two-step approach. Results from the proposed method was also comparable to the reference results when average false positives per scan were within [1, 4]. When small amount of noise ($N_0 = 1 \times 10^5$) was added, the performance of end-to-end detector remained almost the same, whereas the separately trained detectors' performance was obviously decreased. The performance of the end-to-end detector further deteriorated when the noise level increased, but its advantage over the separately trained detector was maintained.

The mean FROC scores are listed in Table 1. It could be noted that end-to-end detector had a higher FROC score when $N_0 = 1 \times 10^5$ compared to the noiseless situation. It indicated that the noise had little influence on the detector, and the gain of score was due to normal detector performance noises.

Table 1. Mean FROC scores

Noise level	Reference	FBP	Two-step	End-to-end
None	0.636	0.563	0.560	0.608
$N_0 = 1 \times 10^5$	N/A	0.549	0.538	0.615
$N_0 = 5 \times 10^4$	N/A	0.525	0.512	0.587

4.2 Reconstructed Images

One slice from the reconstructed images is shown in Fig. 4, where the contrast to noise ratio (CNR) was calculated for a nodule in the slice. The two-step result had the best visual performance, whereas the end-to-end result had the undersampling streak artifacts. However, the better detection performance of the end-to-end detector indicated the difference between human observer and the computer vision, where the latter could ignore such structured noise for the detection task.

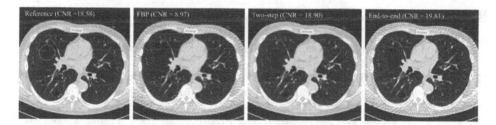

Fig. 4. Reconstructed axial images from different methods. The CNRs were calculated from the nodule within the red circle against the background within the green circle. The display window is [−1400, 200] HU.

Though there existed subtle visual differences between the two-step and end-to-end results except for the streak artifacts, the gain on CNR was significant for the end-to-end result, which could be one of the reasons lead to better detection performance. Note that both two-step and end-to-end results had larger CNR than the reference result. The former was because of the existence of noises in the original images, the latter was because of the gain in contrast.

5 Conclusion and Discussion

In this paper we proposed an end-to-end lung nodule detection system for under-sampled CT data, where a reconstruction sub-network and a detection sub-network were trained end-to-end to maximize the detection performance. The end-to-end methods achieved comparable performance with the detector trained on the fully-sampled data and had a significant gain over two-step methods. The proposed method is general and could be easily applied to other detection tasks and other modalities in medical imaging.

Although the training relied on simulation data, its robustness against moderate noise was also validated in the simulation. The results indicated that if the simulation does not significantly bias from the reality, the trained neural network should be generalizable enough to assure acceptable performance on real data.

Training-from-scratch had the potential to reach better solution than the current fine-tuning scheme, but it was too time consuming because of the heavy computational load of the training of reconstruction network, which required the entire slice as input and could not be broken into patches.

It is acknowledged that neither the reconstruction nor the detection sub-networks were carefully chosen or optimized in the current study. But the advantage of the end-to-end method should be maintained with different reconstruction or detection modules, since the solution to the two-step method could be further optimized in the end-to-end framework. We are actively working with more advanced detection and reconstruction neural networks [10].

References

1. Kalra, M.K., Maher, M.M., Toth, T.L., et al.: Strategies for CT radiation dose optimization. Radiology **230**(3), 619–628 (2004)
2. Greenspan, H., van Ginneken, B., Summers, R.M.: Guest editorial deep learning in medical imaging: Overview and future promise of an exciting new technique. IEEE Trans. Med. Imaging **35**(5), 1153–1159 (2016)
3. Adler J. and Oktem O. Learned primal-dual reconstruction. arXiv preprint, arXiv:1707. 06474 (2017)
4. Sun, J., Li, H., Xu, Z., et al.: Deep ADMM-net for compressive sensing MRI. Adv. Neural Inf. Process. Syst. **29**, 10–18 (2016)
5. Bojarski M., Testa D. D., Dworakowski D., et al. End to end learning for self-driving cars. arXiv preprint, arXiv:1604.07316 (2016)
6. Graves, A., Jaitly, T.: Towards end-to-end speech recognition with recurrent neural networks. In: Proceedings of the 31st International Conference on Machine Learning (ICML-2014), pp. 1764–1772. PMLR, Beijing, China (2014)
7. Armato, S.G., McLennan, G., Bidaut, L., et al.: The lung image database consortium (LIDC) and image database resource initiative (IDRI): a completed reference database of lung nodules on CT scans. Med. Phys. **38**(2), 915–931 (2011)
8. De Wit, J., Hammack, D.: 2nd place solution for the 2017 national datasicence bowl. http://juliandewit.github.io/kaggle-ndsb2017/. Accessed 1 Mar 2018

9. Setio, A.A.A., Traverso, A., de Bel, T., et al.: Validation, comparison, and combination of algorithms for automatic detection of pulmonary nodules in computed tomography images: the luna16 challenge. Med. Image Anal. **42**, 1–13 (2017)
10. Zhu, W., Liu, C., Fan, W. and Xie, X., Deeplung: Deep 3d dual path nets for automated pulmonary nodule detection and classification. arXiv preprint arXiv:1801.09555 (2017)

CT Image Enhancement Using Stacked Generative Adversarial Networks and Transfer Learning for Lesion Segmentation Improvement

Youbao Tang[1(✉)], Jinzheng Cai[1,2(✉)], Le Lu[1], Adam P. Harrison[1], Ke Yan[1], Jing Xiao[3], Lin Yang[2], and Ronald M. Summers[1]

[1] National Institutes of Health Clinical Center, Bethesda, MD 20892, USA
youbao.tang@nih.gov
[2] University of Florida, Gainesville, FL 32611, USA
[3] Ping An Insurance Company of China, Shenzhen 510852, China

Abstract. Automated lesion segmentation from computed tomography (CT) is an important and challenging task in medical image analysis. While many advancements have been made, there is room for continued improvements. One hurdle is that CT images can exhibit high noise and low contrast, particularly in lower dosages. To address this, we focus on a preprocessing method for CT images that uses stacked generative adversarial networks (SGAN) approach. The first GAN reduces the noise in the CT image and the second GAN generates a higher resolution image with enhanced boundaries and high contrast. To make up for the absence of high quality CT images, we detail how to synthesize a large number of low- and high-quality natural images and use transfer learning with progressively larger amounts of CT images. We apply both the classic GrabCut method and the modern holistically nested network (HNN) to lesion segmentation, testing whether SGAN can yield improved lesion segmentation. Experimental results on the DeepLesion dataset demonstrate that the SGAN enhancements alone can push GrabCut performance over HNN trained on original images. We also demonstrate that HNN + SGAN performs best compared against four other enhancement methods, including when using only a single GAN.

Keywords: CT image enhancement · Lesion segmentation · Stacked generative adversarial networks · Transfer learning

1 Introduction

There are many useful and important applications in medical image analysis, *e.g.*, measurement estimation [1], lung segmentation [2], disease classification[3],

---

Y. Tang and J. Cai—Equal contribution.

Y. Shi et al. (Eds.): MLMI 2018, LNCS 11046, pp. 46–54, 2018.
https://doi.org/10.1007/978-3-030-00919-9_6

lesion segmentation [4], etc. Accurate lesion segmentation from computed tomography (CT) scans plays a crucial role in computer aided diagnosis (CAD) tasks, *e.g.*, quantitative disease progression, tumor growth evaluation after treatment, pathology detection and surgical assistance. Quantitative analysis of tumor extents could provide valuable information for treatment planning. Manual lesion segmentation is highly tedious and time consuming, motivating a number of works on automatic lesion segmentation [4–6]. However, as more and more elaborately designed segmentation methods are proposed, performance improvement may plateau. In particular, CT images are often noisy and suffer from low contrast due to radiation dosage limits, as shown in the first row of Fig. 1. The collection of datasets more massive than currently available may provide the means to overcome this, but this eventuality is not guaranteed, particularly given the labor involved in manually annotating training images. We take a different tack, and instead leverage the massive amounts of data already residing in hospital picture archiving and communication systems (PACS) to develop a method to enhance CT images in a way that benefits lesion segmentation.

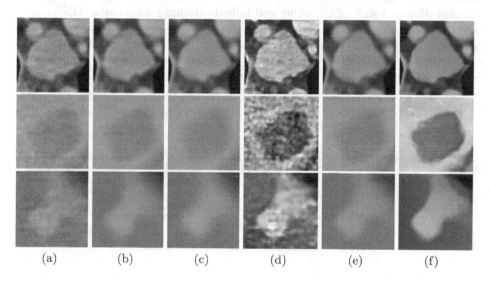

| (a) | (b) | (c) | (d) | (e) | (f) |

Fig. 1. Three examples of CT image enhancement results using different methods on original images (a), BM3D (b), DnCNN (c), single GAN (d), our denoising GAN (e), and our SGAN (f).

Figure 1 presents some examples of current efforts at image enhancement. As Fig. 1(a) demonstrates, classic denoising methods, such as BM3D [7], can preserve image details while introducing very few artifacts. With the recent explosive development of deep convolutional neural networks (CNNs), the field has developed many CNN based denoising methods. These include DnCNN [8], which is able to handle denoising with unknown noise levels. However, most of the CNN based methods, including DnCNN [8], use mean squared error (MSE) loss for model optimization, which can blur high-frequency details, *e.g.* edges. See Fig. 1(c) for an example. Moreover, denoising methods do not explicitly address resolution and contrast issues.

To overcome these problems, this paper proposes a novel CT image enhancement method by designing a stacked generative adversarial network (SGAN) model. As such, this work builds off of classic GANs [9], and is partially inspired by work using GANs for super resolution on natural images [10]. Unlike many natural images, CT images are often noisy and suffer from low contrast. Directly enhancing such images may generate undesirable visual artifacts and edges that are harmful for lesion segmentation accuracy. It is challenging to train a single GAN to directly output enhanced images with high resolution and visual quality from the original CT images. See Fig. 1(d) for the results produced by single GAN. One way to address this is to reduce CT image noise before image enhancement. Therefore, our proposed SGAN operates in two GAN stages. As shown in Fig. 1(e), the first GAN reduces the noise from the original CT image. As depicted in Fig. 1(f), the second GAN generates higher resolution images with enhanced boundary and contrast. Based on the enhanced images, the popular segmentation methods of GrabCut and holistically nested networks (HNNs) are used for lesion segmentation. Experimental results on the large scale DeepLesion dataset [11] demonstrate the effectiveness of our SGAN approach. In particular, we demonstrate that when using SGAN-enhanced with GrabCut, we can produce better results than the much more powerful, yet expensive, HNN applied to the original images, confirming our intuition on the value of attending to image quality.

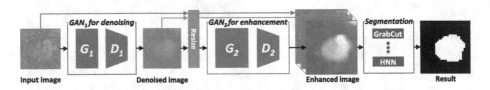

Fig. 2. The pipeline of the proposed method.

2 Methods

Instead of directly performing image enhancement, our SGAN method decomposes enhancement into two sub-tasks, *i.e.*, image denoising followed by enhancement. After SGAN enhancement, either GrabCut or HNN is used for lesion segmentation. Figure 2 depicts the overall workflow of the proposed method. The details of each stage are described below.

2.1 CT Image Enhancement

In [10], generative adversarial networks (GANs) [9] were successfully used for natural-image super resolution, producing high-quality images with more visual details and edges compared to their low-resolution counterparts. For lesion segmentation, if we can improve visual clarity and contrast, particularly at the borders of lesions, the segmentation performance and accuracy may subsequently be improved.

Given a CT lesion image (as shown in Fig. 1(a)), we first generate a denoised version of the input image by employing our first GAN model (consisting of a generator G_1 and a discriminator D_1) that focuses on removing random image noise. The denoised image has the same size as the input image. Although the noise has been reduced in the generated image, as demonstrated in Fig. 1(e), lesions have blurry edges and the contrast between lesion and background regions is generally low. As well, a considerable number of lesions are quite small in size (<10 mm or less than 10 pixels according to their long axis diameters). Human observers typically apply zooming (via commercial clinical PACS workstations) for such lesions. This motivates the use of a second GAN to provide high-resolution enhancement. To solve this issue, our second GAN model, which also contains a generator G_2 and a discriminator D_2, is built upon the denoised image from the first GAN to produce an enhanced high resolution version (as illustrated in Fig. 1(f)). This enhanced high-resolution image provides both clear lesion boundaries and high contrast. Since the three resulting images, *i.e.*, the original, denoised, and enhanced variants, may have complementary information, we concatenate them together into a three-channel image that is fed into the next lesion segmentation stage.

SGAN Architecture. We adapt similar architectures as [10] for the generators and discriminators, where the generator has 16 identical residual blocks and 2 sub-pixel convolutional layers [12], which are used to increase the resolution. Each block contains two convolutional layers with 64 3×3 kernels followed by batch-normalization [13] and ParametricReLU [14] layers. Because it is an easier subtask, a simpler architecture that contains just 9 identical residual blocks is designed for the denoising generator G_1. As well, for a trained model, the method of [10] can only enlarge the input image by fixed amounts. However, in the DeepLesion dataset lesion sizes vary considerably, meaning they have to be enlarged with correspondingly different zooming factors. Therefore the sub-pixel layers are removed in the high-resolution generator G_2. Both G_1 and G_2 are fully convolutional and can take input images of arbitrary size. For the discriminator design, D_1 and D_2, we use the same architecture as [10], which consists of 8 convolutional layers with 3×3 kernels, LeakyReLU activations ($\alpha = 0.2$), and two densely connected layers followed by a final sigmoid layer. The stride settings and kernel numbers of the 8 convolutional layers are $(1, 2, 1, 2, 1, 2, 1, 2)$ and $(64, 64, 128, 128, 256, 256, 512, 512)$, respectively.

Training Data Synthesization. Normally super resolution models are trained with pairs of low- and high-resolution images. While this can be obtained easily in natural images (by down-sampling), physical CT images are imaged by medical scanners at roughly fixed in-plane resolutions of ~ 1 mm per-pixel and CT imaging at ultra-high spatial resolutions does not exist. For the sake of SGAN training, we leverage transfer learning using a large-scale synthesized natural image dataset: DIV2K [15] where all images are converted into gray scale and down-sampled to produce training pairs. For the training of the denoising GAN, we randomly crop 32×32 sub-images from distinct training images of DIV2K. White Gaussian noise at different intensity variance levels $\sigma_i \in (0, 50]$ are added to the cropped images to construct the paired model inputs. For training the image-enhancement GAN, the input images are cropped as 128×128 patches and we perform the following steps: (1) down-sample the cropped image with scale $s \in [1, 4]$, (2) implement Gaussian spatial smoothing with $\sigma_s \in (0, 3]$, (3) execute contrast compression with rates of $\kappa \in [1, 3]$, and (4) conduct up-sampling with the scale s to generate images pairs. To fine-tune using CT images, we process 28,000 training RECIST slices using the currently trained SGAN and select a subset of up to 1,000 that demonstrate visual improvement. The selected CT images are subsequently added to the training for the next round of SGAN fine-tuning. This iterative process finishes when no more visual improvement can be observed.

Model Optimization. A proper loss function needs to be defined for model optimization, which is critical for the performance of our generators. The generators are trained not only to generate high quality images but also to fool the discriminators. Similar to [10], given an input image, x_i $(i = 0, 1)$, this work defines a perceptual loss L_P^i $(i = 1, 2)$ as the weighted sum of a image content loss L_C^i, a feature representation loss L_{VGG}^i and an adversarial loss L_A^i for G_1 and G_2 as

$$L_P^i = L_{DIFF}^i + 10^{-5} L_{VGG}^i + 10^{-3} L_A^i, \tag{1}$$

where i denotes the SGAN stage. Here, L_{DIFF}^i and L_{VGG}^i are computed using the mean square error (MSE) loss function to measure the pixel-wise error and the element-wise error of feature maps between the generated image $G_i(x_i)$ and its ground truth image y_i, respectively. We extract feature maps from five blocks of the VGGNet-16 model [16] pre-trained over ImageNet [17]. The adversarial loss L_A^i is defined using the standard GAN formulation for generators:

$$L_A^i(x_i) = -\log(D_i(G_i(x_i))). \tag{2}$$

The discriminators, on the other hand, are trained to distinguish between real images and enhanced ones, y_i and $G_i(x_i)$, respectively, which can be accomplished by minimizing the following loss:

$$L_D^i(x_i, y_i) = -\log(D_i(y_i)) - \log(1 - D_i(G_i(x_i))) \tag{3}$$

We use the Adam optimizer [18] with $\beta_1 = 0.5$ and a learning rate of 10^{-4} for model optimization. The generator (G_1 or G_2) and discriminator (D_1 or D_2)

are alternatively updated. We train first on the synthesized natural images and then fine-tune using the selected CT images.

2.2 Lesion Segmentation

Because they may contain complementary information, the denoised and enhanced outputs from the SGAN and the original lesion CT image are combined into a three-channel image for lesion segmentation. We investigate two popular segmentation approaches: GrabCut [19] and HNN [20]. The quality of GrabCut's initialization will greatly affect the final segmentation result. For this reason, we construct a high quality *trimap* T using the RECIST diameter marks within the DeepLesion dataset [11]. This produces regions of probable background, probable foreground, background and foreground. Note that unlike the original *trimap* definition [19], we define four region types. With T, we can obtain the lesion segmentation using GrabCut. Since the DeepLesion dataset does not provide the ground truth lesion masks, the GrabCut segmentation results are used as supervision to train the HNN segmentation model until convergence.

3   Experimental Results and Analyses

The DeepLesion dataset [11] is composed of 32, 735 PACS CT lesion images annotated with RECIST long and short diameters. These are derived from 10, 594 studies of 4, 459 patients. All lesions have been categorized into the 8 subtypes of lung, mediastinum, liver, soft-tissue, abdomen, kidney, pelvis, and bone. For quantitative evaluation, we manually segment 1, 000 lesion images as a testing set, randomly selected from 500 patients. The rest serve as a training set. Based on the location of bookmarked diameters, CT region of interests (ROIs) are cropped at two times the extent of the lesion's long diameters, so that sufficient visual context is preserved. Although we do not possess corresponding high quality images in the DeepLesion dataset, we can implicitly evaluate the performance of the proposed SGAN model for CT image enhancement by comparing the segmentation performance with or without enhanced images. Three criteria, *i.e.* Dice similarity coefficient (Dice), precision and recall scores, are used to evaluate the quantitative segmentation accuracy.

Figure 3 shows several visual examples of lesion segmentation results using HNN on original images and their combinations with the images produced by SGAN. From Fig. 3, the segmentation results on the combined images are closer to the manual segmentations than the ones on only original images. This intuitively demonstrates that the enhanced images produced by the SGAN model is helpful for lesion segmentation.

For quantitative evaluation, we test both GrabCut and HNN applied on a variety of image options. Namely, we compare results when the original (OG) images are used, and also when those processed by BM3D [7], DnCNN [8]), a single GAN model (GAN) for enhancement, and the first denoising GAN model of SGAN (GAN$_1$) are used. When enhancement is applied, we concatenate the

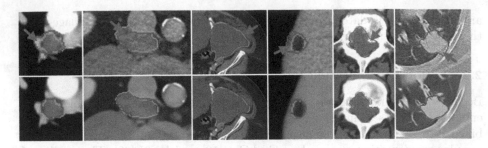

Fig. 3. Visual examples of lesion segmentation produced by HNN from the OG images (1st row) and their combinations with enhanced SGAN images (2nd row). The manual and automatic segmentation boundaries are delineated with green and red curves, respectively. Incorrectly segmented regions when using OG images that are corrected when using SGAN images are highlighted with pink arrows. Best viewed in color.

result with OG images to create a multi-channel input for the segmentation method. From Table 1, we can see that (1) when using any of the enhanced images except the one produced by a single GAN, the Dice performance improves, supporting our intuition on the value of enhancing the CT images prior to segmentation. The possible reason of the worse results when using a single GAN is that it may enhance and introduce some artifacts. (2) Using GAN$_1$ for image denoising produces better Dice scores than using BM3D and DnCNN, suggesting that the adversarial learning strategy is helpful for image denoising while keeping details important for segmentation. (3) Compared with GrabCut, HNN achieves a greater improvement in Dice scores when using the enhanced images, suggesting HNN is able to exploit the complementary information better than GrabCut. (4) Using SGAN for image enhancement produces the largest gain in Dice scores. This confirms that our approach on using a stacked architecture can provide a more effective enhancement than just a blind application of GANs. (5) Most remarkably, the Dice scores of GrabCut with SGAN is greater than just using HNN with OG images. Considering the simplicity of GrabCut, this indicates that focusing attention on improving data quality can sometimes yield larger gains than simply applying more powerful, but costly, segmentation methods. As a result, despite being somewhat neglected in the field, focusing attention on data enhancements can be an important means to push segmentation performance further.

Table 2 lists the Dice scores across lesion types when using HNN on OG and SGAN images. Notably, the segmentation performance over all categories is improved with SGAN images, with abdomen and liver exhibiting the largest improvement. These lesion categories may benefit the most due to their low contrast and blurred boundaries compared to the surrounding soft tissue.

Table 1. The performance of lesion segmentation using GrabCut and HNN with different inputs in terms of recall, precision and Dice score, whose mean and standard deviation are reported.

Input	GrabCut			HNN		
	Recall	Precision	Dice	Recall	Precision	Dice
OG	**0.944±0.096**	0.885±0.107	0.908±0.088	0.933±0.095	0.893±0.111	0.906±0.089
OG+BM3D	0.943±0.105	0.897±0.105	0.910±0.087	0.903±0.108	0.930±0.095	0.912±0.085
OG+DnCNN	0.944±0.101	0.892±0.108	0.909±0.090	0.901±0.114	0.927±0.098	0.910±0.086
OG+GAN	0.944±0.107	0.878±0.112	0.906±0.093	**0.937±0.109**	0.887±0.108	0.906±0.091
OG+GAN_1	0.942±0.102	0.898±0.106	0.910±0.086	0.905±0.104	0.930±0.093	0.913±0.084
OG+SGAN	0.941±0.106	**0.904±0.096**	**0.913±0.085**	0.911±0.097	**0.940±0.091**	**0.920±0.082**

Table 2. Category-wise comparisons of lesion segmentation results using HNN on original images and their combinations with the images produced by SGAN. Mean and standard deviation of Dice score are reported.

Method	Bone	Abdomen	Mediastinum	Liver	
HNN	0.877±0.055	0.909±0.092	0.892±0.076	0.854±0.146	
SGAN+HNN	**0.891±0.061**	**0.927±0.088**	**0.909±0.083**	**0.877±0.142**	
Method	Lung	Kidney	Soft tissue	Pelvis	mDice
HNN	0.912±0.087	0.925±0.056	0.928±0.063	0.911±0.070	0.906±0.089
SGAN+HNN	**0.924±0.073**	**0.938±0.045**	**0.937±0.048**	**0.919±0.080**	**0.920±0.082**

4 Conclusions

We propose an SGAN method to enhance CT images to improve lesion segmentation performance. SGAN divides the task it into two sub-tasks: the first GAN denoises the original CT image while the second generates a high quality image with higher resolution, enhanced boundaries, and higher contrast. Experimental results on the DeepLesion dataset test segmentation performance when GrabCut and HNN are applied on OG and enhanced images. Results demonstrate that SGAN is more effective than four other enhancement approaches, including using a single GAN, in yielding improved segmentation performance, with HNN + SGAN achieving the best performance. Most notably, Grabcut + SGAN outperformed HNN trained on the OG images, despite the latter having orders of magnitude more parameters. This demonstrates that focusing on dataset processing is a crucial research direction in medical imaging analysis.

Acknowledgments. This research was supported by the Intramural Research Program of the National Institutes of Health Clinical Center and by the Ping An Insurance Company through a Cooperative Research and Development Agreement. We thank Nvidia for GPU card donation.

References

1. Tang, Y., Harrison, A.P., et al.: Semi-automatic recist labeling on ct scans with cascaded convolutional neural networks. arXiv:1806.09507 (2018)
2. Jin, D., Xu, Z., et al.: Ct-realistic lung nodule simulation from 3d conditional generative adversarial networks for robust lung segmentation. arXiv:1806.04051 (2018)
3. Tang, Y., Wang, X., et al.: Attention-guided curriculum learning for weakly supervised classification and localization of thoracic diseases on chest radiographs. arXiv:1807.07532 (2018)
4. Cai, J., Tang, Y., et al.: Accurate weakly-supervised deep lesion segmentation using large-scale clinical annotations: Slice-propagated 3d mask generation from 2d recist. arXiv:1807.01172 (2018)
5. Massoptier, L., Casciaro, S.: A new fully automatic and robust algorithm for fast segmentation of liver tissue and tumors from ct scans. Eur. Radiol. **18**(8), 1658 (2008)
6. Christ, P.F., Elshaer, M.E.A., et al.: Automatic liver and lesion segmentation in ct using cascaded fully convolutional neural networks and 3d conditional random fields. MICCA **I**, 415–423 (2016)
7. Dabov, K., Foi, A.: Image denoising by sparse 3-d transform-domain collaborative filtering. IEEE TIP **16**(8), 2080–2095 (2007)
8. Zhang, K., Zuo, W., et al.: Beyond a gaussian denoiser: Residual learning of deep cnn for image denoising. IEEE TIP **26**(7), 3142–3155 (2017)
9. Goodfellow, I., Pouget-Abadie, J., et al.: Generative adversarial nets. In: NIPS, pp. 2672–2680 (2014)
10. Ledig, C., Theis, L., et al.: Photo-realistic single image super-resolution using a generative adversarial network. In: CVPR, pp. 4681–4690 (2017)
11. Yan, K., Wang, X., et al.: Deep lesion graphs in the wild: relationship learning and organization of significant radiology image findings in a diverse large-scale lesion database. In: CVPR, pp. 9261–9270 (2018)
12. Shi, W., Caballero, J., et al.: Real-time single image and video super-resolution using an efficient sub-pixel convolutional neural network. In: CVPR, pp. 1874–1883 (2016)
13. Ioffe, S., Szegedy, C.: Batch normalization: Accelerating deep network training by reducing internal covariate shift. In: ICML, pp. 448–456 (2015)
14. He, K., Zhang, X., et al.: Delving deep into rectifiers: Surpassing human-level performance on imagenet classification. In: ICCV, pp. 1026–1034 (2015)
15. Agustsson, E., Timofte, R.: Ntire 2017 challenge on single image super-resolution: Dataset and study. In: CVPRW, pp. 1122–1131 (2017)
16. Simonyan, K., Zisserman, A.: Very deep convolutional networks for large-scale image recognition. arXiv:1409.1556 (2014)
17. Deng, J., Dong, W., et al.: Imagenet: a large-scale hierarchical image database. In: CVPR, pp. 248–255 (2009)
18. Kingma, D.P., Ba, J.: Adam: A method for stochastic optimization. arXiv:1412.6980 (2014)
19. Rother, C., Kolmogorov, V., et al.: Grabcut: interactive foreground extraction using iterated graph cuts. In: ACM TOG, pp. 309–314 (2004)
20. Xie, S., Tu, Z.: Holistically-nested edge detection. In: ICCV, pp. 1395–1403 (2015)

Deep Learning Based Inter-modality Image Registration Supervised by Intra-modality Similarity

Xiaohuan Cao[1,2], Jianhuan Yang[1], Li Wang[2], Zhong Xue[3], Qian Wang[4], and Dinggang Shen[2(✉)]

[1] School of Automation, Northwestern Polytechnical University, Xi'an, China
[2] Department of Radiology and BRIC,
University of North Carolina at Chapel Hill, Chapel Hill, NC, USA
dgshen@med.unc.edu
[3] Shanghai United Imaging Intelligence Co., Ltd., Shanghai, China
[4] School of Biomedical Engineering, Institute for Medical Imaging Technology,
Shanghai Jiao Tong University, Shanghai, China

Abstract. Non-rigid inter-modality registration can facilitate accurate information fusion from different modalities, but it is challenging due to the very different image appearances across modalities. In this paper, we propose to train a non-rigid inter-modality image registration network, which can directly predict the transformation field from the input multimodal images, such as CT and MRI. In particular, the training of our inter-modality registration network is supervised by intra-modality similarity metric based on the available paired data, which is derived from a pre-aligned CT and MRI dataset. Specifically, in the training stage, to register the input CT and MR images, their similarity is evaluated on the *warped MR image* and *the MR image that is paired with the input CT*. So that, the intra-modality similarity metric can be directly applied to measure whether the input CT and MR images are well registered. Moreover, we use the idea of dual-modality fashion, in which we measure the similarity on both CT modality and MR modality. In this way, the complementary anatomies in both modalities can be jointly considered to more accurately train the inter-modality registration network. In the testing stage, the trained inter-modality registration network can be directly applied to register the new multimodal images without any paired data. Experimental results have shown that, the proposed method can achieve promising accuracy and efficiency for the challenging non-rigid inter-modality registration task and also outperforms the state-of-the-art approaches.

1 Introduction

Non-rigid inter-modality image registration is an active topic in medical image analysis, as it allows for the use of the complementary multimodal information provided by different imaging protocols. The technique is of great importance in many clinical applications such as image-guided intervention, disease diagnosis and treatment planning. For example, in prostate cancer radiation therapy, Computed Tomography

Y. Shi et al. (Eds.): MLMI 2018, LNCS 11046, pp. 55–63, 2018.
https://doi.org/10.1007/978-3-030-00919-9_7

(CT) is necessary for dose planning since it provides precise tissue density information. While Magnetic Resonance (MR) imaging has high soft-tissue contrast, which is more convenient to accurately delineate pelvic organs, *i.e.*, the bladder, prostate and rectum, as shown in Fig. 1. In this case, the registration of pelvic CT and MRI is necessary to effectively fuse the information from two modalities. Additionally, since CT and MRI cannot be scanned simultaneously in practice, due to inevitable physiological phenomenon, such as bladder filling/emptying and irregular rectal movement, local deformations of main pelvic organs cannot be well compensated when only performing linear registration. Thus, this poses a typical *non-rigid inter-modality* image registration problem.

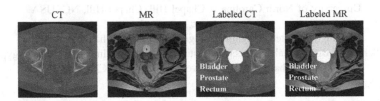

Fig. 1. An example of the multimodal images: pelvic CT and MR images from the same subject after affine registration. Local deformations are obvious in bladder, prostate and rectum

As shown in Fig. 1, CT and MR image have very different image appearances and deformed anatomies. Thus, the inter-modality registration is naturally a more challenging task compared with intra-modality registration, since it is hard to define an effective similarity metric to guide local matching across modalities [1]. Traditionally, mutual information (MI), along with its variants [2], is a popular way to tackle the inter-modality registration problem. However, MI is a good *global* similarity metric, which has limited power to accurately conduct *local* matching, since the insufficient voxel number in local regions makes the intensity distribution less robust when calculating MI.

For the task of non-rigid registration, compared with the traditional optimization-based registration algorithms, deep-learning-based registration methods have drawn much more attention recently. Generally, two kinds of guidance can be applied to train the non-rigid registration network: (1) using *the "ground-truth" transformation fields* [3], or (2) guided by *image similarity metrics* [4]. However, as the *"ground-truth"* transformation fields cannot be manually produced in practice, this guidance is often derived from existing registration algorithms, hence affecting the effective modeling of the registration task and eventually affecting its performance.

Instead, *image similarity metric* is attractive to supervise the training of the registration networks [4]. Since this metric relieves the need of "ground-truth" transformation fields, some works regard it as "unsupervised/self-supervised" learning based registration. Specifically, the network can be trained by maximizing the image similarity (or minimizing the image dissimilarity). In this way, the network can learn to register the images automatically. However, these methods are mainly proposed for *intra-modality* registration, as many effective similarity metrics can be applied, such as cross-correlation (CC), sum of square distance (SSD), *etc*. While the *inter-modality* registration cannot be well tackled due to the lack of effective similarity metrics, which can robustly and accurately measure local matching across different modalities.

In this paper, we propose to train a *non-rigid inter-modality* registration network by using the *intra-modality* similarity guidance, which can directly predict the transformation field from the input CT and MRI in the testing stage. Particularly, we take advantages of the pre-aligned CT and MRI dataset, in which each pair of CT and MRI are carefully registered as *paired data*. Under the help of these *paired data*, the effective *intra-modality* similarity metric can be elegantly transferred to train our *inter-modality* registration network. Specifically, the input CT and MR images (which are not aligned) have their respective counterpart images, *i.e.*, the input CT has a paired-MR image and the input MR image has a paired-CT image. Then, in order to register the input MRI to the input CT, our *inter-modality* registration network can be trained by the similarity guidance calculated on the *warped input MRI* and the *paired-MRI of the input CT*. So that we can directly employ any effective *intra-modality* similarity metric, while it definitely measures whether the input CT and MRI are well registered. Generally, this framework is straightforward and can be extended to any inter-modality registration tasks. The main contributions can be summarized as follows.

(1) Instead of directly defining the similarity across modalities, we elegantly use the *intra-modality* similarity metric to effectively train an *inter-modality* registration network, by taking advantages from the pre-aligned CT and MRI dataset. In testing stage, this network can be flexibly used to predict the transformation field for any to-be-registered CT and MRI, without the need of the paired data.
(2) In order to accurately and robustly train the non-rigid inter-modality registration network, we deploy the similarity guidance on *dual manner*, where the similarity guidance is derived from *not only* the MR modality, *but also* the CT modality. In this way, the complementary anatomies can be jointly considered to effectively train this network. Additionally, the smoothness constraints are also introduced during training, in order to produce the topology-preserving transformation field.
(3) Compared with the traditional optimization-based algorithms, we provide a flexible and applicable solution for the challenging non-rigid inter-modality registration problem, particularly without iterative optimization and parameter tuning in the testing stage, which has high potential to be applied in real applications.

2   Method

In this paper, we propose to train a deep regression network to model the non-rigid inter-modality registration $\mathcal{M} : (I_{CT}, I_{MR}) \Rightarrow \phi$ in a patch-wise manner. The *input* 3D patches (I_{CT}, I_{MR}) are extracted from the to-be-registered CT and MR images, which have been already registered using affine transformation in preprocessing. The *output* is the transformation field ϕ that has the same center with the input patches. As illustrated by Fig. 2, we deploy a 3D spatial transformation layer $\mathcal{T}$ in the network to warp the moving image by ϕ, while the registration network $\mathcal{M}$ aims to maximize the similarity (*i.e.*, minimize the dissimilarity) between the fixed and the warped moving images.

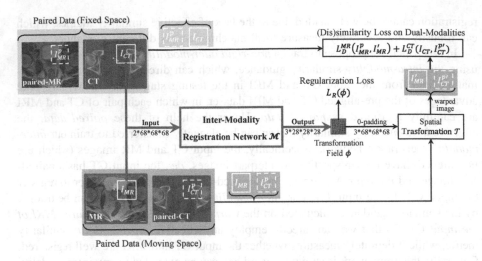

Fig. 2. The flowchart of our proposed deep learning based non-rigid inter-modality registration method. Note that, in the testing stage, only the red paths are invoked, and the input CT and MR images can be directly registered without the need of their paired data

Concerning the difficulty to define image similarity between modalities, we here propose a novel method to adopt the intra-modality similarity based on the *paired data* available in the training stage. That is, the input CT image (I_{CT}) has a paired-MR image (I_{MR}^p) for training, and similarly the input MR image (I_{MR}) has a paired-CT image (I_{CT}^p). The preparation for the paired training data will be detailed in Sect. 3. When registering the input CT and MR images, instead of measuring the similarity between I_{CT} and the warped MR image I'_{MR}, we train the deep network under the supervision of the similarity between I_{MR}^p and I'_{MR}, as well as between I_{CT} and $I_{CT}^{p'}$.

After the network is trained, we can apply it in the testing stage. In particular, by inputting the new CT and MR images, the transformation field between them can be directly obtained through the registration network $\mathcal{M}$, without the need of any paired data. Note that, in Fig. 2, only the red paths are needed in the testing stage.

2.1 Loss Function Based on Intra-modality Similarity

Intuitively, the deep network is trained by minimizing the loss function. For the registration task, we aim to minimize the image dissimilarity (or to maximize the image similarity). To train the inter-modality registration network, the loss can be defined as:

$$L = L_D(I_{CT}, \mathcal{T}(\phi, I_{MR})) + L_R(\phi), \tag{1}$$

where L_D measures the image dissimilarity between the fixed CT image I_{CT} and the warped MR image $I'_{MR} = \mathcal{T}(\phi, I_{MR})$. Here, $\mathcal{T}$ represents the operator of the 3D spatial transformation. L_R favors the smoothness of the estimated transformation field. Since it is difficult to define L_D based on the inter-modality images, we propose to define the intra-modality metric L_D on the paired data. Thus, the loss function can be re-defined as:

$$L = \frac{1}{2}L_D^{CT}\left(I_{CT}, \mathcal{T}\left(\phi, I_{CT}^p\right)\right) + \frac{1}{2}L_D^{MR}\left(I_{MR}^p, \mathcal{T}\left(\phi, I_{MR}\right)\right) + L_R(\phi). \qquad (2)$$

Here, the loss terms L_D^{CT} and L_D^{MR} provide the supervision in the *dual manner* to jointly guide the training of the registration network. The complementary anatomical details from the two modalities can be fused for better training.

Following Eq. (2), we can calculate the dissimilarity between the images of the same modality, which is much more reliable than the inter-modality metric. Specifically, we use the normalized cross-correlation (NCC) to define L_D:

$$L_D = 1 - NCC(I, I') = 1 - \left\langle \frac{I - \bar{I}}{\|I - \bar{I}\|_2}, \frac{I' - \bar{I}'}{\|I' - \bar{I}'\|_2} \right\rangle, \qquad (3)$$

where, I and I' are the fixed and the warped moving images of the same modality. $\|\cdot\|_2$ is the L_2-norm and $\langle \cdot, \cdot \rangle$ is the inner product.

We here adopt NCC for two reasons. (1) It is a robust measure when dealing with the intra-modality images that may potentially have some noises and intensity inconsistency. (2) It can be implemented as a simple convolution operation, which is flexible to be embedded into the convolutional neural network (CNN) for effective forward and backward propagations during training. Notice that other differentiable similarity metrics can also be applied.

Additionally, the smoothness of ϕ is also important to obtain a topology-preserving transformation field. Thus, the regularization term $L_R(\phi)$ is also introduced into the loss function to train the network. Specifically, the regularization is defined as:

$$L_R(\phi) = \left\| \lambda_1 \nabla^2 \phi^2 + \lambda_2 \phi^2 \right\|, \qquad (4)$$

where ∇^2 is the Laplacian operator. The two scalars are empirically set ($\lambda_1 = 0.5$ and $\lambda_2 = 0.01$) to attain the smoothness constraint for the transformation field.

2.2 Inter-modality Registration Network

Figure 3 shows the detailed architecture of our *non-rigid inter-modality registration network* $\mathcal{M}$. The input are two patches extracted from CT and MR images of the size $68 \times 68 \times 68$, and the output is the 3D patch of the transformation field of the size $28 \times 28 \times 28$, which has the same center with the input patches. The size of the output patch is smaller than that of the input in order to enclose sufficient neighborhood information and also provide a sufficient receptive field for the local matching.

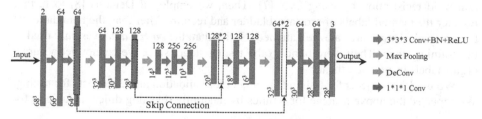

Fig. 3. Detailed architecture of $\mathcal{M}$: the non-rigid inter-modality registration network

The architecture of the registration network is based on U-net [5]. The encoding path includes two times down-sampling, and the decoding path contains two times up-sampling. We use $3 \times 3 \times 3$ kernels in the convolutional layer without padding, followed by batch normalization (BN) and ReLU. The final convolutional layer applies $1 \times 1 \times 1$ kernels without any additional operation, since the output transformation field includes both positive and negative values. Skip connections are also applied.

2.3 Spatial Transformation Layer

The spatial transformation layer [6] needs to be applied to warp the moving image by ϕ, such that the loss L_D can be evaluated. Mathematically, the 3D spatial transformation operation $\mathcal{T}$ with tri-linear interpolation can be defined as

$$I'(x) = \mathcal{T}(\phi(x), I) = \sum_{y \in \mathcal{N}(x + \phi(x))} I(y) \prod_{d \in \{i,j,k\}} (1 - |x_d + \phi(x_d) - y_d|), \qquad (5)$$

where I' is warped from I by ϕ, x represents the voxel location, $\mathcal{N}(x + \phi(x))$ is the 8-voxel cubic neighborhood around the location $x + \phi(x)$. d indicates three directions in 3D image space. Similar to [6], the gradient of $\mathcal{T}$ with respect to the location x can be obtained by the partial derivatives of Eq. (5). Notice that, different from [6], $\mathcal{T}$ here is only used to smoothly propagate the gradient from L_D to the network $\mathcal{M}$. No parameters will be updated in $\mathcal{T}$.

3   Experimental Results

The experimental dataset was collected from 15 prostate cancer patients, each with a CT image and a MR image. To evaluate the registration performance, the prostate, bladder and rectum in both CT and MRI are manually labeled by physicians. In preprocessing, intra-subject linear registration of CT and MRI was performed. Then, inter-subject linear registration was applied to roughly align all the images to a common space. Next, all the images were cropped to the same size ($218 \times 196 \times 100$) with the same resolution ($1 \times 1 \times 1$ mm^3). Finally, we flipped all the subjects along the x-axis to augment the dataset. Note that, the image was cropped for effectively conducting the experiments, and the three main pelvic organs were well included after cropping.

In the training stage, we prepared the *paired data* by fine-tuning the roughly aligned CT and MRI of the same subject. Particularly, we used the manual ground-truth labels of the three pelvic organs for highly accurate registration. We first performed non-rigid registration by using SyN [7]. Then, we employed Demons [8] to further register the manual labels of prostate, bladder and rectum. After that, the boundaries of the anatomical structures are well aligned. Notice that, the *paired data* was only used in the training stage. They were blind to the testing stage, since we cannot get accurate organ labels in practice then.

We used 12 subjects for training, 1 subject for validation and 2 subjects for testing. We repeated the above scheme for 5 times by randomly selecting different subjects for testing and validation. For each training subject, we have 2 image pairs considering the flipped data. We extracted 9.4 K patch samples from each image pair. Totally, there were 225 K patch samples for training. Our proposed method was implemented based on Pytorch, and the network was trained on an Nvidia TitanX GPU. We employed the stochastic gradient decent (SGD) strategy with the learning rate starting at 0.01 and decreasing by 0.5 every 4 epochs. The batch size was set to 2. We stopped training when the validation loss did not decrease significantly. In this paper, the training took ~ 40 h. In the testing stage, it took only 15 s to complete the registration between new CT and MR images.

3.1 Registration Results

Dice Similarity Coefficient (DSC) and Average Surface Distance (ASD) are used to evaluate the registration performance based on the ground-truth labels. Affine registration implemented by FLIRT [9] with the cost function of MI was used as the baseline. Herein, we also compared with SyN [7] due to its outstanding performance on non-rigid registration tasks, and it can also be used for inter-modality registration by using MI in the ANTs toolbox.

To demonstrate the importance of evaluating the intra-modality similarity in the proposed dual-manner, we also implemented our method with only one single-modality measure: either CT modality or MR modality was used to train the inter-modality registration network. We delete the respective loss term in Eq. (2) for single-modality measure and remove the weight ½ in front of the remaining term. All other settings are kept the same for fair comparison.

Table 1 shows the registration performance of our proposed method and all other methods under comparison. We can observe that only affine registration cannot well align the pelvic organs, as the local deformations on bladder, prostate and rectum cannot be effectively compensated. The registration performance can be improved for SyN. Furthermore, the results are much improved for the registration network even trained by the single-modality loss function. This indicates that, the *intra-modality*

Table 1. Comparison of DSCs (%) and ASDs (mm) on three pelvic organs after performing non-rigid registration based on **SyN** and the proposed deep learning based methods, where the network was trained by using the **single-modality** similarity and the **dual-modality** similarity, respectively. **Affine** registration results are used as the baseline.

Metric	Organ	Affine (MI)	SyN (MI)	Single-modality		Dual-modality
				CT	MR	Proposed
DSC (%)	Bladder	85.7 ± 5.3	87.4 ± 4.9	89.8 ± 3.6	90.3 ± 4.0	**90.5 ± 3.8**
	Prostate	81.9 ± 4.7	84.3 ± 3.5	86.1 ± 3.3	85.9 ± 4.1	**87.3 ± 4.2**
	Rectum	79.4 ± 5.1	81.8 ± 4.7	83.6 ± 5.0	84.2 ± 4.3	**85.4 ± 4.5**
ASD (mm)	Bladder	1.83 ± 0.71	1.69 ± 0.63	1.51 ± 0.57	1.47 ± 0.51	**1.23 ± 0.43**
	Prostate	1.91 ± 0.55	1.75 ± 0.41	1.63 ± 0.40	1.72 ± 0.42	**1.58 ± 0.36**
	Rectum	2.28 ± 0.68	2.06 ± 0.62	1.94 ± 0.43	1.83 ± 0.44	**1.44 ± 0.40**

similarity can make the network aware of the inter-modality registration task. The best performance was achieved by the network trained on the intra-modality similarity in *dual manner*. By fusing complementary details from both modalities, the performance of the inter-modality registration can be boosted. An example of the registration results can be visualized in Fig. 4. In general, our proposed methods can effectively solve the challenging non-rigid inter-modality registration problem using deep learning.

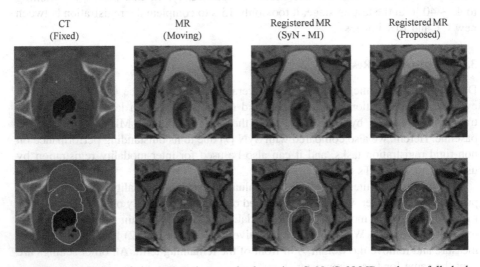

| CT | MR | Registered MR | Registered MR |
| (Fixed) | (Moving) | (SyN - MI) | (Proposed) |

Fig. 4. Visualization of the registration results by using SyN (SyN-MI) and our full dual-modality learning method (Proposed). Orange: manual CT contours of 3 organs. Blue: manual (2nd column) or registered (3rd and 4th columns) MR contours of 3 organs

4   Conclusion

We proposed a deep learning based *non-rigid inter-modality* registration framework, in which the similarity metric on intra-modality images is elegantly transferred to train an inter-modality registration network. Moreover, in order to use the complementary anatomies from both modalities, the dissimilarity loss is calculated in dual manner on MR modality and CT modality, respectively, to more robustly train the network. We conducted CT and MR registration and achieved promising performance on both efficiency and accuracy. The proposed framework can be easily extended and applied to other inter-modality registration tasks.

References

1. Cao, X., et al.: Region-adaptive deformable registration of ct/mri pelvic images via learning-based image synthesis. IEEE Trans. Image Process. **27**(7), 3500–3512 (2018)
2. Pluim, J.P., Maintz, J.A., Viergever, M.A.: Mutual-information-based registration of medical images: a survey. IEEE Trans. Med. Imaging **22**(8), 986–1004 (2003)

3. Cao, X. et al.: Deformable image registration using cue-aware deep regression network. IEEE Trans. Biomed. Eng. (2018)
4. de Vos, B.D., et al.: End-to-end unsupervised deformable image registration with a convolutional neural network. In: Cardoso, M.J., Arbel, T., Carneiro, G., Syeda-Mahmood, T., Tavares, J.M.R.S., Moradi, M., Bradley, A., Greenspan, H., Papa, J.P., Madabhushi, A., Nascimento, J.C., Cardoso, J.S., Belagiannis, V., Lu, Z. (eds.) DLMIA/ML-CDS -2017. LNCS, vol. 10553, pp. 204–212. Springer, Cham (2017). https://doi.org/10.1007/978-3-319-67558-9_24
5. Ronneberger, O., Fischer, P., Brox, T.: U-Net: Convolutional Networks for Biomedical Image Segmentation. In: Navab, Nassir, Hornegger, Joachim, Wells, William M., Frangi, Alejandro F. (eds.) MICCAI 2015. LNCS, vol. 9351, pp. 234–241. Springer, Cham (2015). https://doi.org/10.1007/978-3-319-24574-4_28
6. Jaderberg, M., Simonyan, K., Zisserman, A.: Spatial transformer networks. In: Advances in Neural Information Processing Systems (2015)
7. Avants, B.B., et al.: Symmetric diffeomorphic image registration with cross-correlation: evaluating automated labeling of elderly and neurodegenerative brain. Med. Image Anal. 12(1), 26–41 (2008)
8. Vercauteren, T., Pennec, X., Perchant, A., Ayache, N.: Non-parametric Diffeomorphic Image Registration with the Demons Algorithm. In: Ayache, N., Ourselin, S., Maeder, A. (eds.) MICCAI 2007. LNCS, vol. 4792, pp. 319–326. Springer, Heidelberg (2007). https://doi.org/10.1007/978-3-540-75759-7_39
9. Jenkinson, M., Smith, S.: A global optimisation method for robust affine registration of brain images. Med. Image Anal. 5(2), 143–156 (2001)

Regional Abnormality Representation Learning in Structural MRI for AD/MCI Diagnosis

Jun-Sik Choi, Eunho Lee, and Heung-Il Suk[⊠]

Department of Brain and Cognitive Engineering, Korea University, Seongbuk-gu, Republic of Korea
hisuk@korea.ac.kr

Abstract. In this paper, we propose a novel method for MRI-based AD/MCI diagnosis that systematically integrates voxel-based, region-based, and patch-based approaches in a unified framework. Specifically, we parcellate a brain into predefined regions by using anatomical knowledge, *i.e.*, template, and find complex nonlinear relations among voxels, whose intensity denotes the volumetric measure in our case, within each region. Unlike the existing methods that mostly use a cubical or rectangular shape, we regard the anatomical shape of regions as atypical forms of patches. Using the complex nonlinear relations among voxels in each region learned by deep neural networks, we extract a *regional abnormality representation*. We then make a final clinical decision by integrating the regional abnormality representations over a whole brain. It is noteworthy that the regional abnormality representations allow us to interpret and understand the symptomatic observations of a subject with AD or MCI by mapping and visualizing them in a brain space individually. We validated the efficacy of our method in experiments with baseline MRI dataset in the ADNI cohort by achieving promising performances in three binary classification tasks.

1 Introduction

As the population becomes older, dementia has been emerging as one of the most serious social issues around the world. Of various diseases that cause dementia, the Alzheimer's Disease (AD) is the most prevalent in elderly subjects. In the meantime, it is reported that more than 30% of subjects with amnestic Mild Cognitive Impairment (MCI), situated in between cognitively normal and dementia in the symptomatic spectrum of AD, progress to AD within five years [12]. Although there is no medicine or treatment to cure the disease itself yet, it is expected to develop pharmaceutical solutions that may be effective when treating properly in the early stage of AD. In this regard, it has been of great importance to identify subjects with AD or MCI as early as possible. With the advances in imaging technologies, imaging-based AD/MCI diagnosis has been of great interest in the field and machine learning is playing the pivotal roles

© Springer Nature Switzerland AG 2018
Y. Shi et al. (Eds.): MLMI 2018, LNCS 11046, pp. 64–72, 2018.
https://doi.org/10.1007/978-3-030-00919-9_8

to make an optimal decision by analyzing complicated or latent patterns inherent in images. From a machine learning perspective, it is paramount to extract a well-designed or target-task relevant features to enhance performances. Suk *et al.* [9] divided methods for imaging-based feature extraction into three categories: voxel-based approach, region-based approach, and patch-based approach. A voxel-based approach basically uses voxel intensities, the most fine-grained information, but mostly suffers from the high dimensionality problem [8]. A region-based approach considers the structurally or functionally predefined brain regions and extract representative features, *e.g.*, mean volume, from each region [6]. While this approach greatly reduces the dimension of a feature space, due to the limitation of coarse-grained information, it is generally vulnerable to catch small or subtle pathological changes. In the meantime, a patch-based approach tries to find relations among voxels within the predefined-form of a patch, thus combining the merits of the voxel-based and region-based approaches. But, a patch is generally shaped in a cubical or rectangular form by manual [10].

In this paper, we propose a novel framework that systemically combines the above-mentioned three different approaches. Specifically, we parcellate a brain into predefined regions (region-based approach), and discover complex nonlinear relations among voxels (voxel-based approach) within a patch whose form is determined by the anatomical shape of each region (patch-based approach). Note that in our method a patch is atypically shaped by the forms of regions, rather than cubical or rectangular [3]. Using the complex voxel-relations in each region learned by deep neural networks, we extract regional abnormality representations. We then make a final clinical decision by integrating the regional abnormality representations over a whole brain. The morphological changes in a pathologic brain, *i.e.*, a region's atrophy, possibly caused by AD, would be small and subtle in multiple subparts of a region or spanning over multiple regions. In this regard, the rationale of our method is that by discovering the complex relations among voxels within a region, where an intensity of a voxel denotes the volumetric information, it would be possible to detect small and subtle changes, which generally cannot be detectable from the mean volume of a region. Further, by regarding the regional abnormalities as high-level information extracted from each region, we can build a robust and *generalized* classifier without suffering from an overfitting problem. Last but not least, our regional abnormality representation provides intuitive interpretation and understanding of the pathological status of regions, thereby allowing to make connections to symptomatic observations of a subject.

2   Materials and Preprocessing

We used 1.5T T1-weighted MRI data of 801 subjects in the ADNI cohort publicly available[1]. Specifically, we considered the baseline dataset, consisted of 229 Cognitively Normal (CN), 374 MCI, and 198 AD subjects. The MCI subjects were further categorized into 214 stable MCI (sMCI), 160 progressive MCI

---

[1] 'http://www.loni.ucla.edu/ADNI'.

(pMCI) depending on whether they progressed to AD in 18 months. The MR images were preprocessed by applying the prevalent procedures of Anterior Commissure (AC)-Posterior Commissure (PC) correction, skull-stripping, and cerebellum removal. Specifically, we used MIPAV software[2] for AC-PC correction, resampled images to $256 \times 256 \times 256$, and applied N3 algorithm for intensity inhomogeneity correction. Then, the MR images were segmented into three tissue types of gray matter, white matter, and cerebrospinal fluid with FAST in FSL package[3]. The segmented images were then parcellated into 93 regions by warping each subject's brain to Kabani *et al.*'s atlas [4]. Finally, we acquired the regional volumetric maps, so-called the RAVENS maps [2], by using a tissue preserving image warping method. To focus on the effect of brain atrophy possibly caused by neural death due to AD, we only used gray matter densities. It is worth mentioning that the voxel intensities in our RAVENS maps encode volume prior to warping.

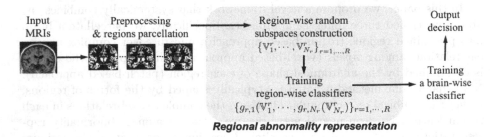

Fig. 1. Overall framework of the proposed method for AD/MCI diagnosis. For the notations, refer to the main contents.

3 Proposed Method

In this section, we describe a novel method of representing local region-wise abnormalities and identifying a global brain-wise neurodegenerative disorder. Figure 1 illustrates the overall framework of our method. Given a set of structural MRIs (sMRI), we first preprocess them as described in Sect. 2 to obtain region-wise volumetric maps by parcellating the RAVENS maps. Then, for each of the regions, we construct random subspaces, which are defined with a number of randomly selected voxels within the region. By regarding only intensities of the voxels, *i.e.*, volumetric measures in our case, in each subspace, a deep neural network is trained to learn the multi-level nonlinear relations among the voxels and to output the regional abnormality in probability. The regional abnormalities of each region are then averaged over the region's random subspaces, which are then fed into a classifier that integrates the regional abnormalities over a whole brain to identify a subject with AD or MCI.

---

[2] Available at 'http://mipav.cit.nih.gov/clickwrap.php'.
[3] Available at 'http://fsl.fmrib.ox.ac.uk/fsl/fslwiki/'.

3.1   Regional Abnormality Representation

From a clinical perspective, it is of paramount importance to understand which parts of a brain are pathologic and how different brain regions are related to the final clinical decision and symptomatic observations. In this regard, we formulate the task of brain disorder identification as two cascaded classification problems, *i.e.*, region-wise and brain-wise classifications.

Note that the voxel intensity after our preprocessing denotes a quantitative volumetric measure - the very fine-grained information that can be extracted from an input image. However, due to the unfavorable high-dimensional nature of an MR image and a limited number of training samples available, it is ultimately challenging to train a feature extractor and/or a classifier for brain disorder diagnosis with such voxel-level information directly. To this end, we propose a novel method of utilizing the fine-grained voxel-level information without suffering from overfitting. Basically, we combine the voxel-based and region-based approaches within a unified framework. In order to make a final brain-level decision, we exploit region-level information, which is estimated from their respective voxel-level information.

Assume that we partition a brain into R number of regions and there are V_r number of voxels in the r-th region, $r \in \{1, \ldots, R\}$. For each region, we learn an abnormality representation function from the voxel-level volumetric measures. Specifically, we propose to utilize the potential nonlinear relations among the voxels within a region to better represent the clinical state of a region. This approach is comparable to the previous region-based methods [7] that mostly considered the mean volume of regions.

When considering the number of voxels, it is still prohibitive to jointly consider all the voxels within a region simultaneously. In order to lessen this challenge, we first preselect voxels that show statistical significance, *i.e.*, small p-values, in group comparison, and then exploit a random subspace method, which has been used for random forest, Support Vector Machine (SVM). That is, given a set of voxels of the r-th region, we randomly resample the voxels and construct N_r number of voxel sets[4], $\mathcal{V}_r \equiv \{\mathbb{V}_i^r\}_{i=1,\ldots,N_r}$. Regarding the number of voxel sets, we set N_r proportional to the total number of voxels in the r-th region in order to take into account the difference in size among regions.

Based on the random voxel sets $\mathcal{V}_r$ of a region r, we define its regional abnormality representation function $G_r(\mathcal{V}_r)$ via deep neural network [1], which has a great power of discovering nonlinear relations among input variables, *i.e.*, volumetric measures in our case. That is, we train a set of deep neural networks, $\{g_{r,i}(\mathbb{V}_i^r)\}_{i=1,\ldots,N_r}$, one for each voxel set $\mathbb{V}_i^r$, such that each neural network

---

[4] As for the cardinality of a voxel set $|\mathbb{V}_i^r|$, we empirically determined and set it equal to all the sets. In our experiments, we set 200.

outputs the target class probabilities, *e.g.*, AD vs. CN or MCI vs. CN, by taking the volumetric measure of voxels in each random subspace as input. From a set of voxel sets $\mathcal{V}_r \equiv \{\mathbb{V}_i^r\}_{i=1,\ldots,N_r}$ and the respective deep neural networks $\{g_{r,i}(\mathbb{V}_i^r)\}_{i=1,\ldots,N_r}$, we draw a consensus vector for the r-th region by taking the average of the output probabilities as follows:

$$G_r(\mathcal{V}_r) = \frac{1}{N_r}\sum_{i=1}^{N_r} g_{r,i}(\mathbb{V}_i^r).\tag{1}$$

It is noteworthy that this region-wise abnormality representation function in Eq. (1) can be regarded as '*weak classifier*' for the target task by considering voxel-level information of the corresponding region only. Further, when regarding each voxel set $\mathbb{V}_i^r$ as an instance of the r-th region, this method can be thought of *multi-instance learning*.

Finally, we use one of the elements in the consensus vector for abnormality representation $a(r)$ of the r-th region. Specifically, in different classification scenarios, we regard the output probability of the most serious state in the AD progression spectrum as abnormality representation. That is, in AD vs. CN or MCI vs. CN classification, the output probability of AD or MCI is regarded as the abnormality representation[5], respectively.

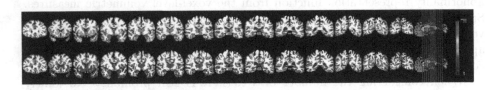

Fig. 2. Example of a regional abnormality map of a subject with AD (top) and a cognitively normal subject (bottom). We have colored over the preselected voxels based on their p-values in group comparison between AD and CN.

One of the main advantages in our regional abnormality representation is that it gives natural interpretation or understanding of the state of an individual's brain in terms of neurodegenerative pathology. That is, we can map and visualize the abnormality representations in a brain space, as presented in Fig. 2, which we call as '*regional abnormality map.*' It is then straightforward to interpret the status of different brain regions and further make potential relations with symptomatic observations. In the meantime, our abnormality representation can be comparable to the regional mean volume, commonly used in the previous methods [8]. Although both have a single scalar value for a region, from an information perspective, the regional mean volume is low-level information while our abnormality representation is high-level information. Thus, it is believed that the multivariate analysis over a brain with our high-level information be more useful to generalize the power of a classifier, and thus improve a clinical accuracy.

---

[5] Since the output probabilities in deep neural networks sum to one, it is enough to consider only one value in binary classification.

3.2   Brain-Wise Feature Extraction and Classifier Learning

In order to make a clinical decision in a brain-wise manner, it is necessary to integrate the distributed region-wise high-level information across a brain. For the information integration, we simply concatenate the regional abnormality representations into a vector as follows:

$$\mathbf{a} = [a(1) \cdots a(r) \cdots a(R)]^{\top} \in \mathbb{R}^{R}. \tag{2}$$

For the M number of training samples, $i.e.$, subjects in our case, we extract the respective feature vectors $\{\mathbf{a}_s\}_{s=1,\ldots,M}$ as described in Sect. 3.1 and in Eq. (2). From the pairs of extracted imaging features and the subjects' clinical label, $i.e.$, $\{(\mathbf{a}_s, l_s)\}_{s=1,\ldots,M}$, we train a linear SVM for making a clinical decision.

4   Experimental Settings and Results

4.1   Experimental Settings

In our experiments, we considered three binary classification problems: AD vs CN, MCI vs. CN, and pMCI vs. sMCI. In the MCI vs. CN classification, we labeled both pMCI and sMCI as MCI. Due to the limited number of samples, we applied a 10-fold cross-validation technique in each binary classification problem. For performance comparison, we took the average of the 10 cross-validation results.

Specification of Our Method In constructing random voxel sets of a region r, we first conducted voxel-wise statistical significance test between target groups, $i.e.$, AD vs. CN, MCI vs. CN, and pMCI vs. sMCI, and then discarded voxels whose p-value was higher than 0.05. From the remaining voxels $\mathbb{R}^r$, we randomly selected 200^6 voxels for a single voxel set and repeated this process to construct $N_r = Round\left(|\mathbb{R}^r|/200\right) \times 3$ number of voxel sets. Thus, for different regions, there were different numbers of voxel sets by reflecting the difference in size among regions.

For each random voxel set, we built a three-layer neural network with an architecture of '200(input)-350(hidden)-60(hidden)-2(output).' In order for better network training, we pretrained our network with greedy layer-wise pretraining by using stacked denoising auto-encoders [11], and then fine-tuned the whole network parameters simultaneously by stochastic gradient descent with a mini-batch size of 50. We also applied a dropout rate of 0.5 for hidden layers,

---

[6] In our exhaustive experiments, we varied this value in $\{100, 200, 300, 400\}$ and obtained low performance with 100 but reasonably higher performance with the other values. Thus, by concerning computational complexity, we set the lowest value, $i.e.$, 200, at the end.

a learning rate of 0.003, a momentum of 0.9, and an epoch of 120. Regarding a linear SVM, we performed a 5-fold nested cross-validation with the soft-margin parameter $C \in \{10^{-5}, 10^{-4}, \cdots, 10^{5}\}$. We used the public packages of 'DeepLearnToolbox'[7] and 'libsvm'[8] for our experiments.

Comparative Methods In order to present the efficacy and validity of our method, we conducted various experiments by comparing with the existing methods. Specifically, we considered three different methods characterized as follows:

- Regional Mean Volume (RMV) [7]: This method used a simple low-level mean volume feature for each region while our method uses a high-level abnormality representation.
- Hierarchical Feature Fusion (HFF) [5]: This method gradually integrates features from a number of cubical local patches extracted from a GM density map. For computational efficiency, we resized GM density maps into 64×64 and extracted patches of $11 \times 11 \times 11$ in size by following Liu *et al.*'s work.
- Regional Abnormality Representation with Random Forest (RF-RAR): A random forest classifier, which exploits random subspace and ensemble methods during training, is used for regional abnormality representation, same as our method. By reflecting the difference in size among regions, we set the number of trees proportional to the size of regions, *i.e.*, $Round\left(\left|\mathbb{R}^r\right|/200\right) \times 100$. The maximum depth of a tree was set to 12 and a Gini index was used as an impurity function.

For all the competing methods, we used a linear SVM for the brain-wise classification.

4.2   Results and Discussion

Table 1 presents the performance of the competing methods in four different metrics, commonly considered in AD/MCI diagnosis. It is remarkable that our method achieved very promising results in all three tasks. Specifically, in tasks of MCI vs. CN and pMCI vs. sMCI, which are of high importance for proper clinical treatments, our method obtained an accuracy of 89.22% (MCI vs. CN) and 88.52% (pMCI vs. sMCI), and an AUC of 0.9573 (MCI vs. CN) and 0.9568 (pMCI vs. sMCI). To our knowledge, these are of the highest performances reported in the literature [8] for these classification tasks over the ADNI dataset.

Our proposed method clearly outperformed the competing methods in all three binary classification tasks with a large margin. In comparison between RF-RAR and our method, both of which use regional abnormality representations for AD/MCI identification. However, while RF-RAR represents regional abnormality based on the low-level voxel intensities (*i.e.*, volumetric measure), our method used the complex nonlinear relations among voxels (*i.e.*, high-level

---

[7] 'https://github.com/rasmusbergpalm/DeepLearnToolbox'.
[8] 'https://www.csie.ntu.edu.tw/~cjlin/libsvm/'.

Table 1. Performance comparison on three different classification tasks

Tasks	Methods	Accuracy (%)	Sensitivity (%)	Specificity (%)	AUC
AD vs. CN	RMV [7]	86.64 ± 4.81	84.36	88.61	0.9283
	HFF [5]	90.18 ± 5.25	91.54	90.61	0.9620
	RF-RAR	85.01 ± 5.14	81.23	88.22	0.8516
	Ours	**92.75 ± 6.06**	**91.89**	**93.47**	**0.9804**
MCI vs. CN	RMV [7]	64.80 ± 6.14	72.67	51.94	0.6949
	HFF [5]	81.14 ± 10.22	97.08	48.18	0.8352
	RF-RAR	65.51 ± 3.66	90.92	23.99	0.6687
	Ours	**89.22 ± 4.13**	**93.33**	**82.55**	**0.9573**
pMCI vs. sMCI	RMV [7]	60.33 ± 10.62	49.38	68.48	0.6518
	HFF [5]	64.75 ± 14.83	22.22	89.57	0.6355
	RF-RAR	78.07 ± 3.13	60.00	91.96	0.7576
	Ours	**88.52 ± 5.65**	**87.50**	**89.22**	**0.9568**

information) learned by deep neural networks. Based on the performance in Table 1, we can see the effect of learning nonlinear relations among voxels, thus the validity of high-level feature representations. Comparing to the hierarchical feature fusion method [5], which uses cubical patches for local feature representation and gradually combines the informative patches to form atypical form of a patch over a whole brain, our method obtained superior performance in all metrics. Further, since our method defines a patch based on anatomical knowledge, it is advantageous in interpreting the regional abnormality by making relations with any symptomatic observation in a subject.

5   Conclusion

In this work, we proposed a novel method that systematically integrates voxel-based, region-based, and patch-based approaches in a unified framework. From a machine learning perspective, our method exploits a random subspace method, nonlinear feature representation with deep neural networks, and ensemble method to enhance classification performance. We compared our results with the counterpart methods by conducting experiments on the ADNI dataset and validated the effectiveness of our proposed method by outperforming those methods with a large margin.

Acknowledgement. This work was partially supported by Basic Science Research Program through the National Research Foundation of Korea (NRF) funded by the Ministry of Science, ICT & Future Planning (NRF-2015R1C1A1A01052216); and also by the Bio & Medical Technology Development Program of the NRF funded by the Korean government, MSIP (2016941946).

References

1. Bengio, Y.: Learning deep architectures for AI. Found. Trends® Mach. Learn. **2**(1), 1–127 (2009)
2. Davatzikos, C., Genc, A., Xu, D., Resnick, S.M.: Voxel-based morphometry using the RAVENS maps: methods and validation using simulated longitudinal atrophy. NeuroImage **14**(6), 1361–1369 (2001)
3. Fan, Y., Shen, D., Gur, R.C., Gur, R.E., Davatzikos, C.: Compare: classification of morphological patterns using adaptive regional elements. IEEE Trans. Med. Imaging **26**(1), 93–105 (2007)
4. Kabani, N.J.: 3D anatomical atlas of the human brain. NeuroImage **7**, P-0717 (1998)
5. Liu, M., Zhang, D., Shen, D.: Hierarchical fusion of features and classifier decisions for Alzheimer's disease diagnosis. Hum. Brain Mapp. **35**(4), 1305–1319 (2014)
6. Liu, S., et al.: Multimodal neuroimaging feature learning for multiclass diagnosis of Alzheimer's disease. IEEE Trans. Biomed. Eng. **62**(4), 1132–1140 (2015)
7. Möller, C., et al.: Alzheimer disease and behavioral variant frontotemporal dementia: automatic classification based on cortical atrophy for single-subject diagnosis. Radiology **279**(3), 838–848 (2016)
8. Rathore, S., Habes, M., Iftikhar, M.A., Shacklett, A., Davatzikos, C.: A review on neuroimaging-based classification studies and associated feature extraction methods for Alzheimer's disease and its prodromal stages. NeuroImage **155**, 530–548 (2017)
9. Suk, H.I., Lee, S.W., Shen, D., Initiative, A.D.N., et al.: Hierarchical feature representation and multimodal fusion with deep learning for AD/MCI diagnosis. NeuroImage **101**, 569–582 (2014)
10. Tong, T., Wolz, R., Gao, Q., Guerrero, R., Hajnal, J.V., Rueckert, D., et al.: Multiple instance learning for classification of dementia in brain MRI. Med. Image Anal. **18**(5), 808–818 (2014)
11. Vincent, P., Larochelle, H., Lajoie, I., Bengio, Y., Manzagol, P.A.: Stacked denoising autoencoders: learning useful representations in a deep network with a local denoising criterion. J. Mach. Learn. Res. **11**(Dec), 3371–3408 (2010)
12. Ward, A., Tardiff, S., Dye, C., Arrighi, H.M.: Rate of conversion from prodromal Alzheimer's disease to Alzheimer's dementia: a systematic review of the literature. Dement. Geriatric Cognit. Disorders Extra **3**(1), 320–332 (2013)

Joint Registration And Segmentation Of Xray Images Using Generative Adversarial Networks

Dwarikanath Mahapatra[1(✉)], Zongyuan Ge[2],
Suman Sedai[1], and Rajib Chakravorty[1]

[1] IBM Research Australia, Melbourne, VIC, Australia
{dwarim,ssedai}@au1.ibm.com, rajib.chakravorty@gmail.com
[2] Monash University, Melbourne, VIC, Australia
zongyuan.ge@monash.edu

Abstract. Medical image registration and segmentation are complementary functions and combining them can improve each other's performance. Conventional deep learning (DL) based approaches tackle the two problems separately without leveraging their mutually beneficial information. We propose a DL based approach for joint registration and segmentation (JRS) of chest Xray images. Generative adversarial networks (GANs) are trained to register a floating image to a reference image by combining their segmentation map similarity with conventional feature maps. Intermediate segmentation maps from the GAN's convolution layers are used in the training stage to generate the final segmentation mask at test time. Experiments on chest Xray images show that JRS gives better registration and segmentation performance than when solving them separately.

1 Introduction

Image registration and segmentation are essential steps of many medical image analysis pipelines. Registration is important for atlas building, correcting deformations and monitoring pathological changes over time. Segmentation is crucial for disease identification, pathology localization and measuring organ function. Accurate segmentation improves registration while accurate registration improves segmentation. Hence a joint registration and segmentation (JRS) framework is expected to improve both over solving them separately. Earlier works combining registration and segmentation have used active contours [17] or Graph cuts [9]. Active contours are iterative, time consuming and may get stuck in local optima, while graph cuts require high computation time. We propose a deep learning (DL) based JRS method that uses generative adversarial networks (GANs) for simultaneous registration and segmentation.

Previous DL based segmentation methods (e.g. brain MRI [13] and lung CT [4]), have used variants of FCN [8] or UNets [12]. DL based approaches for registration have used convolution neural network (CNN) regressors to estimate deformation field [1,10], or combined them with reinforcement learning

© Springer Nature Switzerland AG 2018
Y. Shi et al. (Eds.): MLMI 2018, LNCS 11046, pp. 73–80, 2018.
https://doi.org/10.1007/978-3-030-00919-9_9

[7]. These approaches still use a conventional model to generate the transformed image from the deformation field which increases computation time and does not fully utilize the generative capabilities of DL methods. RegNet [15] and DIR-Net [16] are among the first methods to achieve registration in a single pass but are limited by reliance on spatially corresponding patches to predict transformations. Finding corresponding patches is challenging in low contrast medical images and adversely affects the registration task. Rohe et al. [11] propose SVF-Net trained using reference deformations obtained by registering *previously segmented* regions of interest (ROIs).

Our proposed JRS method is different from existing methods as: (1) we combine registration and segmentation in a single DL framework, which eliminates the need to train a separate segmentation network; (2) registration is driven by segmentation and vice-versa; and '(3) we do not require explicit segmentation of ROIs as in [11], relying instead on segmentation masks generated on the fly from the GAN and use it for registration. We demonstrate its effectiveness for intra-patient lung registration over multiple visits. Our DL approach has the advantage of fast image registration without using conventional time consuming methods, and we outperform DL based registration and segmentation methods, as well as conventional JRS approaches.

2   Methods

In our proposed JRS architecture, the generator network, G, takes three input images: (1) reference image (I^{Ref}), (2) floating image (I^{Flt}) to be registered to I^{Ref}, and (3) I^{Ref}_{Seg}, the segmentation mask of I^{Ref} indicating the organ to be segmented. The outputs of G are: (1) I^{Trans}, the registered image (transformed version of I^{Flt}); (2) I^{Trans}_{Seg}, the segmentation mask of I^{Trans}; and (3) $I^{Def-Recv}$ the recovered deformation field. The discriminator network compares all the three outputs with their corresponding training data to determine if they are real or not. During testing only the generator network is used.

2.1   Joint Registration and Segmentation Using GANs

GANs [3] are generative models trained in an adversarial setting. The generator G outputs a desired image type while a discriminator D outputs a probability of the generated image matching the training data. The training database has chest Xray images and the corresponding masks of the two lungs. To generate training data the images are first translated in the left, right, top or bottom direction with a displacement range of $\pm[25, 40]$ pixels. The translated images are rotated by different angles in the range $\pm[20, 180]°$ at equal steps of $5°$. Finally the rotated images are subjected to local elastic deformation using B-splines with the pixel displacements in the range of $\pm[1, 15]$. We denote this deformation field as $I_{Def-App}$, the applied deformation field. The transformations are such that when applied to the corresponding segmentation masks, the Dice Metric (DM) between the original and transformed mask has values less than 0.70. This is done to ensure that the transformed images are significantly different from the original images and truly test algorithm performance. The original images are I^{Ref} and the transformed images are I^{Flt}. Applying synthetic deformations allows us to: (1) accurately quantify the registration error; and (2) determine the similarity between I^{Trans} and I^{Ref}. G is a feed-forward CNN whose parameters θ_G are,

$$\widehat{\theta} = \arg \min_{\theta_G} \frac{1}{N} \sum_{n=1}^{N} l^{JRS} \left(G_{\theta_G}(I^{Flt}), I^{Ref}, I^{Flt}, I_{Seg}^{Ref} \right), \qquad (1)$$

where the loss function l^{JRS} combines content loss (Eq. 2) and adversarial loss (Eq. 3), and $G_{\theta_G}(I^{Flt}) = I^{Trans}$. The content loss is,

$$l_{content}(I^{Trans}, I^{Ref}, I_{Seg}^{Ref}, I_{Seg}^{Trans}) = NMI + [1 - SSIM] + VGG. \qquad (2)$$

NMI denotes normalized mutual information between I^{Ref} and I^{Trans} and is suitable for multimodal and unimodal deformable registration. $SSIM$ denotes structural similarity index metric (SSIM) based on edge distribution [19] and quantifies landmark correspondence between different images. $SSIM \in [0, 1]$ with higher values indicating greater similarity. VGG is the $L2$ distance between two images using all the multiple feature maps obtained from a pre-trained $VGG16$ network [14]. Note that we extract all the feature maps from all convolution layers of VGG16. This sums up to $64 \times 2 + 128 \times 2 + 256 \times 2 + 512 \times 3 + 512 \times 3 = 3968$ feature maps. The feature maps are of different dimensions due to multiple max pooling steps. Using all feature maps ensures we are comparing information from multiple scales, both coarse and fine, and thus improves robustness. All feature maps are normalized to have values between $[0, 1]$.

2.2 Deformation Field Consistency

CycleGANs [21] learn mapping functions $G : X \rightarrow Y$ and $F : Y \rightarrow X$, between image sets $X = I^{Flt}$ and $Y = I^{Ref}$. Adversarial discriminators D_X differentiate between images x and registered images $F(y)$, and D_Y distinguishes between y and $G(x)$. G registers I^{Flt} to I^{Ref} while F registers I^{Ref} to I^{Flt}. Due to space constraints we refer the reader to [21] for details of CyclicGan implementation. In addition to the content loss (Eq. 2) we have: (1) an adversarial loss; and (2) a cycle consistency loss to ensure transformations G, F do not contradict.

The adversarial loss is an important component to ensure that the generated outputs are plausible. In previous works the adversarial loss was based on the similarity of generated image to training data distribution. Since our generator network has three outputs we have additional terms for the adversarial loss. The first term matches the distribution of I^{Trans} to I^{Flt} and is given by:

$$L_{cycGAN}(G, D_Y) = E_{y \in p_{data}(y)} [\log D_Y(y)] + E_{x \in p_{data}(x)} [\log (1 - D_Y(G(x)))], \quad (3)$$

We retain notations X, Y for conciseness. There also exists $L_{cycGAN}(F, D_X)$, the corresponding adversarial loss for F and D_X.

The second component of the adversarial loss incorporates segmentation information by calculating the logarithm of the dice metric (DM) between the generated mask I_{Seg}^{Trans} during each training step, and I_{Seg}^{Ref} the segmentation mask of I^{Ref}. DM is a normalized metric between $[0, 1]$ and acts like a probability measure similar to those in Eq. 3 The third adversarial loss term is the mean square error between $I^{Def-App}$ and $I^{Def-Recv}$, the applied and recovered deformation fields. The final adversarial loss is

$$L_{adv} = L_{cycGAN}(G, D_{IRef}) + L_{cycGAN}(F, D_{IFlt}) + \log DM(I_{Seg}^{Ref}, I_{Seg}^{Trans}) \\ + \log\left(1 - MSE_{Norm}(I^{Def-App}, I^{Def-Recv})\right), \tag{4}$$

where MSE_{Norm} is the MSE normalized to $[0, 1]$, and $1 - MSE_{Norm}$ ensures that similar deformation fields give a corresponding higher value.

Cycle consistency loss ensures that for each $x \in X$ the reverse deformation should bring x back to the original image, i.e. $x \to G(x) \to F(G(x)) \approx x$. Similar constraints also apply for mapping F and y. This is achieved using,

$$L_{cyc}(G, F) = E_x \|F(G(x)) - x\|_1 + E_y \|G(F(y)) - y\|_1, \tag{5}$$

Thus the full objective function is

$$L(G, F, D_{IFlt}, D_{IRef}) = L_{adv} + l_{content} + \lambda L_{cyc}(G, F) \tag{6}$$

where $\lambda = 10$ controls the contribution of the two objectives. The optimal parameters are given by:

$$G^*, F^* = \arg\min_{F,G} \max_{D_{IFlt}, D_{IRef}} L(G, F, D_{IFlt}, D_{IRef}) \tag{7}$$

G (Fig. 1(a)) employs residual blocks having two convolution layers with 3×3 filters and 64 feature maps, followed by batch normalization and ReLU activation. G also outputs the segmentation mask which is fed back for training. F (to ensure cycle consistency) has a similar architecture. The discriminator D (Fig. 1 (b)) determining the similarity between I^{Trans} and I^{Ref} has eight convolutional layers with the kernels increasing by a factor of 2 from 64 to 512 . Leaky ReLU is used and strided convolutions reduce the image dimension when the number of features is doubled. The resulting 512 feature maps are followed by two dense layers and a final sigmoid activation. We do not use max pooling in any layer as we want the input and output images to have the same size.

2.3 Obtaining Segmentation Mask

The segmentation mask is obtained by concatenating the feature maps of different convolution layers which function as activation maps highlighting informative parts of the image [20]. This is similar to the approach by UNet [12] which adds skip connections between corresponding layers of the upsampling and downsampling path to get the final segmentation map. Since our generator network has

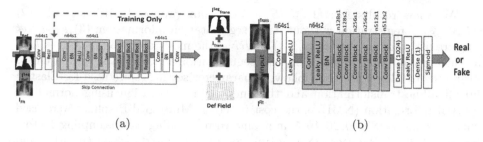

(a)   (b)

Fig. 1. (a) Generator Network; (b) Discriminator network. $n64s1$ denotes 64 feature maps (n) and stride (s) 1 for each convolutional layer.

no downsampling steps we do not add any skip connections. Instead we take the feature maps of each convolution layer, normalize its values to $[0,1]$, add them and finally employ Otsu's thresholding to get a segmentation mask. Note that since this mask is generated at each iteration and its similarity with I_{Seg}^{Ref} is being calculated, the feedback is used to update the network weights. Thus, after convergence the segmentation mask thus obtained is an accurate segmentation of the image. We *do not* use a weighted combination similar to [20] because the weights are also being updated.

3   Experiments

Our registration method was tested on the NIH ChestXray14 dataset [18] with $112,120$ frontal-view X-rays from $30K$ patients with 14 disease labels (multiple-labels for each image). Since the original dataset is designed for classification studies, we selected samples and applied the following steps to make it suitable for validating registration experiments.

1. 30 patients each from all the 14 disease classes were selected, giving a total of $14 \times 30 = 420$ different patients. Care was taken to ensure that all the patients had multiple visits (minimum 3 visits and maximum 8 visits.
2. For each set of patient images the left and right lung were manually outlined. We manually annotate corresponding region of disease activity for a particular patient. In some cases there were multiple disease labels for a single patient and each pathology was outlined by the expert. Consequently one image may have multiple labels.
3. In total we had 420 reference images from 420 patients and 1087 floating images (excluding the reference images) across multiple visits of all patients.

Our method was implemented in TensorFlow. We use Adam [5] with $\beta_1 = 0.93$ and batch normalization. The ResNet of G was initialized using mean square error and learning rate of 0.001. Subsequently the final GAN was trained with 10^5 update iterations at learning rate 10^{-3}. Training and test was performed on a NVIDIA Tesla K40 GPU with 12 GB RAM.

We show results for: (1) $JRS - Net$ - our proposed JRS network; (2) JRS_{NoSeg} - registration without using segmentation information; (3) $FlowNet$ - the registration method of [1]; (4) $DIRNet$ the method of [16]; (5) $GC - JRS$ a conventional joint registration and segmentation method using graph cuts ([9]); and (6) Elastix [6]. The following parameter settings were used for Elastix: initial affine transformation and then non rigid registration using normalized mutual information (NMI) as the cost function. Multi grid B-splines were used with spacing of $80, 40, 20, 10, 5$ mm and corresponding downsampling factors being $4, 3, 2, 1, 1$. Average training time for an augmented dataset (rotation and translation) with $98, 000$ images is 36 h. Affine registration was applied only for Elastix and not the other methods.

3.1   Results on NIH dataset

The image acquired on the first visit is I^{Ref} and images acquired on subsequent visits are I^{Flt}. I_{Seg}^{Ref} is obtained by manual delineation. For subsequent visits I_{Seg}^{Flt} is obtained by our algorithm. This highlights our JRS algorithm's advantages since the trained model can be applied to different applications using a single manual annotation. The total registration error (TRE) and segmentation overlap measures such as Dice Metric (DM) and 95% Hausdorff Distance (HD_{95}) are calculated before and after registration to quantify each method's efficacy. Intra-patient registration and segmentation results for the lung are summarized in Table 1. We use the UNet trained on the SCR [2] database to segment both lungs from the NIH dataset. The average values for normal images ($DM = 84.9$, $HD = 8.9$) and diseased images ($DM = 84.0$, $HD = 9.3$) is inferior than those reported in Table 1 for $JRS - Net$.

In the example case of patient 5, from day 0 to day 5 had no pathologies in the lung, and hence these 6 images are considered non-diseased. However, infiltration was detected for visits on days 6, 7 and these images were considered diseased. Figure 2 shows results for non-diseased images where I^{Ref} was day 0 image and I^{Flt} was day 3 image. Figure 3 shows the corresponding results for diseased case where I_{Flt} is from day 6. Superimposed contours $(I_{Seg}^{Flt}, I_{Seg}^{Ref})$ on I^{Ref} (Figs. 2(c), 3(c)) clearly show the difference in lung positions and size on

Table 1. *Intra-patient* image registration results for **left and right lung** using different methods on the NIH-14 database. *Time* indicates computation time in seconds.

	Normal Images							Diseased Images						
	Bef. Reg	After Registration						Bef. Reg	After Registration					
		JRS Net	JRS $_{NoSeg}$	DIR Net	Flow Net	GCJRS	Elastix		JRS Net	JRS $_{NoSeg}$	DIR Net	Flow Net	GCJRS	Elastix
DM(%)	78.9	89.3	85.2	84.8	83.5	85.6	82.1	79.1	88.9	85.0	84.4	83.1	85.2	81.5
HD_{95}(mm)	12.9	6.9	8.4	8.7	9.8	8.0	10.8	11.8	7.3	8.6	8.9	10.1	8.8	11.5
TRE	13.3	7.6	8.9	9.5	10.6	8.9	11.5	12.9	7.9	9.4	9.7	11.0	9.3	12.1
Time(s)		0.5	0.4	0.6	0.5	0.6	21		0.5	0.4	0.6	0.5	53	21

different days due to different acquisition positions. The green and red contours should coincide for ideal registration and results show $JRS - Net$ outperforms all other methods (despite diseased images showing more artificats than normal images) by including segmentation information in the registration task. Segmentation output from UNet is shown in Figs. 2(g), 3(g) using a super imposed yellow contour which demonstrates the superior performance of JRS over conventional segmentation methods.

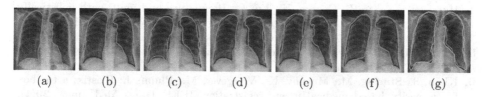

(a)   (b)   (c)   (d)   (c)   (f)   (g)

Fig. 2. Results for normal lung Xray images from NIH dataset (patient 5). (a) I_{Flt} with I_{Flt}^{Seg} (green); (b) I_{Ref} with I_{Ref}^{Seg} (red) and I_{Flt}^{Seg} before registration; Superimposed registered mask obtained using: (c) $JRS - Net$; (d) $DIR - Net$; (e) $GC - JRS$; (f) Elastix. (g) Segmentation masks of I^{Flt} - manual ground truth (red), $JRS - Net$ (green) and $UNet$ (yellow).

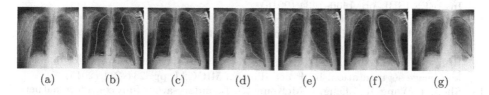

(a)   (b)   (c)   (d)   (e)   (f)   (g)

Fig. 3. Results for diseased lung Xray images from NIH dataset (patient 5). (a) (b) I_{Flt} with I_{Flt}^{Seg} (green); (b) I_{Ref} with I_{Ref}^{Seg} (red) and I_{Flt}^{Seg} before registration; Superimposed registered mask obtained using: (c) $JRS - Net$; (d) $DIR - Net$; (e) $GC - JRS$; (f) $Elastx$; (g) Segmentation masks of I^{Flt} - manual ground truth (red), $JRS - Net$ (green) and $UNet$ (yellow).

4   Conclusion

We have proposed a novel deep learning framework for joint registration and segmentation of lung xray images. Generative adversarial networks are used to register a floating image to a reference image. A simultaneous segmentation of the registered image is achieved by fusing the outputs of the different convolution layers in the GAN. The registration is driven by segmentation information, hence truly integrating registration and segmentation. Experimental results show our joint approach performs better than existing methods that solve registration and segmentation separately. The method's effectiveness is demonstrated on lung xray images of normal and healthy patients with multiple clinical visits.

References

1. Dosovitskiy, A., Fischer, P., et. al.: Flownet: Learning optical flow with convolutional networks. In: Proceedings of IEEE ICCV, pp. 2758–2766 (2015)
2. van Ginneken, B., Stegmann, M., Loog, M.: Segmentation of anatomical structures in chest radiographs using supervised methods: a comparative study on a public database. Med. Imag. Anal. 10(1), 19–40 (2006)
3. Goodfellow, I., et al.: Generative adversarial nets. In: Proceedings of NIPS, pp. 2672–2680 (2014)
4. Harrison, A., Xu, Z., George, K., Lu, L.: Progressive and multi-path holistically nested neural networks for pathological lung segmentation from ct images. In: Proceedings of MICCAI, pp. 621–629 (2017)
5. Kingma, D., Ba, J.: Adam: a method for stochastic optimization. In: arXiv preprint arXiv:1412.6980 (2014)
6. Klein, S., Staring, M., Murphy, K., Viergever, M., Pluim, J.: Elastix: a toolbox for intensity based medical image registration. IEEE Trans. Med. Imag. 29(1), 196–205 (2010)
7. Liao, R., et al.: An artificial agent for robust image registration. In: AAAI, pp. 4168–4175 (2017)
8. Long, J., Shelhamer, E., Darrell, T.: Fully convolutional networks for semantic segmentation. In: Proceedings of CVPR, pp. 3431–3440 (2015)
9. Mahapatra, D., Sun, Y.: Joint registration and segmentation of dynamic cardiac perfusion images using mrfs. In: Proceedings of MICCAI, pp. 493–501 (2010)
10. Miao, S., Z.J. Wang, Y.Z., Liao, R.: Real-time 2d/3d registration via cnn regression. In: IEEE ISBI, pp. 1430–1434 (2016)
11. Rohe, M., Datar, M., Heimann, T., Sermesant, M., Pennec, X.: SVF-Net: Learning deformable image registration using shape matching. In: Proceedings of MICCAI, pp. 266–274 (2017)
12. Ronneberger, O., Fischer, P., Brox, T.: U-net: Convolutional networks for biomedical image segmentation. In: Proceedings of MICCAI, pp. 234–241 (2015)
13. Shen, H., Wang, R., Zhang, J., McKenna, S.: Boundary-aware fully convolutional network for brain tumor segmentation. In: Proceedings of MICCAI, pp. 433–441 (2017)
14. Simonyan, K., Zisserman., A.: Very deep convolutional networks for large-scale image recognition. CoRR absarXiv:1409.1556 (2014)
15. Sokooti, H., de Vos, B., Berendsen, F., Lelieveldt, B., Isgum, I., Staring, M., et al.: Nonrigid image registration using multiscale 3d convolutional neural networks. In: MICCAI, pp. 232–239 (2017)
16. de Vos, B., Berendsen, F., Viergever, M., Staring, M., Isgum, I.: End-to-end unsupervised deformable image registration with a convolutional neural network. In: arXiv preprint arXiv:1704.06065 (2017)
17. Wang, F., Vemuri, B., Eisenschenk, S.: Joint registration and segmentation of neuroanatomic structures from brain mri. J Acad. Radiol. 12(9), 1104–1111 (2006)
18. Wang, X., Peng, Y., Lu, L., Lu, Z., Bagheri, M., Summers, R., et al.: Chestx-ray8: Hospital-scale chest x-ray database and benchmarks on weakly-supervised classification and localization of common thorax diseases. In: Proceedings of CVPR (2017)
19. Wang, Z., et al.: Image quality assessment: from error visibility to structural similarity. IEEE Trans. Imag. Proc. 13(4), 600–612 (2004)
20. Zhou, B., Khosla, A., Lapedriza, A., Oliva, A., Torralba, A.: Learning deep features for discriminative localization. In: Proceedings of CVPR, pp. 2921–2929 (2016)
21. Zhu, J., park, T., Isola, P., Efros, A.: Unpaired image-to-image translation using cycle-consistent adversarial networks. In: arXiv preprint arXiv:1703.10593 (2017)

SCCA-Ref: Novel Sparse Canonical Correlation Analysis with Reference to Discover Independent Spatial Associations Between White Matter Hyperintensities and Atrophy

Gerard Sanroma[✉], Loes Rutten-Jacobs, Valerie Lohner, Johanna Kramme,
Sach Mukherjee, Martin Reuter, Tony Stoecker, and Monique M. B. Breteler

German Center for Neurodegenerative Diseases (DZNE), Bonn, Germany
gerard.sanroma-gueell@dzne.de

Abstract. White matter hyperintensities (WMH) and atrophy are common findings in neurodegenerative diseases as well as healthy aging. However, it is not clear whether their co-occurrence is due to shared risk factors. Previous work has analyzed univariate associations between individual brain regions but not joint patterns over multiple regions. We propose a new method that jointly analyzes all the regions to discover spatial association patterns between WMH and atrophy. Univariate analyses typically correct for shared risk factors at the level of individual WMH and atrophy variables. Our method incorporates a novel correction strategy at the level of the entire pattern over multiple regions. Furthermore, we enforce sparsity to yield interpretable results. Results in a cohort of 703 participants from the Rhineland Study reveal two consistent spatial association patterns. Correction of individual variables did not yield qualitatively different patterns. Our proposed multi-variate correction strategy yielded different patterns thus, suggesting that it might be more appropriate for multi-variate analysis.

Keywords: WMH · Atrophy · CCA · Rhineland Study

1 Introduction

White matter hyperintensities (WMH), as seen in Fluid Attenuated Inversion Recovery (FLAIR) images, and brain atrophy are common findings in neurodegenerative diseases and normal aging. However, it is not clear whether their concomitant presence is due to shared risk factors or whether the presence of WMH promotes atrophy independently. Understanding the relationships between both manifestations may help understand their effects on cognitive decline [9].

Previous works found associations between WMH and atrophy [2,6,9,12]. In some cases, the associations disappeared after correcting for shared risk factors

© Springer Nature Switzerland AG 2018
Y. Shi et al. (Eds.): MLMI 2018, LNCS 11046, pp. 81–88, 2018.
https://doi.org/10.1007/978-3-030-00919-9_10

[2,6], while in others it remained [9,12]. These works analyzed the relation-ships independently across regions, thus failing to capture potential interactions between them. Moreover, many of the approaches measured global WMH load, which does not allow to capture region-specific associations [2,6,9]. The above limitations may be responsible for the inability to find associations, especially in healthy aging, where the pathological burden is lower.

We develop a novel method based on canonical correlation analysis (CCA) to find associations between WMH and atrophy that jointly analyzes all the regions to capture their potential interactions. Instead of correcting for the effects of shared risk factors at each individual variable, as commonly done in univari-ate analysis, we propose to correct for the shared risk factors at the level of the discovered patterns, which might be more suitable for multi-variate analysis. Moreover, our proposed method enforces sparsity to yield sharp spatial patterns, thus we name it Sparse Canonical Analysis with Reference (SCCA-ref). To lever-age the full potential of SCCA-ref, we propose a novel parcellation method to measure regional WMH burden that allows us to discover region-specific associ-ations whilst controlling the effective spatial resolution of the analysis. We use our method to discover associations between WMH and atrophy in a cohort of 703 healthy participants of the Rhineland Study [8].

2   Method

2.1   Classical CCA for Joint Analysis of WMH and Atrophy

Let $\mathbf{X_h} \in \mathbb{R}^{N \times m_h}$, $\mathbf{X_a} \in \mathbb{R}^{N \times m_a}$ be two matrices containing measures of regional WMH burden and brain atrophy of N participants, respectively. Each row of $\mathbf{X_h}$ contains the WMH burden in m_h different regions (Sect. 2.3 describes how to obtain these measures). Similarly, each row of $\mathbf{X_a}$ contains the volumes of m_a brain anatomical structures corrected by head size, representative of atrophy.

CCA aims at finding a latent representation, denoted as $\mathbf{y} = \mathbf{Xw}$, of both datasets so that they are maximally correlated. That is:

$$\max \frac{\mathbf{y_h}^\top \mathbf{y_a}}{\|\mathbf{y_h}\|_2 \|\mathbf{y_a}\|_2} = \max_{\mathbf{w_h}, \mathbf{w_a}} \frac{\mathbf{w_h}^\top \mathbf{R_{h,a}} \mathbf{w_a}}{\sqrt{\mathbf{w_h}^\top \mathbf{R_{h,h}} \mathbf{w_h} \mathbf{w_a}^\top \mathbf{R_{a,a}} \mathbf{w_a}}}, \tag{1}$$

where $\mathbf{w_h} \in \mathbb{R}^{m_h}$ and $\mathbf{w_a} \in \mathbb{R}^{m_a}$ are vectors of parameters governing the lin-ear projection of each dataset and $\mathbf{R_{h,a}} = \mathbf{X_h}^\top \mathbf{X_a}/N$ is the empirical cross-covariance (the data should be zero-centered). To improve numerical stability and generalization to unseen data, empirical auto-covariances can be substituted by their regularized versions $\tilde{\mathbf{R}}_{\mathbf{h,h}} = \mathbf{R_{h,h}} + \lambda_h I$, where λ_h is a small constant and I is the identity matrix (similarly for $\mathbf{R_{a,a}}$).

Alternatively, Eq. (1) can be formulated as follows:

$$\max_{\mathbf{w_h}, \mathbf{w_a}} \mathbf{w_h}^\top \mathbf{R_{h,a}} \mathbf{w_a}$$
$$\text{subject to} \quad \mathbf{w_h}^\top \tilde{\mathbf{R}}_{\mathbf{h,h}} \mathbf{w_h} = \mathbf{w_a}^\top \tilde{\mathbf{R}}_{\mathbf{a,a}} \mathbf{w_a} = 1 . \tag{2}$$

which can be readily solved by eigenvalue decomposition. This approach does not allow to enforce sparsity to limit the number of regions involved in the spatial patterns and, more importantly, does not allow to include a reference.

2.2 SCCA-Ref

Let $\mathbf{z}_i \in \mathbb{R}^N$ $(i = 1 \ldots)$ be sets of reference values we want our discovered patterns to be invariant to, such as age (e.g., $\mathbf{z}_1$) and blood pressure (e.g., $\mathbf{z}_2$). We extend Sparse CCA formulation [5] to allow for reference as follows:

$$
\begin{aligned}
\max_{\mathbf{w_h}, \mathbf{w_a}} \quad & \mathbf{w_h}^\top \mathbf{R}_{h,a} \mathbf{w_a} \\
\text{subject to} \quad & \mathbf{w_h}^\top \tilde{\mathbf{R}}_{h,h} \mathbf{w_h} \le 1, \ \mathbf{w_a}^\top \tilde{\mathbf{R}}_{a,a} \mathbf{w_a} \le 1 \\
& \|\mathbf{w_h}\|_1 \le c_h, \ \|\mathbf{w_a}\|_1 \le c_a \\
& \tfrac{1}{\sqrt{N}} \mathbf{w_h}^\top \mathbf{X_h}^\top \mathbf{z}_i = 0, \ \tfrac{1}{\sqrt{N}} \mathbf{w_a}^\top \mathbf{X_a}^\top \mathbf{z}_i = 0, \ \forall i,
\end{aligned}
\tag{3}
$$

where $\|\mathbf{w}\|_1 = \sum_i |w_i|$ denotes the L1-norm responsible for inducing the sparsity with constants c_h, c_a controlling its amount. To solve for both $\mathbf{w_h}$ and $\mathbf{w_a}$, we follow and alternating optimization strategy, where one vector, e.g., $\mathbf{w_h}$, is optimized while keeping the other fixed (and vice-versa) until convergence.

The latter set of constraints in Eq. (3) enforces the discovered spatial association patterns between WMH and atrophy to be uncorrelated with the references such as age and blood pressure. That is, the amount of atrophy and WMH load represented by these patterns remain constant throughout age and blood pressure values, and therefore they are independent of shared risk factors. The reference signals $\mathbf{z}_i$ need to be zero-centered and normalized to unit L2-norm, $\|\mathbf{z}_i\|_2^2 = 1, \forall i$. Note also, that the unit-variance equality constraints in Eq. (2) have been substituted by inequality constraints in Eq. (3) in order to maintain the convexity of the problem. Note that both options are equivalent in practice, because the correlation increases with the variance and therefore the value of these constraints in the solution will always be 1. We follow an alternating optimization strategy using the convex optimization package CVXPY [10].

The solution to Eq. (3) yields the main spatial association pattern between WMH and atrophy, denoted as $\mathbf{w_h}^{(1)}$ and $\mathbf{w_a}^{(1)}$, respectively. We find the subsequent uncorrelated patterns, denoted as $\mathbf{w_h}^{(2)}$ and $\mathbf{w_a}^{(2)}$, via the deflation technique [5]. A recent related work by Qi et al. [11] allow the discovered components to be *correlated* to a reference signal. Note that we take the opposite approach in order to discover associations independent of shared risk factors. Also, the approach by Qi et al. does not allow for sparsity.

2.3 Regional WMH Burden

We propose a parcellation approach to obtain the regional WMH load that defines each parcel based on two elements: a depth element determining its position relative to the ventricles and cortex, and an angular element determining its spatial extent. For a given point i, the depth coordinate is defined as the normalized distance between the ventricles and the cortex, i.e., $d_i^{\text{norm}} = d_i^{\text{vent}} / (d_i^{\text{vent}} + d_i^{\text{ctx}})$, where d_i^{vent} and d_i^{ctx} are the distances from i to the closest point in the ventricles and cortex, respectively. These distances can be easily obtained via the *distance transform*. The normalized distance ranges from 0 in the surface of the ventricles to 1 in the surface of the cortex, and can be used to divide this space into equidistant intervals (shell-like) in a way adapted to the anatomy of each individual. The angular element determining the spatial extent of the parcel is obtained by projecting the set of FreeSurfer cortical parcels [1] from the cortex down to the ventricles following the gradient of the normalized distance map. Figure 1 shows the subdivisions into depth and angular elements on an example image. The final parcels used to count the WMH load are obtained by the intersection of the depth and angular elements. Recently, another method used a similar approach to define the regions [4]. Instead of using the normalized distance as proposed here, they used a more complex approach based on the solution of the Laplace equation. They used 4 depth and 9 angular subdivisions while we use higher amount for a finer characterization.

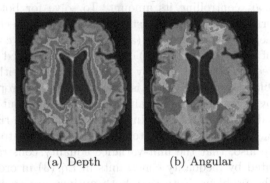

(a) Depth   (b) Angular

Fig. 1. The depth element defines an anatomically-adapted subdivision of the space between ventricles and cortex. The angular element defines the spatial extent.

3   Experiments

We present experiments of discovering spatial associations between WMH and atrophy in 703 participants of the Rhineland Study, aged 30 to 95. The Rhineland Study is a population-based study in the Bonn area (Germany) aiming to identify determinants of neuro-degenerative diseases [8].

Study participants underwent T1 (MPRAGE) and FLAIR scanning at a 3T Siemens Prisma scanner. BIANCA tool [7] was used to segment the WMH from FLAIR scans, using 17 manually annotated scans as training. We obtained regional WMH burden for $m_h = 680$ regions resulting of the intersection between 10 depth levels and 68 FreeSurfer cortical parcels [1] (see Sect. 2.3). Regional WMH was corrected for total brain volume (TBV) and arranged in the data matrix $\mathbf{X_h} \in \mathbb{R}^{N \times m_h}$. T1 scans were processed with the FreeSurfer *aseg* pipeline [3] and $m_a = 39$ structural volumes were selected, including various sub-cortical structures, ventricles, cerebellum (cortex and white matter) and brainstem. Structural volumes were corrected for estimated total intra-craneal volume (eTIV) and arranged in the data matrix $\mathbf{X_a} \in \mathbb{R}^{N \times m_a}$.

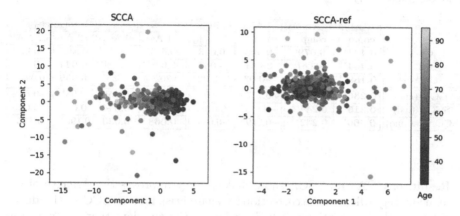

Fig. 2. Scatter plots with the projection of each participant onto the two main components for the methods SCCA and SCCA-ref with color-coded age.

We evaluate the contribution of each component of our method by comparing our full method, named SCCA-ref, with two degraded versions, namely without reference (SCCA) and without sparsity (CCA). SCCA and CCA consists on the elimination of the latter, and the latter two constraints in Eq. (3), respectively.

As references we use age and mean arterial pressure (MAP), which are common risk factors for WMH and atrophy. We compare the proposed strategy of eliminating the references from the discovered patterns, as implemented by the latter constraint in Eq. (3), with the strategy of eliminating the references a priori from the individual variables, denoted as *(ind)*, by correcting each variable for age and MAP (as done with TBV and eTIV).

To explore the distribution of the participants w.r.t. the discovered components, Fig. 2 shows scatter plots of the two main components (i.e., $\mathbf{w}^{(1)}$ and $\mathbf{w}^{(2)}$ for each modality). In contrast to SSCA, SSCA-ref components are less related to age. Moreover, in both methods, the components are uncorrelated among them, meaning that they are expressed independently in the population.

Table 1 shows quantitative results by each method for the main two components on independent test sets of 3-fold cross-validation experiments (regularization parameters were selected by nested cross-validation in the training set). The first two columns show the strength of the associations between WMH and atrophy for each component (high correlations are better). The next two columns show the independence between the two components for each modality (low correlations are better). The last four columns show the independence of each component w.r.t. the references (low correlations are better).

Table 1. Pearson correlation coefficients indicating the strength of the spatial association between WMH and atrophy for each component (columns 1, 2), the independence of the components across modalities (cols. 3, 4) and the independence of the spatial associations to the reference signals (cols. 5–8). The last three rows show results with individual variables corrected for age and MAP before optimization. Bold indicates favourable results. Significant correlations at $p = 0.05$ and $p = 0.001$ are denoted with $\star$ and $\star\star$, respectively.

	Strength Assoc.		Indep. Comp.		Indep. wrt References			
	comp. 1	comp. 2	WMH	Atrophy	c1 Age	c1 MAP	c2 Age	c2 MAP
CCA	**0.424****	**0.079***	**0.008**	**0.033**	−0.633**	−0.19**	0.032*	**−0.027**
SCCA	**0.464****	0.067	**0.041**	**0.062**	−0.608**	−0.199**	**0.044**	**−0.042**
SCCA-ref	**0.189****	**0.188****	−0.03	−0.02	0.202**	0.095*	**0.059**	0.091*
CCA (ind)	**0.236****	**0.253****	−0.177**	**0.0**	**0.027**	**0.055**	0.08*	**−0.029**
SCCA (ind)	**0.315****	**0.244****	−0.091*	0.049*	**0.051**	**0.044**	**0.053**	**−0.018**
SCCA-ref (ind)	**0.366****	**0.242****	−0.319**	−0.083*	**0.068**	**0.033**	0.196**	0.125

Results of CCA and SCCA show that sparsity improves the strength of the associations regardless of the correction for shared risk factors. SCCA-ref reduced considerably the associations with the references in the data that was not originally corrected for age and MAP (third row). However, the strength of the WMH-Atrophy associations was also weaker (but still significant) because the share of age and MAP was removed from these associations. In the data corrected a priori, there were no significant differences between SCCA-ref and SCCA. This is probably because the constraints in SCCA-ref did not influence too much the optimization due to using individually corrected variables. Figure 3 shows the spatial association maps between WMH ($\mathbf{w_h}$) and atrophy ($\mathbf{w_a}$) overlaid on a template image, for the first and second components.

Comparison of CCA and CCA (ind) shows similar patterns regardless the individual variables are corrected for shared risk factors or not. The first component reveals an association between lower peri-ventricular WMH load, smaller ventricles and larger thalamus, putamen and cerebellum. The second component captures an association between larger peri-ventricular and lower frontal WMH load with a prominently asymmetric atrophy in the left hemisphere (larger ventricle, smaller thalamus and putamen). SCCA patterns are similar but sparser, which helps identify the important structures. Interestingly, a different ordering of the patterns arise when correcting only at the pattern level (i.e., SCCA-ref). The first SCCA-ref component reveals an asymmetric left atrophy associated with higher peri-ventricular and lower frontal WMH load, similarly as the first component in the previous case. The second SCCA-ref component captures an association between high peri-ventricular WMH load with enlargement of ventricles and shrinkage of the cerebellum.

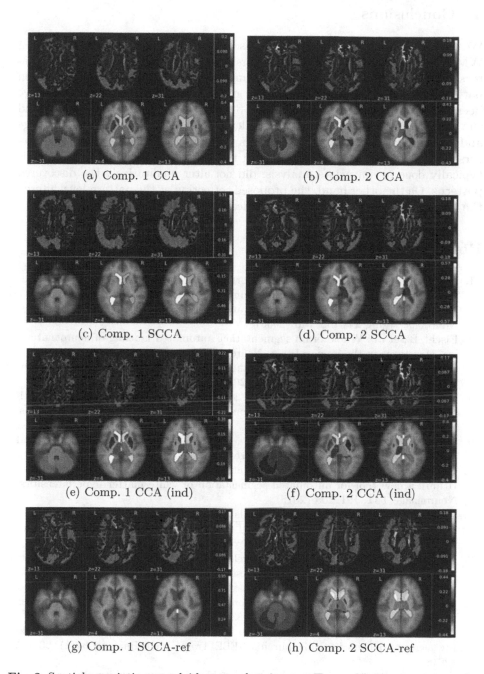

(a) Comp. 1 CCA

(b) Comp. 2 CCA

(c) Comp. 1 SCCA

(d) Comp. 2 SCCA

(e) Comp. 1 CCA (ind)

(f) Comp. 2 CCA (ind)

(g) Comp. 1 SCCA-ref

(h) Comp. 2 SCCA-ref

Fig. 3. Spatial associations overlaid on template images. Top and bottom rows in each subfigure show WMH and atrophy maps, respectively. Red (blue) indicates association with higher (lower) WMH loads and volumes.

4   Conclusions

We have presented a method for the discovery of spatial associations between WMH and atrophy that allows for sparsity and correction of shared risk factors at the pattern level. The different methods found 2 consistent association patterns containing interactions among different regions that would not have been detected with univariate analysis. Sparser associations were stronger and the proposed correction at the pattern level reduced the associations with age and MAP when the individual variables were uncorrected for shared risk factors. Correcting for shared risk factors at the level of the individual variables, as typically done in univariate analysis, did not alter qualitatively the discovered patterns. On the other hand, the proposed correction at the pattern level altered the order of the discovered patterns, reflecting a shift in their importance.

References

1. Dale, A.M., Fischl, B., Sereno, M.I.: Cortical surface-based analysis. I. Segmentation and surface reconstruction. Neuroimage 9(2), 179–194 (1999)
2. Du, A.T., et al.: Age effects on atrophy rates of entorhinal cortex and hippocampus. Neurobiol. Aging 27, 733–740 (2006)
3. Fischl, B., et al.: Whole brain segmentation: automated labeling of neuroanatomical structures in the human brain. Neuron 33(3), 341–355 (2002)
4. Sudre, C.H., et al.: Bullseye's representation of cerebral white matter hyperintensities. J. Neuroradiol. 45(2), 114–122 (2017)
5. Witten, D.M., Tibshirani, R., Hastie, T.: A penalized matrix decomposition, with applications to sparse principal components and canonical correlation analysis. Biostatistics 10(3), 515–534 (2009)
6. Korf, E.S.C., White, L.R., Scheltens, P., Launer, L.J.: Midlife blood pressure and the risk of hippocampal atrophy. Hypertension 44, 29–34 (2004)
7. Griffanti, L., et al.: BIANCA (Brain Intensity AbNormality Classification Algorithm): a new tool for automated segmentation of white matter hyperintensities. Neuroimage 141, 191–205 (2016)
8. Breteler, M.M.B., Wolf, H.: The Rhineland study: a novel platform for epidemiologic research into alzheimer disease and related disorders. Alzheimer's & Dement. 10(4), 520 (2014)
9. Breteler, M.M.B., et al.: Cognitive correlates of ventricular enlargement and cerebral white matter lesions on magnetic resonance imaging. Rotterdam Study. Stroke 25(6), 1109–1115 (1994)
10. Diamond, S., Boyd, S.: CVXPY: a python-embedded modeling language for convex optimization. J. Mach. Learn. Res. 17(83), 1–5 (2016)
11. Qi, S.: Multimodal fusion with reference: searching for joint neuromarkers of working memory deficits in Schizophrenia. IEEE Trans. Med. Imaging 37(1), 93–105 (2018)
12. den Heijer, T., et al.: Association between blood pressure, white matter lesions, and atrophy of the medial temporal lobe. Neurology 64, 263–267 (2005)

Synthesizing Dynamic MRI Using Long-Term Recurrent Convolutional Networks

Frank Preiswerk[1](✉), Cheng-Chieh Cheng[1], Jie Luo[1,2], and Bruno Madore[1]

[1] Brigham and Women's Hospital, Harvard Medical School, Boston, MA, USA
frank@bwh.harvard.edu
[2] Graduate School of Frontier Sciences, The University of Tokyo, Tokyo, Japan

Abstract. A method is proposed for converting raw ultrasound signals of respiratory organ motion into high frame rate dynamic MRI using a long-term recurrent convolutional neural network. Ultrasound signals were acquired using a single-element transducer, referred to here as 'organ-configuration motion' (OCM) sensor, while sagittal MR images were simultaneously acquired. Both streams of data were used for training a cascade of convolutional layers, to extract relevant features from raw ultrasound, followed by a recurrent neural network, to learn its temporal dynamics. The network was trained with MR images on the output, and was employed to predict MR images at a temporal resolution of 100 frames per second, based on ultrasound input alone, without any further MR scanner input. The method was validated on 7 subjects.

1 Introduction

Ultrasound (US) and Magnetic Resonance Imaging (MRI) signals are highly complementary. MRI is based on magnetic and RF fields and can achieve diversified soft-tissue contrasts, while US imaging is based on longitudinal pressure waves and offers a high temporal resolution, convenient and relatively low cost approach to diagnostic imaging. Efforts have been made to combine these two very different modalities, for US-MRI image fusion [1], as well as prospective motion compensation in MRI [2], using brightness mode (B-mode) ultrasound. A potentially useful idea in the context of image-guided intervention would be to learn the appearance of free-breathing MRI images during a training stage, then estimate them later on when MRI scanning may not be available anymore, for example after the patient left the MRI suite. Whether on the same day or a different day, the ability to generate MRI contrast based solely on US signals alone would be helpful as the patient proceeds to other diagnostic and/or therapy device(s), to continue generating MRI-like images even as the patient lies in a positron-emission tomography (PET) scanner or a radiotherapy device, for example. To this end, the approach introduced in [3] and the publicly-available software[1] was considerably expanded here to allow the rapid synthesizing of

---

[1] https://github.com/fpreiswerk/OCMDemo.

© Springer Nature Switzerland AG 2018
Y. Shi et al. (Eds.): MLMI 2018, LNCS 11046, pp. 89–97, 2018.
https://doi.org/10.1007/978-3-030-00919-9_11

MRI contrast using a long-term recurrent convolutional network inspired from the video-recognition work in [4].

An MR-compatible single-element ultrasound transducer [5] and a 3D-printed capsule, collectively referred to here as an 'organ-configuration motion' (OCM) sensor, acquired amplitude mode (A-mode) US signals of respiratory organ motion. In contrast to the conventional 2D spatial interpretation of US signals through delay-and-sum beamforming, the OCM's A-mode signals were not spatially encoded but provided a high temporal resolution signature of abdominal configuration, sensitive over a region in the area of sensor placement. Fast OCM signals (100 fps) can be correlated with slower-rate MRI acquisitions (1 fps), to estimate fast synthetic MR images of respiratory organ motion at the rate of the OCM signals (100 fps). This could be done using kernel density estimation (KDE) [6,7] to model this relationship in a non-parametric way, as data is acquired during online learning, as proposed in [3,8]. KDE is well suited for online learning, because there is no separation into training and inference stage. However, this comes at computational cost, as the time complexity at inference depends on the size of the dataset. In [3], an image reconstruction time of 45 ms for a single 2D MR image was reported using such KDE approach, on a relatively-small database accumulated over 2 min of hybrid OCM-MRI data. Furthermore, the inter-fraction variability of OCM signals was reported to be significant, which would presumably prevent any removal/re-attachment of an OCM probe, and confuse the KDE-based processing. As a result, any scenario involving the use of MRI+OCM data acquired on a given day to supplement, for example, radiotherapy treatments performed on a different day could not be considered, as the removal and re-attachment of the sensor days later would destroy the ability to generate accurate MR images from OCM signals. Lastly, due to the curse of dimensionality being a limiting factor in kernel methods, a small subset of depth values had to be pre-selected in the OCM traces in [3], as a trade-off between information vs. dimensionality of the data. Recently, artificial neural networks have become state-of-the-art models for computer vision (CV) and natural language processing (NLP) [9]. Feed-forward architectures, most notably convolutional neural networks (CNNs) [10] are used to automatically extract hierarchical features from (labeled) data, while recurrent networks (RNNs), typically based on long-short term memory (LSTM) units [11], allow temporal structures to be learned from data. We propose to use a combined CNN-LSTM model, called a long-term recurrent convolutional network (LRCN) [4], to learn the relationship between OCM sensor data and fully reconstructed MR images end-to-end. Our method improves on all the aforementioned challenges associated with KDE; By directly learning a mapping between OCM signals and MR images, the computational cost of image reconstruction is shifted from inference time to the training stage. Hence, the computational cost of image reconstruction becomes independent of the training set size. Our approach can therefore, in principle, be scaled to estimating several planes at once, i.e., 4D-MRI, at a high temporal rate. Our pre-processing step, closely related to Doppler processing, makes OCM signals more robust against signal changes that have little to do with physiological motion, and more to do with inconsequential details on exact sensor placement and/or anatomy. As a consequence, the Doppler-like pre-processing may help avoid registration steps when removing and re-attaching OCM sensors. Lastly, the curse of dimensionality is defeated since, unlike kernel methods, the proposed method does not rely on a high-dimensional similarity measure to be evaluated between any new OCM signal and all signals from the training set.

2   Materials and Methods

Hybrid OCM-MRI data were acquired on 7 subjects following informed consent using an IRB-approved protocol. Scanning was performed on a Siemens Verio 3T system, using a T1-weighted spoiled gradient echo MRI sequence with two-fold parallel imaging acceleration and 5/8 partial-Fourier acceleration. The US transducer at the heart of the OCM sensor was either a 5 MHz (subjects 1–4) or 1 MHz (subjects 5 and 6) MR-compatible transducer (Imasonics). The transducer was enclosed in a custom 3d-printed capsule that allowed for quick and easy attachment to the skin, regulation of pressure through a screwable lid (see Fig. 1), and retention of water-based US gel for acoustic coupling. The 1 MHz transducer employed in later subjects achieved greater signal penetration; nevertheless, both 5 MHz and 1 MHz OCM signals appeared equally appropriate for our purpose.

The OCM data acquisition was synchronized with the scanner's repetition rate, TR = 10 ms, using dedicated hardware and minor modifications to the MRI pulse sequence: At the beginning of each TR interval, the scanner was programmed to generate an optical synchronization pulse, which was then converted to a TTL voltage pulse using dedicated hardware. These pulses were used to trigger the OCM acquisition, at the rate of exactly one OCM trace acquisition per TR interval, thus precisely synchronizing the MRI and OCM streams of data. The purpose of such synchronization was two-fold: to allow MRI and OCM data to be unambiguously located on a common time axis, and to avoid the OCM sensor being fired during an MRI acquisition window, which would have caused artifacts in the MRI images. A total of 60 k-space lines and corresponding OCM signals were acquired per image. Individual OCM traces u were sampled at $f_s = 100$ MS s^{-1} for $t_s = 200\,\mu$s, yielding $D = f_s \cdot t_s = 20e^3$ samples per trace. The window from index 1000 to 8000 was retained for further processing, and downscaled to $d = 560$ samples. MR images of the breathing liver in the sagittal plane were acquired at a rate of 0.85 fps. Figure 1 gives an overview of the OCM sensor and data.

Preprocessing of OCM Signals and MR Images: Raw (magnitude) OCM signals $u(s,t)$ are highly sensitive to physiological motion along t (the repeat index, as OCM traces are repeatedly acquired every TR = 10 ms), but unfortunately, they tend to also prove highly sensitive to mostly unimportant details along s (the sampling index) relating to sensor placement and underlying anatomy. In the process to separate the former from the latter, OCM signals

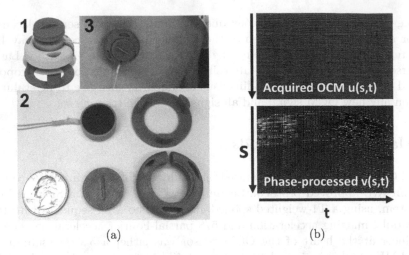

(a)   (b)

Fig. 1. (a) 3d model rendering (1) and Individual parts (2) of an OCM sensor. The US transducer (a 1 MHz version is depicted in (a)) was fitted into a 3d-printed capsule of our own design (green parts), which housed water-based gel for acoustic coupling and allowed for the pressure onto the skin to be adjusted by twisting the screw-like lid (3). Two-sided tape on the bottom was used for adhesion on the skin. (b) Visualization of unprocessed signals u and phase-processed versions v over a 3 s window. Respiratory motion is more pronounced in phase-processed signals (bright/dark pixels correspond to traces acquired during inspiration/expiration, respectively).

were first transformed into a complex entity:

$$\hat{u}(s,t) = \mathcal{F}_s^{-1}(\Omega(\mathcal{F}_s(u(s,t)))) = |u(s,t)|(\cos\theta(s,t) + i\sin\theta(s,t)), \qquad (1)$$

where $\mathcal{F}_s$ is the discrete Fourier transform along s, and Ω is a Fermi filter that cancels negative as well as very high frequencies ($>10 \cdot f_0$, where f_0 is the transducer center frequency). In analogy with Doppler ultrasound, we shall now consider $\theta(s,t)$, the complex angle of $\hat{u}(s,t)$ for further analysis. Variations along s have more to do with the object itself rather than how the object moves; for this reason the signal evolution along t, i.e., from trace to trace, was more closely linked to internal organ motion than variations along t. In particular, from $\theta(s,t)$, speed can be computed according to

$$v(s,t) = \alpha \cdot \frac{d\theta(s,t)}{dt} = \alpha \cdot \frac{\theta(s,t) - \theta(s,t-1)}{2}, \qquad (2)$$

with $\alpha = \frac{0.5 \cdot \lambda}{360}$, where λ is the wavelength in mm. Figure 1b visualizes u and v. We denote the vector of signals of a single timestep t, over the whole signal depth $s = \{1, \ldots, d\}$, as $\mathbf{v}(t) := [v(1,t), \ldots, v(d,t)]^T$. For further processing, OCM signals were rearranged as $X_t := [\mathbf{v}(t-n+1), \ldots, \mathbf{v}(t)]$, combining the most recent signal history of length $n = 300$ (3 s) in the form of a 2d image patch. This format proved well suited as input to the neural network described in the next section. Instead of explicitly modeling all pixels of the MR image domain (i.e., the model output dimension), we exploit correlations between pixels by compressing the images first, using Principal Component Analysis (PCA); 10 principal components are retained and used as target variables y_t for the neural network. This compression from size $192\,\mathrm{px} \times 192\,\mathrm{px}$ into a vector of 10 principal components for each image allows to significantly reduce the number of parameters in our model, at the cost of an acceptable loss of high-frequency image content.

2.1   Network Architecture

In [3], KDE is used to compute the expectation of unknown MR images I_t, given new OCM signals X_t and a database of previously seen data $D_t = \{I_\tau, U_\tau | \tau < t\}$,

$$\mathbb{E}_{I \sim p(I|X)}[I_t|X_t, D_t] \tag{3}$$

From a learning theory perspective, our motivation to replace KDE with a neural network to solve Eq. 3 is guided by the following result from calculus of variations. We can view a neural network as any function f, granted the network is sufficiently powerful. Learning then becomes equivalent to choosing the best function according to the variational problem

$$f^* = \underset{f}{\operatorname{argmin}} \, \mathbb{E}_{I,X \sim p_{data}} \, ||I_t - f(X)||^2, \tag{4}$$

which has a solution at

$$f^*(X) = \mathbb{E}_{I \sim p_{data}(I|X)}[I]. \tag{5}$$

In the hypothetical case where infinitely many samples are available, Eq. 4 implies that the mean squared error loss leads to an optimal estimate of Eq. 3, so long as f^* is part of the class of functions we optimize over. In practice, of course, a limited amount of data is available, and regularization techniques are typically applied. The major difference to non-parametric approaches, including KDE, is that a set of fixed model parameters is obtained. If the number of neurons is treated as a constant, the time complexity of a single prediction equals $O(1)$, while a single prediction using KDE has complexity $\mathcal{O}(Nd)$, where N is the number of OCM training samples in D, and d is their dimensionality.

Inspired by recent work in image captioning and related tasks in video analysis, a long-term recurrent convolutional network (LRCN) [4] architecture is used to learn the mapping $f(\cdot)$ from signals X_t to MR images, $f(X_t) = \mathbf{y}_t$. The network consists of convolutional layers, $\phi_\tau(\cdot)$, followed by recurrent layers $\psi_\upsilon(\cdot)$, $f_{\tau,\upsilon}(X_t) = \psi_\upsilon(\phi_\tau(X_t))$, both with their respective set of parameters (τ, υ). For brevity, we omit these parameters from here on. Figure 2a shows an overall picture of the network. The purpose of the convolutional layers is to extract features over the spatial dimension, s (i.e., columns), from input signals X_t. To this end, 1-d convolutions are applied along s; each output feature map corresponds to one 1-d filter applied along s to all columns of the

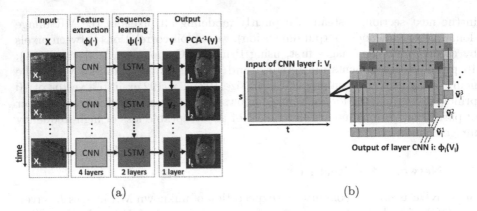

(a)   (b)

Fig. 2. (a) Overview of unrolled long-term recurrent convolutional network (LRCN) structure. 1-d convolutional layers extract image features from the input, and recurrent layers learn the temporal evolution of transformed features, using LSTM units. A densely-connected layer maps to 10 PCA coefficient outputs, y_i used to reconstruct the final image $\hat{I}_t$. (b) Detailed view of a 1-d convolutional layer. Convolutions are applied along the spatial dimension s only, transforming all columns to a vector $\mathbf{v}$. Colors green, blue and yellow represent different feature maps, i.e. learned kernels. A dense output layer transforms the LSTM outputs into a vector of principal components, and the inverse PCA transform (PCA^{-1}) restores the final image.

input. Thus, the output of convolutional layer $\phi_i(\cdot)$ is a set of k_i row vectors $V_i = [\{\tilde{\mathbf{v}}_i^1\}^T, \ldots, \{\tilde{\mathbf{v}}_i^{k_i}\}^T]$ (another image), each row being a convolved version of all columns in V_{i-1} (see Fig. 2b). Down at the last convolutional layer l, $k_l = 1$, so its output $V_i = \{\tilde{\mathbf{v}}_i\}^T$ represents one-dimensional encoding of the signal evolution over the n time steps contained in X_t. It is now the task of the following recurrent layers to learn how this encoding evolves over time. Recurrent layer i transforms its input according to $\psi_i(V_i, h_{t-1})$, where h_{t-1} is its internal state from the previous time step. Through this recurrence, coupled with an internal memory state, recurrent units are able to learn from the arbitrarily distant past, if necessary. Long-short term memory (LSTM) units [11] are used here in all recurrent layers. Finally, a densely-connected output layer at depth L maps V_{L-1} to final outputs $\mathbf{y} = g(WV_{L-1})$, with weight matrix W and linear activation $g(\cdot)$. For all experiments, the network structure was set to 4 convolutional layers with 64, 32, 16 and 1 output channels, respectively, followed by 2 recurrent layers with 10 output channels each. Both convolutional and recurrent units use *tanh* activations. The network architecture is depicted in Fig. 2b. Not shown in the figure are average pooling operations (pool size 2) between all convolutional layers, as well as are dropout layers (rate 0.2) active during training on all convolutional layers.

3   Results and Discussion

Each of the 7 datasets was separated into a training set of 60 s (100 MR images of size 192 × 192 px with 100 corresponding OCM signal histories of 300 × 560 px) and a test set of 30 s (50 MR images with OCM signals). For each subject, a separate LRCN model was trained on the training set and evaluated on the test set. The mean squared error loss function was employed to optimize the 28, 471 trainable parameters of each of the 7 networks, using the Adam optimizer (learning rate 0.001, β_1=0.9, β_2=0.999) over 1000 epochs. Training time was below 5 min per dataset on an NVIDIA Titan X GPU. Code and sample data is available online.[2] Figure 3a compares MRI reconstructions from the test set with their ground-truth. High-speed MRI reconstructions at the rate of OCM signals are best appreciated in video format (see Footnote 2). We used publicly available code and data from [3] for the KDE approach to compare the two methods, as shown by the M-mode image in Fig. 3b. In [3], a CPU reconstruction time of 45 ms per frame for a single plane was reported using KDE, on 2 min of data. Using LRCN on the CPU, with the same hardware used in [3], one reconstruction took only 4 ms, for LRCN forward pass and PCA reconstruction combined. This amounts to a 10-fold speedup compared to KDE. On the GPU (NVIDIA Titan X), an additional factor of two was gained, with a reconstruction time of 2 ms (20 faster than KDE on CPU). Moreover, the reconstruction cost of the proposed LRCN method is constant, while KDE would become even slower with increasing size of the training set. This speedup might enable multi-plane real-time image synthesis in the future. We performed a pixel-wise sum of squared error (SSE) analysis between KDE, LRCN and ground-truth images, to link our LRCN results to the quantitative validation for KDE in [3]. For the dataset presented in Fig. 3(b), the average SSE per image was slightly higher with LRCN, but comparable (39.0 ± 12 for LRCN vs. 33.9 ± 7 for KDE), which can be explained by the loss of information resulting from working in PCA subspace of the original MR images. In conclusion, the intriguing possibility of compressing the imaging capabilities of an MRI machine into small OCM sensors using machine learning could lead to promising image-guided therapy applications, such as real-time motion imaging for radiotherapy and biopsy needle guidance, even outside the MR bore.

---

[2] https://github.com/fpreiswerk/OCM-LRCN.

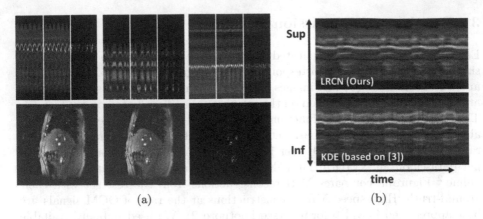

(a)   (b)

Fig. 3. (a) Top row: M-mode display of all 50 test images of subjects 1–3. Reconstruction, ground-truth (in PCA space) and difference images side-by-side. Bottom row: Random image from subject 1 from test set, ground-truth (in PCA space) and difference image. (b) Comparison of LRCN vs. KDE approach [3], where an average error of 1 pixel was reported through manual validation by a radiologist. LRCN-based reconstructions are smoother but comparable.

Acknowledgement. Support from grants NIH P41EB015898, R03EB025546, R01CA149342, and R21EB019500 is duly acknowledged. GPU hardware was generously donated by NVIDIA Corporation.

References

1. Petrusca, L., et al.: Hybrid ultrasound/magnetic resonance simultaneous acquisition and image fusion for motion monitoring in the upper abdomen. Investig. Radiol. **48**(5), 333–340 (2013)
2. Feinberg, D.A., Giese, D., Bongers, D.A., Ramanna, S., Zaitsev, M., Markl, M., Günther, M.: Hybrid ultrasound MRI for improved cardiac imaging and real-time respiration control. Magn. Reson. Med. **63**(2), 290–296 (2010)
3. Preiswerk, F., et al.: Hybrid MRI-ultrasound acquisitions, and scannerless real-time imaging. Magn. Reson. Med. (2016)
4. Donahue, J., et al.: Long-term recurrent convolutional networks for visual recognition and description. CoRR abs/1411.4389 (2014)
5. Schwartz, B.M., McDannold, N.J.: Ultrasound echoes as biometric navigators. Magn. Reson. Med. **69**(4), 1023–1033 (2013)
6. Nadaraya, E.A.: On estimating regression. Theory Probab. & Its Appl. **9**(1), 141–142 (1964)
7. Watson, G.S.: Smooth regression analysis. Sankhyā: Indian J. Stat., Ser. A **26**, 359–372 (1964)
8. Preiswerk, F., et al.: Hybrid Utrasound and MRI Acquisitions for High-Speed Imaging of Respiratory Organ Motion. In: Navab, Nassir, Hornegger, Joachim, Wells, William M., Frangi, Alejandro F. (eds.) MICCAI 2015. LNCS, vol. 9349, pp. 315–322. Springer, Cham (2015). https://doi.org/10.1007/978-3-319-24553-9_39

9. LeCun, Y., Bengio, Y., Hinton, G.: Deep learning. Nature **521**(7553), 436–444 (2015)
10. LeCun, Y., Bottou, L., Bengio, Y., Haffner, P.: Gradient-based learning applied to document recognition. Proc. IEEE **86**(11), 2278–2324 (1998)
11. Hochreiter, S., Schmidhuber, J.: Long short-term memory. Neural Comput. **9**(8), 1735–1780 (1997)

Automatically Designing CNN Architectures for Medical Image Segmentation

Aliasghar Mortazi$^{(\boxtimes)}$ and Ulas Bagci

Center for Research in Computer Vision (CRCV), University of Central Florida,
Orlando, FL, USA
a.mortazi@knights.ucf.edu, ulasbagci@gmail.com

Abstract. Deep neural network architectures have traditionally been designed and explored with human expertise in a long-lasting trial-and-error process. This process requires huge amount of time, expertise, and resources. To address this tedious problem, we propose a novel algorithm to optimally find hyperparameters of a deep network architecture automatically. We specifically focus on designing neural architectures for medical image segmentation task. Our proposed method is based on a policy gradient reinforcement learning for which the reward function is assigned a segmentation evaluation utility (i.e., dice index). We show the efficacy of the proposed method with its low computational cost in comparison with the state-of-the-art medical image segmentation networks. We also present a new architecture design, *a densely connected encoder-decoder CNN*, as a strong baseline architecture to apply the proposed hyperparameter search algorithm. We apply the proposed algorithm to each layer of the baseline architectures. As an application, we train the proposed system on cine cardiac MR images from Automated Cardiac Diagnosis Challenge (ACDC) MICCAI 2017. Starting from a baseline segmentation architecture, the resulting network architecture obtains the state-of-the-art results in accuracy without performing any trial-and-error based architecture design approaches or close supervision of the hyperparameters changes.

Keywords: Policy gradient · Reinforcement learning · *DenseCNN*
Cardiac MRI segmentation

1 Introduction

Deep learning based segmentation algorithms play a key role in medical applications [1–3]. However, designing highly accurate and efficient deep segmentation networks is not trivial. It is because manual exploration of high-performance deep networks requires extensive research by close supervision of human expert (from several months to several years) and huge amount of time and resources due to training time of networks. Considering that the choice of architecture

© Springer Nature Switzerland AG 2018
Y. Shi et al. (Eds.): MLMI 2018, LNCS 11046, pp. 98–106, 2018.
https://doi.org/10.1007/978-3-030-00919-9_12

and hyperparameters affects the segmentation results, it is extremely important to select the optimal hyperparameters. In this study, we address this pressing problem by developing a proof of concept optimization algorithm for network architecture design, specifically for medical image segmentation problems.

Our proposed method is generic and can be applied to any medical image segmentation task. As a proof concept study, we demonstrate its efficacy by automatically segmenting heart structures from cardiac magnetic resonance imaging (MRI) scans. Our motivation comes from the fact cardiac MRI plays a significant role in quantification of cardiovascular diseases (CVDs) such that radiologists need to measure the volume of heart and its substructures in association with the cardiac function. This requires a precise segmentation algorithm available in the radiology rooms.

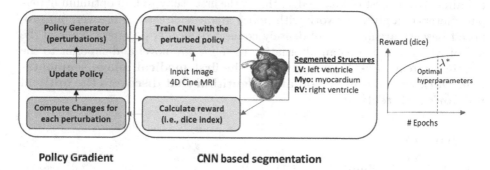

Fig. 1. Overview of proposed method. First, the policy is initialized randomly and then P perturbation are generated. The network is trained with each perturbation and reward from each perturbation is calculated. The policy will be updated accordingly and the process will be repeated until no significant changes in the reward. Reward is simply set as dice coefficient for evaluating how good the segmentation is.

In recent years, the CNN based deep learning algorithms become the natural choice for medical image segmentation tasks. However, the state-of-the-art CNN-based segmentation methods have very similar fixed network architectures and they all have been designed with a trial-and-error basis. SegNet [2], Cardiac-Net [3], and U-Net [1] are some of the notable approaches from the literature. To design such networks, experts have often large number of choices involved in design decisions, and manual search process is significantly guided by intuition. To address this issue, there is a considerable interest recently for designing the network architecture automatically. Reinforcement Learning (RL) [4] and evolutionary based algorithms [5] are proposed to search the optimum network hyperparameters. Such methods are computationally expensive and require a large number of processors (as low as 800 GPUs in Google's network search algorithm [4]) and may not be doable for a widespread and more general use. Instead, in this paper, **we propose a very efficient search algorithm for network optimization based on a policy gradient (PG) algorithm.** PG is one of the successful algorithms in robotics field [6] for learning system design parameters. Another example is by Zoph and Le [4] where authors used LSTM (long short term memory) to learn the hyperparameters of the CNN and the PG was used to learn the parameters of the LSTM. Learning parameters of LSTM need considerable amount of resources as it is discussed in [4]. Unlike that indirect parameter estimation, in this paper we propose a PG algorithm to directly learn network hyperparameters. Our proposed approach is inspired by [6] and it has been adapted to deep network architecture design for performing image segmentation tasks with high accuracy. In this study, to make the whole system economical to implement for wide range of applications, search space is significantly restricted.

The overview of the proposed method is illustrated in Fig. 1. The hyperparameters of the network are considered as policies to be learned during PG training. To our best of knowledge, this is the first study to find optimum hyperparameters of a given network with policy gradient directly. Moreover, our proposed baseline architecture of densely connected encoder-decoder CNN and the use of *Swish* function as an alternative to *ReLU* are novel and superior to the existing systems. **Lastly, our study is the first medical image segmentation work with a fully automated algorithm that discovers the optimal network architecture.**

2   Methods

2.1   Policy Gradient

Policy gradient is a class of reinforcement learning (RL) algorithms and relied on optimization of parametrized policies with respect to a expected return (reward) [7]. Unlike other RL methods (such as Q-Learning), the PG learns the policy function directly to maximize receiving rewards. In our setting, we consider each hyperparameter of the network as a policy, which can be learned during network training. Assume that we have a policy $\pi_0 = \{\theta_1, \theta_2, \ldots, \theta_N\}$, indicating the hyperparameters of the network, where N is the number of hyperparameters (dimensions). Our objective is to learn these hyperparameters (i.e., policies) by maximizing a receiving reward. In segmentation task, this reward can be anything measuring the goodness of segmentations such as dice index and Hausdorff distances. Once we randomly initialize hyperparameters, we generate new policies by randomly perturbing the policies in each dimension. Note that each dimension represents an exploration space for hyperparameters such as filter width, height, and etc. Let $P(\pi_0) = \{\pi_1, \pi_2, \ldots, \pi_p\}$ be p random perturbation generated near π_0, represented as $\pi_i = \pi_0 + \Delta_i$ for $i \in \{1, 2, \ldots, p\}$. For each random perturbation, $\Delta_i = \{\delta^1, \delta^2, \ldots, \delta^N\}$, we assume that δ^d is randomly chosen from $\{-\epsilon^d, 0, +\epsilon^d\}$ for every $d \in \{1, 2, \ldots, N\}$ where epsilon is derivative of a function $\mathbf{y}$ with respect to $\mathbf{x}$ (Later we will define $\mathbf{x}$ and $\mathbf{y}$ for each dimension in Sect. 2.3).

The network is trained with these p generated policies, and reward (segmentation outcome) is obtained for each policy. Finally, the maximal reward (i.e., highest dice coefficient) is determined to set the optimal network architecture hyperparameters accordingly. To estimate the partial derivative of the policy function for each dimension, each perturbation is grouped to non-overlapping categories of negative perturbation, zero perturbation, and positive perturbation: C_-^d, C_0^d, and C_+^d such that $\pi_i^d \in \{C_-^d, C_0^d, C_+^d\}$. The perturbations are generated to make sure each category has approximately $p/3$ members. Then, the absolute reward for each category is calculated as a mean of all the rewards $Ave^d = \{Ave_-^d, Ave_0^d, Ave_+^d\}$ for each dimension d. Based on this average reward, the initial policy is updated accordingly:

$$\pi_{0,new}^d = \begin{cases} \pi_0^d - \epsilon^d \text{ if } & Ave_-^d > Ave_0^d \text{ and } & Ave_-^d > Ave_+^d \\ \pi_0^d + 0 \text{ if } & Ave_0^d \geq Ave_-^d \text{ and } & Ave_0^d \geq Ave_+^d \\ \pi_0^d + \epsilon^d \text{ if } & Ave_+^d > Ave_0^d \text{ and } & Ave_+^d > Ave_-^d \end{cases} \tag{1}$$

The pseudo-code for policy gradient is given in Algorithm 1.

Algorithm 1 Policy Gradient's algorithm

1: Initialize π_0 randomly
2: **for** e=1:epochs **do**
3:     Generate p randomly perturbation of $P(\pi_0) = \{\pi_1, \pi_2, \ldots, \pi_p\}$
4:     **for** i=1:p **do**
5:         Train network with policy π_i
6:         Calculate reward
7:     **for** d=1:N **do**
8:         $Ave_+^d \leftarrow Average$ rewards for C_+^d
9:         $Ave_0^d \leftarrow Average$ rewards for C_0^d
10:        $Ave_-^d \leftarrow Average$ rewards for C_-^d
11:        **Update** $\pi_{0,new}^d$ based on Equation 1.

2.2 Proposed Base-Architecture for Image Segmentation

As it has been shown in [2,3], the encoder-decoder architecture is well design deep learning architecture for the segmentation tasks. More recently, the densely connected CNN [8] has been shown that connecting different layers lead into more accurate results for detection problem. Based on this recent evidence, a densely connected encoder-decoder is proposed herein as a new CNN architecture and we use this as our baseline architecture to optimize. The proposed baseline architecture is illustrated in Fig. 2. Dense blocks consist of four layers, each layer includes convolution operation following by batch normalization operation (BN) and *Swish* activation function [9] (unlike commonly used ReLU). Also, a concatenation operation is conducted for combining the feature maps (through direction (axis) of the channels) for the last three layers. In other words, if the input to l^{th} layer is $\mathbf{X}_l$, then the output of lth layer can be represented as:

$$F(\mathbf{X}_l) = Conv(BN(Swish(\mathbf{X}_l))), \tag{2}$$

where $Swish(x) = xSigmoid(\beta x)$ and as it is discussed in [9], the **Swish** was shown to be more powerful than ReLu since parameter β can be learned during training to control the interpolation between linear function ($\beta = 0$) and ReLu function ($\beta \approx \infty$). Since we are doing concatenation before each layer (except the first one), so the output of each layer can be calculated only by considering the input and output of first layer as:

$$F(\mathbf{X}_l) = F(\overset{l'=l-1}{\underset{l'=0}{\|}} F(\mathbf{X}_{l'})) \quad for \quad l \geq 1 \quad and \quad l = \{1, 2, \ldots, L\}, \quad (3)$$

where $\|$ is the concatenation operation. For initialization $F(\mathbf{X}_{-1})$ and $F(\mathbf{X}_0)$ are considered as ϕ and $\mathbf{X}_1$, respectively, which ϕ is an empty set and there are L layers inside each block.

The decoder part of the CNN consists of three dense blocks and two transition layers. The decoder transition layers can be *average pooling* or *max pooling* and decrease the size of the image by half. In the encoder part, we have same architecture as decoder part except that the transition layers are bilinear interpolation (i.e., unpooling). Each of the decoder transition doubles the size of the feature maps and at the end of this part, we obtain features maps as the same size as input images. Finally, the output of the decoder is passed through a convolution and softmax to produce the probability map. *Adam optimizer* with a learning rate of 0.0001 is selected for training and *Cross Entropy* is used as a loss function. The other hyperparameters of network such as number of filters, filter heights, and widths for each layer are discussed in next section.

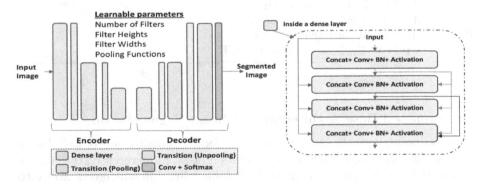

Fig. 2. Details of the baseline architecture. We combine encoder-decoder based segmentation network with densely connected architecture as a novel segmentation network, which has less parameters to tune and more accurate. Concat: concatenation, BN: batch normalization, and conv: convolution.

2.3   Learnable Hyperparameters

Following hyperparameters are learned automatically with our proposed architecture search algorithm: number of filters, filter height, and filter width for each layer. Additionally, type of pooling layer was considered as learnable hyperparameters in our setting. Totally, there are 76 parameters (N) to be learned: 3 parameters (filter size, height, and weight) for each of 25 layers (last layer has fixed number of filters), and 2 additional hyperparameters (average or max pooling) for down-sampling layers. More specifically:

- **Number of filters:** The number of filters (NF) for each layer is chosen from function $y_{NF} = 16x_{NF} + 16$ which $x_{NF} = \{1, 2, \ldots, 12\}$.
- **Filter height:** The filter height (FH) for each layer is chosen from function $y_{FH} = 2x_{FH} + 1$ which $x_{FH} = \{0, 1, \ldots, 5\}$.
- **Filter width:** The filter width (FW) for each layer is chosen from function $y_{FW} = 2x_{FW} + 1$ which $x_{FW} = \{0, 1, \ldots, 5\}$.
- **Pooling functions:** The pooling layer is chosen from function $y_{poolimg} = x_{pooling}$ which $x_{pooling} = \{0, 1\}$ which '0' represents max pooling and '1' represents average pooling.

The number of generated perturbation p is considered as 42 (experimentally) and in order to decrease the computational cost, each network is trained for 50 epochs, which is adequate to determine a stable reward for the network. The average of dice index for the last 5 epochs on the held-out validation set is considered as reward for the reinforcement learning.

3   Experiments and Results

Dataset: We used Automatic Cardiac Diagnosis Challenge (ACDC-MICCAI Workshop 2017) data set for evaluation of the proposed system. This dataset is composed of 150 cine-MR images including 30 normal cases, 30 patients with myocardium infarction, 30 patients with dilated cardiomyopathy, 30 patients with hypertrophic cardiomyopathy, and 30 patients with abnormal right ventricle (RV). While 100 cine-MR images were used for training, the remaining 50 images were used for testing. We have applied data augmentation methods, as described in Table 1, prior to training. The MR images were obtained using two MRI scanners of different magnetic strengths (1.5T and 3.0T). Cine MR images were acquired in breath hold (and gating) with a SSFP sequence in short axis. A series of short axis slices cover the LV from the base to the apex, with a thickness of 5 mm (or sometimes 8 mm) and sometimes an inter-slice gap of 5 mm. The spatial resolution goes from 1.37 to 1.68 mm^2/pixel and 28 to 40 volumes cover completely or partially the cardiac cycle.

Implementation details: We calculated dice index (DI) and Hausdorff distance (HD) to evaluate segmentation accuracy (blind evaluation through challenge web page on the test data). The quantitative results for LV (left ventricle), RV, and Myo (myocardium) as well as mean accuracy (Ave.) are shown in Table 2. Twenty images were randomly selected out of the 100 training images as validation set. After finding optimized hyperparameters, the network with

Table 1. Data augmentation.

Data augmentation	
Methods	Parameters
Rotation	$k \times 45, k\,\varepsilon[-1,1]$
Scale	$\varepsilon[1.3, 1.5]$
Training images	
# of images	Image size
8470	200×200

learned hyperparameters was trained fully with the augmented data. The augmentation was done with in-plane rotation and scaling (Table 1). The number of images increased by factor of five after augmentation.

Post-processing: To have a fair comparison with other segmentation methods, which often use post-processing for improving their segmentation results, we also applied post-processing to refine (improve) the overall segmentation results of all compared methods. We presented our results with and without post-processing in Table 2. Briefly, a 3D fully connected Conditional Random Field (CRF) method was used to refine the segmentation results, taking only a few additional milliseconds. The output probability map of the CNN is used as unary potential and a Gaussian function was used as pairwise potential. Finally, a connected component analysis was applied for further removal of isolated points.

Comparison to other methods: The performances of the proposed segmentation algorithm in comparison with state-of-the-art methods are summarized in Table 2. The *DenseCNN* (with *ReLu* and with *Swish*) is the densely connected encoder-decoder CNN designed by experts, and its use in segmentation tasks recently appeared in some few applications, but never used for cardiac segmentation before. Filter sizes were all set to 3×3 in *DenseCNN* and growth rates were considered as 32, 64, 128, 128, 64, and 32 for each block from beginning to the end of the network, respectively. Also, the average pooling is chosen as the pooling layer. These values were all found after trial-error and empirical experiences, guided by expert opinions as dominant in this field. The 2D U-Net, as one of the state of the arts, is the original implementation of the U-Net architecture proposed by Ronneberger et al. in [1] was used for comparison too. Although we apply our algorithm into 2D setting for efficiency purpose, one can apply it to 3D architectures once memory and other hardware constraints are solved. The details of the learned architecture with the proposed method is shown in Fig. 3.

We obtained the final architecture design in 10 days of continuous training of a workstation with 15 GPUs (Titan X). Unlike the common CNN architecture designs (expert approach), which requires months or even years of trial-and-error and experience guided search, the proposed search algorithm found optimal (or near-optimal) segmentation results compared to the state of the art segmentation architectures within days.

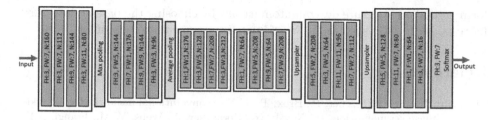

Fig. 3. Details of the optimally learned architecture by the proposed method. Note that connections among layers inside of each block are same as dense layers.

Table 2. DI and HD for all methods and substructures.

Methods		2D-UNET	DenseCNN (ReLU)	DenseCNN	Proposed	Proposed+CRF
DI	LV	0.904	0.913	0.922	0.921	**0.928**
	RV	0.868	0.826	0.834	0.857	**0.868**
	MYO	0.847	0.832	0.845	0.838	**0.849**
	Ave.	0.873	0.857	0.867	0.872	**0.882**
HD (mm)	LV	9.670	9.15	8.937	8.99	**8.90**
	RV	14.37	16.35	16.31	14.27	**14.13**
	MYO	12.13	11.32	11.28	10.70	**10.66**
	Ave.	12.06	12.27	13.02	11.32	**11.23**

4   Discussions and Conclusion

We proposed a new deep network architecture to automatically segment cardiac cine MR images. Our architecture design was fully automatic and based on policy gradient reinforcement learning. After baseline network was structured based on densely connected encoder-decoder network, the policy gradient algorithm automatically searched the hyperparameters of this network, achieving the state of the art results. **Note that our hypothesis was to show that it was possible to design CNN automatically for medical image segmentation with similar or better performance in accuracy, and much better in efficiency. It is because expert-design networks require extensive trial-and-error experiments and may take even years to design.** Our study has opened a new venue for designing a segmentation engine within a short period of time. Our study has some limitations due to its proof of concept nature. One interesting way to extend the proposed model will be to learn hyperparameters conditionally in each layer (unlike independent assumption of the layers). With the availability of more hardware sources, one may explore many more hyperparameters, such as ability to put more layers than basic model, defining skip-connections, and exploring different activation functions instead of ReLU and other default ones. One may also avoid increasing search space and still perform a good architecture design automatically by choosing the base-architecture more powerful ones such as the **SegCaps** (i.e., segmentation capsules) [10].

References

1. Ronneberger, O., Fischer, P., Brox, T.: U-Net: convolutional networks for biomedical image segmentation. In: Navab, N., Hornegger, J., Wells, W.M., Frangi, A.F. (eds.) MICCAI 2015. LNCS, vol. 9351, pp. 234–241. Springer, Cham (2015). https://doi.org/10.1007/978-3-319-24574-4_28
2. Badrinarayanan, V., Kendall, A., Cipolla, R.: Segnet: a deep convolutional encoder-decoder architecture for image segmentation, arXiv preprint arXiv:1511.00561 (2015)
3. Mortazi, A., Karim, R., Rhode, K., Burt, J., Bagci, U.: *CardiacNET*: segmentation of left atrium and proximal pulmonary veins from MRI using multi-view CNN. In: Descoteaux, M., Maier-Hein, L., Franz, A., Jannin, P., Collins, D.L., Duchesne, S. (eds.) MICCAI 2017. LNCS, vol. 10434, pp. 377–385. Springer, Cham (2017). https://doi.org/10.1007/978-3-319-66185-8_43
4. Zoph, B., Le, Quoc V.: Neural architecture search with reinforcement learning, arXiv preprint arXiv:1611.01578 (2016)
5. Stanley, K.O., D'Ambrosio, D.B., Gauci, J.: A hypercube-based encoding for evolving large-scale neural networks. Artif. Life **15**(2), 185–212 (2009)
6. Kohl, N., Stone, P.: Policy gradient reinforcement learning for fast quadrupedal locomotion, In: 2004 IEEE International Conference on Robotics and Automation, Proceedings. ICRA 2004, vol. 3. IEEE (2004)
7. Sutton, R.S., McAllester, D.A., Singh, S.P., Mansour, Y.: Policy gradient methods for reinforcement learning with function approximation. Adv. Neural Inf. Process. Syst. 1057–1063 (2000)
8. Huang, G., Liu, Z., Weinberger, K.Q., van der Maaten, L.: Densely connected convolutional networks, arXiv preprint arXiv:1608.06993
9. Ramachandran, P., Zoph, B., Le, Q.V.: Searching for activation functions (2017)
10. LaLonde, R., Bagci, U.: Capsules for object segmentation, arXiv preprint arXiv:1804.04241 (2018)

Rotation Invariance and Directional Sensitivity: Spherical Harmonics versus Radiomics Features

Adrien Depeursinge[1,2(✉)], Julien Fageot[1], Vincent Andrearczyk[2], John Paul Ward[3], and Michael Unser[1]

[1] Biomedical Imaging Group, Ecole Polytechnique Fédérale de Lausanne (EPFL), Lausanne, Switzerland
[2] Institute of Information Systems, University of Applied Sciences Western Switzerland (HES-SO), Sierre, Switzerland
adrien.depeursinge@hevs.ch
[3] Department of Mathematics, North Carolina A&T State University, Greensboro, NC, USA

Abstract. We define and investigate the Local Rotation Invariance (LRI) and Directional Sensitivity (DS) of radiomics features. Most of the classical features cannot combine the two properties, which are antagonist in simple designs. We propose texture operators based on spherical harmonic wavelets (SHW) invariants and show that they are both LRI and DS. An experimental comparison of SHW and popular radiomics operators for classifying 3D textures reveals the importance of combining the two properties for optimal pattern characterization.

Keywords: Radiomics · 3D texture · Spherical harmonics · Wavelets

1 Introduction

Radiomics aims at establishing potential links between radiological image content and disease phenotypes [1]. Its potential for personalized medicine is enormous, thanks to the ability to accurately identify disease subtypes and responders to therapy in a noninvasive fashion. Its success fully relies on the relevance of extracted quantitative image measures for characterizing the manifestation of disease under the form of local tissue alterations (i.e. 3D texture) observed in Computed Tomography (CT), Magnetic Resonance Imaging (MRI) and Positron Emission Tomography (PET). The tissue alterations can be diverse, including necrosis, angiogenesis, fibrosis, cell proliferation (e.g. densification and higher metabolism) [2]. The latter induce corresponding imaging signatures in terms of 3D low-level patterns (e.g. blobs, intersecting surfaces and curves, Fig. 1). Such patterns are characterized by discriminative directional properties and have arbitrary 3D orientations. As a consequence, optimal radiomics image operators must combine Local Rotation Invariance (LRI) with Directional Sensitivity (DS) [3].

© Springer Nature Switzerland AG 2018
Y. Shi et al. (Eds.): MLMI 2018, LNCS 11046, pp. 107–115, 2018.
https://doi.org/10.1007/978-3-030-00919-9_13

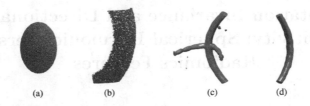

(a)   (b)   (c)   (d)

Fig. 1. 3D low-level patterns associated with biomedical tissue architectures. The latter include ellipsoid blobs (a), tumor or organ walls (b), and diverse vascular configurations (c), (d). These patterns can have arbitrary orientations in 3D medical images.

In this paper, we first formally define the notion of LRI and discuss how it relates to the DS of operators. We then propose a novel texture operator based on Spherical Harmonic Wavelet (SHW) invariants that can combine the two properties. Second, we qualitatively compare SHW invariants with classic 3D radiomics features in terms of LRI and DS. Finally, we evaluate experimentally the importance of the latter properties for 3D texture classification.

2   Materials and Methods

2.1   Notations

Vectors are written with bold symbols. The Fourier transform of an integrable function $f : \mathbb{R}^3 \to \mathbb{R}$ is $\widehat{f}(\boldsymbol{\omega}) = \int_{\mathbb{R}^3} f(\boldsymbol{x}) e^{j\boldsymbol{\omega}^T \boldsymbol{x}} d\boldsymbol{x}$. It is naturally extended to any square-integrable function in the usual manner. We use spherical coordinates (r, θ, ϕ) in Fourier domain, with radial distance $r \geq 0$, polar angle $\phi \in [0, 2\pi)$, and azimuthal angle $\theta \in [0, \pi)$.

2.2   Local Rotation Invariance and Directional Sensitivity

We follow the framework introduced in [3], where it is proposed that any texture analysis approach can be decomposed into (i) the application of a *texture operator* $\mathcal{G}$ associating to an image $f(\boldsymbol{x})$ a *response map* $h(\boldsymbol{x}) = \mathcal{G}\{f\}(\boldsymbol{x})$ and (ii) the aggregation of the response map information, transforming $h(\boldsymbol{x})$ into a scalar measurement through the use of an *aggregation function*[1] on a Volume Of Interest (VOI). This approach allows focusing on the properties of the texture operator in terms of LRI and DS, which we define as follows.

Definition 1. *A texture operator $\mathcal{G}$ is Locally Rotation Invariant (LRI) if the response map at $\boldsymbol{x}_0$ is not affected by the rotation of the input image around $\boldsymbol{x}_0$. In other terms, if, for any rotation operator $\mathcal{R}$, any $\boldsymbol{x}_0 \in \mathbb{R}^3$, and any input image $f \in L_2(\mathbb{R}^3)$, we have*

$$\mathcal{G}\{f\}(\boldsymbol{x}_0) = \mathcal{G}\{\mathcal{R}_{\boldsymbol{x}_0} f\}(\boldsymbol{x}_0), \tag{1}$$

---

[1] It is worth noting that steps (i) and (ii) are repeated multiple times in Convolutional Neural Networks (CNN).

where $\mathcal{R}_{\boldsymbol{x}_0}$ is a translated version of the rotation operator $\mathcal{R}$ that is centered around $\boldsymbol{x}_0$ instead of the origin $\boldsymbol{0}$ as $\mathcal{R}_{\boldsymbol{x}_0} = \mathcal{T}_{\boldsymbol{x}_0}\mathcal{R}\mathcal{T}_{-\boldsymbol{x}_0}$, with $\mathcal{T}_{\boldsymbol{x}_0}$ is a translation operator by $\boldsymbol{x}_0$.

The LRI is highly desirable for texture analysis, but is antagonist with the will of being sensitive to directional features to avoid mixing blobs, edges and ridges. For instance, it can be shown that a convolutional texture operator of the form $\mathcal{G}\{f\} = g * f$ is LRI if and only if the filter g is isotropic, therefore insensitive to the directional features of the input signal f. It follows that operators combining LRI and DS require using more complex designs such as SHW invariants presented in the next section.

2.3 Spherical Harmonic Wavelets

We design operators combining LRI and DS based on SHW. We use wavelets to characterize the local image information at different scales. The wavelet decomposition is computed efficiently due to the filterbank structure [4]. In what follows, we denote by $\widehat{g}(r)$ the 3-dimensional isotropic wavelet of interest, that only depends on the radius r. In practice, we use the Meyer wavelet [4] known for its good localization in space and frequency. The scale index is $i \in \mathbb{Z}$ and we set $\widehat{g}_i(r) = 2^{2i/3}\widehat{g}(2^i r)$ the wavelet at different scale (the normalization is chosen so that each g_i has norm 1). In what follows, $\mathcal{I} = \{i_{\min}, \dots, i_{\max}\}$ always refer to a finite subset of $\mathbb{Z}$.

The directional information is taken into account using spherical harmonics. The family of spherical harmonics is denoted by $(Y_n^m)_{n \geq 0, m \in \{-n,\dots,n\}}$, where n is called the degree and m the order of Y_n^m. Spherical harmonics form an orthonormal basis for square-integrable functions in the $2D$-sphere $\mathbb{S}^2$. They are defined as [5]

$$Y_n^m(\theta, \phi) = A_n^m P_n^{|m|}(\cos(\theta))e^{jm\phi}, \tag{2}$$

with $A_n^m = (-1)^{(m+|m|)/2}\left(\frac{2n+1}{4\pi}\frac{(n-|m|)!}{(n+|m|)!}\right)^{1/2}$ a normalization constant and $P_n^{|m|}$ the associated Legendre polynomial given for $0 \leq m \leq n$ by [6]

$$P_n^m(x) := \frac{(-1)^m}{2^n n!}(1-x^2)^{m/2}\frac{\mathrm{d}^{n+m}}{\mathrm{d}x^{n+m}}(x^2-1)^n. \tag{3}$$

We consider finitely many degrees, $N \geq 0$ being the maximal degree. In particular, we have $\sum_{n=0}^{N}(2n+1) = (N+1)^2$ harmonics of degree up to N. Note that one can recover any angular pattern when $N \to \infty$. We then combine isotropic wavelets and spherical harmonics to consider filters of the form $(r, \theta, \phi) \mapsto \widehat{g}_i(r)Y_n^m(\theta, \phi)$ in Fourier domain.

SHW Invariants to Local Rotations. Fix an image f. For the scale $i \in \mathcal{I}$, the degree $n \in \{0, \dots, N\}$, and the order $m \in \{-n, \dots, n\}$, we set the texture measurement scalar $c_{i,n,m}(f) := \langle \widehat{f}, \widehat{g}_i Y_n^m \rangle$ and vector $\boldsymbol{c}_{i,n}(f) = (c_{i,n,m})_{|m| \leq n}$. Here, $\boldsymbol{c}_{i,n}(f)$ contains the spectral information for the degree n, once we have projected the $3D$ image on the sphere using the isotropic wavelet $\widehat{g}$ at scale i. We set

$$\alpha_{i,n}(f) = \frac{\|c_{i,n}(f)\|_2^2}{2n+1} = \frac{1}{2n+1} \sum_{-n \le m \le n} |c_{i,n,m}|^2, \tag{4}$$

that represents the spherical energy of the image, centered around $\mathbf{0}$, and averaged on the $(2n+1)$ components of $\mathbf{c}_{i,n}$, for the degree n and at scale i. The quantities (4) represent the directional information of the image of interest f at the location $\mathbf{x}_0 = \mathbf{0}$. The texture operators are defined by sliding the image to different center $\mathbf{x}_0 \in \mathbb{R}^3$. For $i \in \mathcal{I}$ and $n \le N$, we set

$$h_{i,n}(\mathbf{x}_0) = \mathcal{G}_{i,n}\{f\}(\mathbf{x}_0) = (\alpha_{i,n}(f(\cdot - \mathbf{x}_0)))^{1/2}. \tag{5}$$

Here, $h_{i,n}$ is a new image (i.e. response map) that can be interpreted as follows. It extracts the energy contained in the spatial and spherical frequencies corresponding to the degree n, at scale i, for the image f centered around the location $\mathbf{x}_0$. Then, $\mathcal{G}_{i,n}$ is a texture operator in the sense of [3].

Proposition 1. *The texture operators $\mathcal{G}_{i,n}$ are LRI in the sense of Definition 1.*

Proof. We show (1) for $\mathbf{x}_0 = \mathbf{0}$. It is then easily extended by exploiting that $\mathcal{R}_{\mathbf{x}_0} = \mathcal{T}_{\mathbf{x}_0} \mathcal{R} \mathcal{T}_{-\mathbf{x}_0}$. The rotated spherical harmonic $\mathcal{R}Y_n^m$ is in the span of the spherical harmonics of same degree $Y_n^{m'}$; that is, $\mathcal{R}Y_n^m = \sum_{m'=-n}^{n} s_{n,\mathcal{R}}[m,m']Y_n^{m'}$. Because rotations are isometric operators, we have that

$$1 = \|Y_n^m\|_{L_2} = \|\mathcal{R}Y_n^m\|_{L_2} = \left\| \sum_{m'=-n\ldots n} s_{n,\mathcal{R}}[m,m']Y_n^{m'} \right\|_{L_2} = \|s_{n,\mathcal{R}}[m,\cdot]\|_2. \tag{6}$$

Moreover, $\mathcal{R}Y_n^m$ and $\mathcal{R}Y_n^{m'}$ are orthogonal as soon as $m \ne m'$, implying that $\langle s_{n,\mathcal{R}}[m,\cdot], s_{n,\mathcal{R}}[m',\cdot] \rangle = 0$ for $m \ne m'$. In other terms, $S_{n,\mathcal{R}} = (s_{n,\mathcal{R}}[m,m'])_{m,m'}$ is a matrix preserving the Euclidean norm.[2] We then have, using that the rotations commute with the Fourier transform and expanding $\mathcal{R}^*Y_n^m$ where $\mathcal{R}^*$ is the adjoint rotation of $\mathcal{R}$,

$$c_{i,n}(\mathcal{R}f) = \left(\langle \mathcal{R}\widehat{f}, \widehat{g}_i Y_n^m \rangle \right)_m = \left(\langle \widehat{f}, \widehat{g}_i \mathcal{R}^* Y_n^m \rangle \right)_m = (S_{n,\mathcal{R}^*} c_{i,n}(f))_m. \tag{7}$$

Finally, since $S_{n,\mathcal{R}^*}$ preserves the Euclidean norm, we deduce that

$$\mathcal{G}_{i,n}\{\mathcal{R}f\}(\mathbf{0}) = \frac{1}{2n+1}\|c_{i,n}(\mathcal{R}f)\|_2^2 = \frac{1}{2n+1}\|S_{n,\mathcal{R}^*} c_{i,n}(f)\|_2^2$$

$$= \frac{1}{2n+1}\|c_{i,n}(f)\|_2^2 = \mathcal{G}_{i,n}\{f\}(\mathbf{0}). \tag{8}$$

---

[2] The matrix $S_{n,\mathcal{R}}$ is called the steering matrix in the literature [7]. We recovered the well-known property that the steering matrix of spherical harmonics is orthogonal.

In summary, $\mathcal{G}_{i,n}$ incorporates directional information by considering different spherical frequencies defined by the degree n, and taking the norm of the vector $c_{i,n}(f)$ allows extracting the spherical frequencies in a rotation invariant fashion. The latter can qualitatively be interpreted as the spherical Fourier modulus computed for a degree n, at a position x_0 and scale i. This is the main advantage of the proposed method.

To obtain a set of scalar texture measurements, we use the average of the image $\mathcal{G}_{i,n}\{f\}$ over a VOI M as an aggregation function $\mu_{i,n}$ in the sense of [3].

3   Results

3.1   LRI and DS of Popular Radiomics Operators

We provide a qualitative comparison of popular radiomics operators[3] in terms of their DS and LRI. This comparison is presented in Table 1 and includes SHW invariants, aligned Riesz wavelets [8], separable Haar wavelets and Coiflets [4], Laplacians of Gaussians (LoG) and the three main approaches based on Gray-Level Matrices (GLM): Gray-Level Co-occurrence Matrices (GLCM) [9], Gray-Level Run-Length Matrices (GLRLM) [10], Gray-Level Size Zone Matrices (GLSZM) [11]. We refer to [3] for detailed descriptions of the texture operators. We observe that only SHW invariants and can combine LRI with DS. Aligned Riesz wavelets can approximately combine the two properties.

3.2   3D Synthetic Texture Classification

We evaluate the importance of radiomics operators combining directional sensitivity and local rotation invariance on the synthetic RFAI database [12]. The texture images resemble medical tissues observed in CT, MRI and PET, including pronounced directional components. The *Fourier* dataset includes 15 classes built from various synthetic power spectrums (see Fig. 2). There are ten $64 \times 64 \times 64$ instances per class, which are built from randomly selected phase values in the Fourier domain. Two test suites are available. The first one, referred to as *Normal* contains the initial 150 instances. A second one, referred to as *Rotate* includes 150 new instances that underwent random 3D rotations of the initial power spectrum. We use linear Support Vector Machines (SVM) in order to classify adequately the 3D textures, where the cost of errors is optimized in $[10^{-4}; 10^6]$. We use a Leave-One-Out (LOO) cross-validation to evaluate the average classification performance in terms of accuracy. For both *Normal* and *Rotate* test suites, only instances from the *Normal* set are used for training the models. Mirror boundary conditions and average energies of the coefficients were used for all convolutional approaches. Specific settings of the feature groups are listed in the following paragraphs.

---

[3] Considered popular operators are those included in radiomics libraries including pyRadiomics, TexRAD, IBEX, CERR, MAZDA, QIFE, LifeX and QuantImage.

Table 1. Qualitative comparison of popular radiomics operators.

	Directional sensitivity	Invariance to local rotations
SHW invariants	Yes, i.e. in terms of spherical frequencies of a given degree n	Yes (via Proposition 1)
Aligned Riesz wavelets [8]	Yes, i.e. in terms of higher order partial image derivatives	Approximately, via the local alignment of the filters based on the structure tensor
Haar wavelets and Coiflets [4]	Yes. The separable filters are directional and aligned with image axes	No, rotations will redistribute energies among the subbands
LoGs	No. The convolutional texture operator $g(\boldsymbol{x}) = g(\|\boldsymbol{x}\|) = g(r)$ is isotropic	Yes (via isotropy)
GLCMs [9]	No. The texture operators become isotropic when averaged over all image directions	Approximately (via discrete isotropy)
GLRLMs [10]	No. The texture operators become isotropic when averaged over all image directions	Approximately (via discrete isotropy)
GLSZMs [11]	No, the texture operator will mix elongated and circular zones	Approximately (via discrete isotropy)

SHW Invariants. One considers the feature vector $\boldsymbol{\mu} = (\mu_{i,n})_{i \in \mathcal{I}, \, 0 \leq n \leq N}$ from the SHW invariants. The number of features is therefore $|\mathcal{I}| \times (N+1)$, the number of scales $|\mathcal{I}|$ being chosen as 4. Concatenated degrees up to $N = 11$ are tested, resulting in feature vectors of dimensionalities from 4 to 48.

Aligned Riesz wavelets. We compute features from aligned 3D Riesz wavelets as developed in [8] and included in the QuantImage platform[4]. The Meyer isotropic wavelet is used with four scales. The variance of the Gaussian window regularizing the structure tensor is fixed to 1. Separated Riesz orders in [0; 4] are tested, resulting in feature vectors of dimensionalities from 4 to 60.

---

[4] https://radiomics.hevs.ch, as of June 2018.

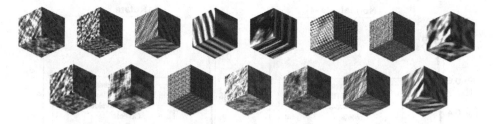

Fig. 2. The 15 classes of the *Fourier* dataset of the RFAI database [12]. Each instance is a 3D image of $64 \times 64 \times 64$ voxels.

Haar wavelets and Coiflets. 3D Separable Haar wavelets and Coiflets [4] are computed using the pyRadiomics toolbox[5] [1]. The pure Lowpass (L) filter is not used, resulting in 7 filters involving the Highpass (H) per scale (i.e. following $x - y - z$ convention: HHH, HLL, LHL, LHH, LLH, HHL, HLH). Coiflets with 1 to 5 Vanishing Moments (VM) were tested, where one VM provided best results. Concatenated scales in [1; 4] are tested, resulting in 7 to 28 features.
Laplacians of Gaussian. 3D LoGs are computed using pyRadiomics [1]. Concatenated variances $\sigma = 1, 1.5, \ldots, 5$ are tested, resulting in 1 to 9 features.
Gray level matrices. GLMs features including GLCMs, GLRLMs and GLSZMs are computed using pyRadiomics [1]. Default values are used. 23 GLCMs features are computed as listed in pyRadiomics' documentation. GLCMs operators with distances in [1; 5] are tested resulting in 23 to 115 features when concatenated. 16 GLRLMs and 16 GLSZMs features are computed using default values.

The classification accuracies with respect to the number of features are reported in Fig. 3 for *Normal* and *Rotate* test suites. SHW invariants provide excellent classification performance for a low number of features (i.e. 16 with $N = 3$). They also showed high generalization abilities with best performance on the *Rotate* dataset. The degradation of classification performance is caused by (i) the use of interpolation for implementing rotations in RFAI and (ii) important boundary effects when using four dyadic wavelet scales on $64 \times 64 \times 64$ images, which are more or less present based on a given rotation. Separable wavelets showed poor generalization on *Rotate*, which is due to their lack of LRI. LoGs, and all GLM designs achieved relatively poor performance on both datasets, which highlights the importance of DS. While LoGs showed excellent generalization on *Rotate*, all GLMs did not perform well on rotated instances. This suggests that approximate LRI via discrete isotropy is not sufficient. Overall, the results strongly support our hypothesis that combining LRI with DS is essential for optimal texture characterization.

We did not included CNNs in the comparison as the number of features largely exceeds the dimensionalities considered here and they require many more

---

[5] https://pyradiomics.readthedocs.io, as of June 2018.

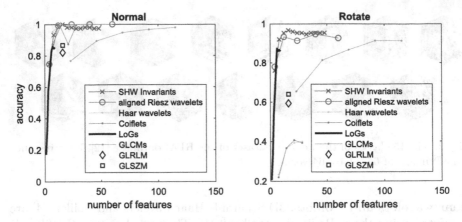

Fig. 3. Classification accuracies with respect to the number of features for both *Normal* and *Rotate* test suites. Chance level accuracy is 0.07.

instances for training. However, it is worth noting that although classical CNNs are DS but not LRI, recent designs such as group equivariant CNNs can approximate LRI [13].

4   Conclusions

We introduced the notions of LRI and DS and their importance for designing optimal radiomics image operators. The difficulty of combining the two properties was highlighted, and we subsequently proposed a simple approach based on SHW invariants to fulfill the two requirements. A qualitative comparison of popular radiomics operators revealed that none of them are able to combine LRI and DS. We demonstrated the importance of these two properties for 3D synthetic texture classification, where the proposed SHW invariants showed improved classification performance on rotated images. We believe that such operators capable of combining LRI and DS will yield optimal performance for radiomics.

Acknowledgments. This work was supported by the Swiss National Science Foundation (grants PZ00P2_154891 and 205320_179069).

References

1. van Griethuysen, J.J.M., et al.: Computational radiomics system to decode the radiographic phenotype. Cancer Res. **77**(21), e104–e107 (2017)
2. Gatenby, R.A., Grove, O., Gillies, R.J.: Quantitative imaging in cancer evolution and ecology. Radiology **269**(1), 8–14 (2013)
3. Depeursinge, A., Al-Kadi, O.S., Mitchell, J.R.: Biomedical Texture Analysis: Fundamentals. Applications and Tools. Elsevier-MICCAI Book series. Academic Press, London (2017)

4. Daubechies, I.: Ten Lectures on Wavelets, vol. 61. SIAM, Philadelphia (1992)
5. Driscoll, J.R., Healy, D.M.: Computing fourier transforms and convolutions on the 2-sphere. Adv. Appl. Math. **15**(2), 202–250 (1994)
6. Abramowitz, M., Stegun, I.: Handbook of Mathematical Functions: with Formulas, Graphs, and Mathematical Tables, vol. 55. Courier Corporation, New York (1964)
7. Ward, J.P., Unser, M.: Harmonic singular integrals and steerable wavelets in $L_2(\mathbb{R}^d)$. Appl. Comput. Harmon. Anal. **36**(2), 183–197 (2014)
8. Dicente Cid, Y., Müller, H., Platon, A., Poletti, P.-A., Depeursinge, A.: 3-D solid texture classification using locally-oriented wavelet transforms. IEEE Trans. Image Process. **26**(4), 1899–1910 (2017)
9. Haralick, R.M.: Statistical and structural approaches to texture. Proc. IEEE **67**(5), 786–804 (1979)
10. Galloway, M.M.: Texture analysis using gray level run lengths. Comput. Graph. Image Process. **4**(2), 172–179 (1975)
11. Thibault, G., et al.: Texture indexes and gray level size zone matrix: application to cell nuclei classification. Pattern Recognit. Inf. Process. 140–145 (2009)
12. Paulhac, L., Makris, P., Ramel, J.-Y.: A solid texture database for segmentation and classification experiments. In: 4th International Conference on Computer Vision Theory and Applications, pp. 135–141 (2009)
13. Andrearczyk, V., Depeursinge, A.: Rotational 3D texture classification using group equivariant CNNs. In submitted to SPIE Medical Imaging (2018)

Can Dilated Convolutions Capture Ultrasound Video Dynamics?

Mohammad Ali Maraci[✉], Weidi Xie, and J. Alison Noble

Department of Engineering Science, University of Oxford, Institute of Biomedical
Engineering, Oxford, UK
mohammad.maraci@eng.ox.ac.uk

Abstract. Automated analysis of free-hand ultrasound video sweeps is
an important topic in diagnostic and interventional imaging, however, it
is a notoriously challenging task for detecting the standard planes, due to
the low-quality data, variability in contrast, appearance and placement
of the structures. Conventionally, sequential data is usually modelled
with heavy Recurrent Neural Networks (RNNs). In this paper, we propose to apply a convolutional architecture (CNNs) for the standard plane
detection in free-hand ultrasound videos. Our contributions are twofolds,
firstly, we show a simple convolutional architecture can be applied to
characterize the long range dependencies in the challenging ultrasound
video sequences, and outperform the canonical LSTMs and the recently
proposed two-stream spatial ConvNet by a large margin (89% versus
83% and 84% respectively). Secondly, to get an understanding of what
evidences have been used by the model for decision making, we experimented with the soft-attention layers for feature pooling, and trained
the entire model end-to-end with only standard classification losses. As
a result, we find the input-dependent attention maps can not only boost
the network's performance, but also indicate useful patterns of the data
that are deemed important for certain structure, therefore provide interpretation while deploying the models.

1 Introduction

In the recent years, breakthroughs of machine learning technique has led significant advances towards analysis and understanding of ultrasound images. Early
related work utilized handcrafted features such as SIFT with Fisher vector encoding to categorize the video frames [1], In [2], sequential Bayesian filtering are
used to predict the visibility, position and orientation of the heart in the video.
In contrast, more recent works [3] have trained the Convolutional Neural Networks (CNNs) to identify the fetal standard scan planes from the 2D ultrasound
data in an end-to-end manner.

Undoubtedly, the CNNs have shown tremendous success on processing 2D
ultrasound images, to further model the sequential data, current image-based
architectures have been extended in three different ways, one is to use a heavy
Recurrent Neural Networks (RNNs) trained with the feature descriptors from a

© Springer Nature Switzerland AG 2018
Y. Shi et al. (Eds.): MLMI 2018, LNCS 11046, pp. 116–124, 2018.
https://doi.org/10.1007/978-3-030-00919-9_14

set of consecutive frames, for instance, in [4], the authors proposed to use a combination of CNNs and RNNs for standard planes detections in fetal ultrasound video, while in [5], the authors focus on the fine-grained analysis of heart, and predict the visibility, viewing plane, location and orientation of the fetal heart; another methods [6] is to apply a two-stream network to capture the spatio-temporal information by incorporating optical flow from the linear sweep fetal ultrasound video, more recent works have tried to apply the 3D convolutional networks, which can ingest and learn both low and high-level representations from the video data directly [7].

Intuitively, taking a set of consecutive frames into account rather than a single frame at any point should always enhance the performance of video analysis. However, there remains a number of considerable challenges for training the aforementioned approaches on freehand ultrasound videos, *firstly*, the amount of annotated medical data is usually limited, to prevent overfitting, strong regularizations or extensive data augmentations are usually required to train heavy models, like 3D CNNs or RNNs, *secondly*, for ultrasound data, due to its visual appearance characteristics, it is difficult to compute the optical flow information.

In contrast, recent research indicates that an alternative, and yet simpler convolutional architecture can reach state-of-the-art accuracy in several sequential modelling tasks, e.g audio synthesis, word-level language modeling, and machine translation [8–10]. This raises the question of whether these successes of convolutional sequence modelling are confined to specific application domains or can we borrow the experience from the success of CNNs.

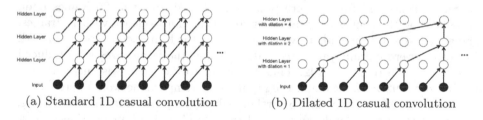

(a) Standard 1D casual convolution   (b) Dilated 1D casual convolution

Fig. 1. Schematic of a stack of standard convolution and the dilated convolution.

In this paper, we proposed to model the challenging ultrasound video data only with convolutional architectures, we explicitly factorize the 3D convolution into two separate and successive operations, namely, 2D spatial convolution and 1D temporal casual convolution. As shown in Fig. 1, we adopt the similar ideas proposed by [8], where 2D CNNs are shared for individual frames and 1D dilated casual convolution for long-range sequence modelling without greatly increasing computational cost, note that, the output from the casual convolution is only conditioned on the past and current time step.

Moreover, it has been shown that focusing on objects of interest rather than the entire image can improve performance in certain applications [11–13], and provide better model interpretation. In this paper, we also try to investigate the efficacy of learning an attention map during training without any additional supervision. The attention module can be seen as a generalization of the widely used global average pooling, where the pooling masks are implicitly inferred based on the input image (instead of averaging).

2 Materials and Methods

2.1 Data and Experimental Setup

The dataset consisted of 353 2D fetal ultrasound videos that were acquired from healthy volunteers by an experienced obstetrician using a Philips HD9 ultrasound machine with a V7-3 transducer, following a predefined free-hand acquisition protocol. Data was acquired while moving the probe from the bottom of the maternal abdomen to the top, thus in each video various parts of the fetal anatomy can be captured. The challenge with this dataset is that there exists a high level of variation and artefacts in the representation of the fetal anatomical parts of interest which are the fetal skull, abdomen and heart.

The duration of videos varied in length and ranged between 240 to 630 total frames. For the frame-wise experiments, all video frames were extracted and labelled manually as abdomen, heart, skull, and background. For the temporal experiments, each video sequence was broken down into smaller sequences of 10 frames long. A sliding window of 2 frames was utilized in this process. For the extended range temporal experiments and to cover longer input sequence, each ultrasound video was initially broken down to 25 frames as opposed to 10. Subsequently, 10 frames were randomly selected from this 25 frames pool, while keeping the frames original order, resulting in a sequence with 10 frames. The ground-truth frame labels were the same as the frame-wise experiment. All the frames were initially pre-processed, such that the frame sizes were reduced from 240×320 to 192×192. Thus the input to the frame-wise network was batch-size $\times 192 \times 192 \times 3$ and the input to the temporal networks were batch-size $\times 10 \times 192 \times 192 \times 3$. To further reduce the probability of over-fitting, training data was randomly augmented through Gaussian-blur, motion-blur, j-peg compression, frame re-sampling, and horizontal flip.

2.2 Network Architecture

In this section, we describe the three different experimented network architectures; (1) the widely used baseline frame-wise classification model, (2) a model composed of CNNs and a uni-directional LSTM model, and (3) a spatio-temporal dilated convolution classification model. For each of these models, we also inserted the attention layers after the last convolutional layer.

Frame-wise Classification Model. Figure 2 shows the architecture of the frame-wise classification model. It is based on the AlexNet architecture, where five convolution (conv) layers are used, with each followed by a batch normalization and ReLU layer. The last conv layer is connected to two fully-connected layers and a linear classifier. After each of the dense fully connected layers of the network, a 60% and 50% dropout was added respectively.

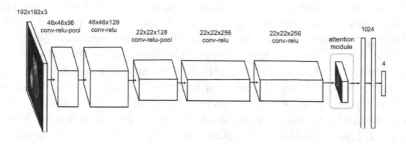

Fig. 2. Frame-wise classification model

Spatio-temporal model based on CNNs and Uni-directional LSTM.
The network architecture is shown in Fig. 3. Overall, it consists of two parts, where the frame-wise information is first extracted and encoded as a single feature vector with 2D CNNs, secondly the feature descriptors from consecutive frames are further fed into unidirectional RNNs (LSTMs). In particular, the input to the model is a short sequence in the form of b × n × w × h × c, where b is the mini-batch size, n is the number of frames in the sequence, and w, h, and c represent width, height and the number of channels of each frame respectively. The network consists of five conv layers and a set of pooling layers, the two fully-connected layers in the base frame-wise network were replaced with a global average pooling layer [14]. Therefore each frame is now represented as single feature vector and passed into LSTM units. The proposed models were trained for detecting the fetal abdomen, heart, skull and the background resulting K = 4 classes with a temporal window of 10 consecutive frames. The temporal models were trained using mini-batch (batch size = 20) and Adam with an initial learning rate of 0.001.

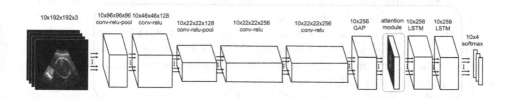

Fig. 3. Spatio-temporal model based on CNNs and LSTMs

Spatio-temporal model based on 1d dilated convolutions. The network architecture for the proposed spatio-temporal dilated convolution (DC) classification model is show in Fig. 4. Similarly, the input to the model is a short sequence in the form of $b \times n \times w \times h \times c$, where b is the mini-batch size, n is the number of frames in the sequence, and w, h, and c represent width, height and the number of channels of each frame respectively. The network architecture is identical to the spatio-temporal LSTM classification network, with the main difference being the use of the 1D dilated causal convolutional layers rather than LSTM units. The last three layers of the network are the 1D conv layers with dilation factors 1, 2, and 4 respectively, allowing the receptive field to grow exponentially [8]. Given d is the dilation factor in a network, in a dilated causal convolution the filter is applied to every d^{th} element in the previous time-step, allowing the model to only condition on the past. We use a similar structure to [8] with L layers of dilated convolutions $l = 1, \ldots, L$ and with the dilations increasing by a factor of two $d \in [2^0, 2^1, \ldots, 2^{L-1}]$. In this paper given the input sequence length, L is set to 3.

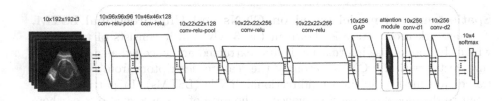

Fig. 4. Spatio-temporal model based on 1D dilated convolution.

2.3 Attention Mask Module

Attention modules have show to increase intractability and enhance the performance of deep neural networks. As a secondary hypothesis, in this paper we have also investigated the soft-attention mechanisms for the ultrasound video analysis.

Take the frame-wise classification CNN model for example, the attention mask layer receives the features maps from the last convolutional layer as input, and output a attention map normalized as a probability distribution, the values on this map is therefore dependent on the appearance of the input images. Ideally, if the input image contains the structure of interest, the model should learn to output higher weights within the regions of interest.

In detail, let $\mathbf{f}_k$ be the output of the last 2D convolution in the network, an attention mask layer filters them with a kernel $\mathbf{q}$ via dot product, yielding a set of corresponding significance e_k. They are then passed to a softmax operator to generate positive weights a_k, where $\sum_k a_k = 1$. Therefore, mathematically

$$e_k = \mathbf{q}^\mathsf{T} \mathbf{f}_k,$$
$$a_k = \frac{exp(e_k)}{\sum_j exp(e_j)}.$$

Afterwards, the feature descriptor for the input image is obtained by pooling with this attentional map, this process can be treated as a generalization of the widely used average pooling, where the weights are naively decided based on the spatial footprint of the feature map.

3   Results

The proposed models were trained for 75 epochs with an initial learning rate of 0.001, while reducing the learning rate every 32 steps by a factor of 10 until training termination. We evaluated the performance of each model in terms of per-class classification accuracy as shown in Table 1. As for a direct comparison, we asked the authors of [6] to run their state-of-the-art models on the test data. The results are presented and discussed in the next section.

Table 1. Classification accuracy (%) for the different network architectures.

Method	Abdomen	Heart	Skull	Background	Mean
Frame-wise	89	87	93	76	86
Frame-wise + spatial attention	86	93	71	92	86
Temporal - dilated convolution					
Base net	82	86	96	76	85
+ temporal attention	77	90	84	98	87
+ extended range (10of25)	90	88	91	85	**89**
+ extended range (10of25) + temporal attention	84	91	96	84	**89**
Temporal LSTM	79	79	78	95	83
Two stream net [6]	80	83	80	94	84

The frame-wise classification accuracy is set as the baseline. As can be seen, in that case the skull classification performed best with 93%, while the background class performed worst at 76%. With the help from attention modules, the performances for the heart class and the background class are boosted, however it has a negative effect on the skull classification accuracy. This can be explained by the fact that the attention module helps to focus on smaller objects in the image. However for larger objects such as the skull, where one of the main features is the skull boundaries, the attention module can have an adverse effect. The attention masks on an example from each class are illustrated on Fig. 5.

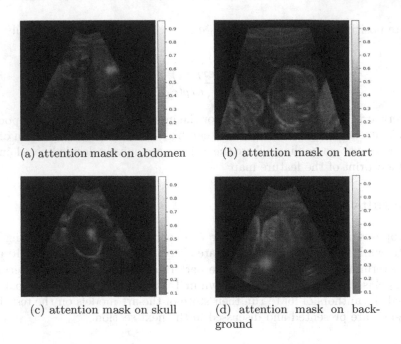

(a) attention mask on abdomen   (b) attention mask on heart

(c) attention mask on skull   (d) attention mask on background

Fig. 5. Attention masked learned during training are overlayed on an example frame from the abdomen class Fig. 5a, heart Fig. 5b, skull Fig. 5c, and the background class Fig. 5d.

The temporal experiment consisted of small video sequences of 10 frames long as the input to the network. For the base temporal network, a mean accuracy of 85% was achieved, which is similar to the frame-wise network with similar per class accuracies. However, adding the attention module to the network improved the mean classification accuracy to 87%. In addition, a similar behaviour to the individual class accuracies as for the frame-wise model is seen where the attention module improves the background class to 98% and heart class to 90%. However, the abdomen and the skull class are again adversely affected.

As the aim of the temporal model is to learn long class dependencies and associations, the range of input sequences was extended by initially selecting sequences of 25 frames, and then randomly selecting 10 frames from these sequences, while keeping the overall order of the frames unchanged. This operation served as the temporal dropout and diversifies the input sequence, meaning the chance of having frames from different classes has been increased. This is labelled as extended range (10of25) in Table 1. As can be seen, this range extension has boosted the mean accuracy to 89%, where, compared to the base temporal net, the abdomen class and background class have had the largest performance gain. Finally, adding the attention module to this network does not significantly change the mean classification accuracy. For completeness, we have reported the results using an LSTM with the same architecture, as well as running the pre-trained two-stream network that holds state-of-art results for this problem on our test dataset. As can be seen from Table 1, our proposed method outperforms both.

4 Discussion and Conclusion

In this paper we have considered the problem of classifying freehand ultrasound video. We have shown how dilated convolutions can be used to model temporal dependencies without hugely increasing the computational cost of training the network, unlike RNNs, 1D dilated convolutions can be efficiently parallelized and trained. Although the fixed input length could potentially be a limiting factor in some applications such as analysis of audio file or natural videos, for ultrasound images it is unlikely that such long dependencies are meaningful or useful since the goal in freehand ultrasound is typically to examine a 3D anatomical object space with arbitrary multiple sweeps of the transducer; thus locally a video may have certain characteristic (anatomical) patterns, but globally, the patterns will differ due to different navigation paths in the object space.

Acknowledgments. The National Institute for Health Research (NIHR) Oxford Biomedical Research Centre, grant BRC-1215-20008, EPSRC grant EP/M013774/1, MRC grant MR/P027938/1, ERC Advanced Grant 694581 (PULSE) and NVIDIA Corporations GPU grant are acknowledged.

References

1. Maraci, M.A., Bridge, C.P., Napolitano, R., Papageorghiou, A., Noble, J.A.: A framework for analysis of linear ultrasound videos to detect fetal presentation and heartbeat. Med. Image Anal. **37**, 22–36 (2017)
2. Bridge, C.P., Ioannou, C., Noble, J.A.: Automated annotation and quantitative description of ultrasound videos of the fetal heart. Med. Image Anal. **36**, 147–161 (2017)
3. Baumgartner, C.F., et al.: Real-time detection and localisation of fetal standard scan planes in 2d freehand ultrasound. CoRR abs/1612.05601 (2016)
4. Chen, H., et al.: Automatic fetal ultrasound standard plane detection using knowledge transferred recurrent neural networks. In: Navab, N., Hornegger, J., Wells, W.M., Frangi, A.F. (eds.) MICCAI 2015. LNCS, vol. 9349, pp. 507–514. Springer, Cham (2015). https://doi.org/10.1007/978-3-319-24553-9_62
5. Huang, W., Bridge, C.P., Noble, J.A., Zisserman, A.: Temporal heartnet: towards human-level automatic analysis of fetal cardiac screening video. In: Descoteaux, M., Maier-Hein, L., Franz, A., Jannin, P., Collins, D.L., Duchesne, S. (eds.) MICCAI 2017. LNCS, vol. 10434, pp. 341–349. Springer, Cham (2017). https://doi.org/10.1007/978-3-319-66185-8_39
6. Gao, Y., Alison Noble, J.: Detection and characterization of the fetal heartbeat in free-hand ultrasound sweeps with weakly-supervised two-streams convolutional networks. In: Descoteaux, M., Maier-Hein, L., Franz, A., Jannin, P., Collins, D.L., Duchesne, S. (eds.) MICCAI 2017. LNCS, vol. 10434, pp. 305–313. Springer, Cham (2017). https://doi.org/10.1007/978-3-319-66185-8_35

7. Carreira, J., Zisserman, A.: Quo vadis, action recognition? a new model and the kinetics dataset. In: 2017 IEEE Conference on Computer Vision and Pattern Recognition (CVPR), pp. 4724–4733. IEEE (2017)
8. Van Den Oord, A., et al.: A generative model for raw audio. arXiv preprint arXiv:1609.03499 (2016)
9. Kalchbrenner, N., Grefenstette, E., Blunsom, P.: A convolutional neural network for modelling sentences. In: ACL (2014)
10. Dauphin, Y.N., Fan, A., Auli, M., Grangier, D.: Language modeling with gated convolutional networks. arXiv preprint arXiv:1612.08083 (2016)
11. Girdhar, R., Ramanan, D.: Attentional pooling for action recognition. CoRR abs/1711.01467 (2017)
12. Yang, J., Ren, P., Chen, D., Wen, F., Li, H., Hua, G.: Neural aggregation network for video face recognition. CoRR abs/1603.05474 (2016)
13. Wang, X., Girshick, R.B., Gupta, A., He, K.: Non-local neural networks. CoRR abs/1711.07971 (2017)
14. Lin, M., Chen, Q., Yan, S.: Network in network. CoRR abs/1312.4400 (2013)

Topological Correction of Infant Cortical Surfaces Using Anatomically Constrained U-Net

Liang Sun[1], Daoqiang Zhang[1(✉)], Li Wang[2], Wei Shao[1], Zengsi Chen[2,3], Weili Lin[2], Dinggang Shen[2], and Gang Li[2(✉)]

[1] College of Computer Science and Technology, Nanjing University of Aeronautics and Astronautics, Nanjing 211106, China
dqzhang@nuaa.edu.cn
[2] Department of Radiology and BRIC, University of North Carolina at Chapel Hill, Chapel Hill, NC 27599, USA
gang_li@med.unc.edu
[3] College of Sciences, China Jiliang University, Hangzhou 310018, China

Abstract. Reconstruction of accurate cortical surfaces with minimal topological errors (i.e., handles and holes) from infant brain MR images is important in early brain development studies. However, infant brain MR images usually exhibit extremely low tissue contrast (especially from 3 to 9 months of age) and dynamic imaging appearance patterns. Thus, it is inevitable to have large amounts of topological errors in the infant brain tissue segmentation results, thus leading to inaccurate surface reconstruction. To address these issues, inspired by recent advances in deep learning methods, we propose an anatomically constrained U-Net method for topological correction of infant cortical surfaces. Specifically, in our method, we first extract candidate voxels with potential topological errors, by leveraging a topology-preserving level set method. Then, we propose a U-Net with anatomical constraints to correct those located candidate voxels. Due to the fact that infant cortical surfaces often contain large handles or holes, it is difficult to completely correct all errors using one-shot correction. Therefore, we further gather these two steps into an iterative framework to correct large topological errors gradually. To our knowledge, this is the first work introducing deep learning for infant cortical topological correction. We compare our method with the state-of-the-art method on infant cortical topology and show the superior performance of our method.

1 Introduction

Reconstruction of accurate cortical surfaces with minimal topological errors from infant MR images is a critical but challenging step in early brain development

This work was supported in part by the National Natural Science Foundation of China(61861130366, 61703301, 61473149), NIH grants (MH100217, MH107815, MH108914, MH109773, MH116225 and MH110274), Zhejiang Provincial Natural Science Foundation of China(LQ18A010003) and China Council Scholarship.

studies [1]. Due to the rapid brain growth and ongoing myelination [2], infant brain MR images typically have extremely low tissue contrast (especially from 3 to 9 months of age), severe partial volume effects, and regionally-heterogeneous, dynamically-changing imaging appearances. Hence, it is inevitable to have many topological errors in brain tissue segmentation. Of note, Even a very small error in segmentation could result in a significant topological defect, thus bring errors for cortical surface reconstruction and subsequent surface-based measurement or analysis.

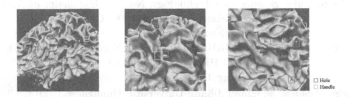

Fig. 1. Illustration of topological errors in infant cortical surfaces.

Topological errors generally include holes and handles. Typically, holes (indicated by blue squares in Fig. 1) incorrectly perforate the cortical surface, while handles (indicated by red squares in Fig. 1) bridge geodetically nonadjacent regions in the cortical surface. Therefore, the purpose of topological correction methods is appropriately to fill the holes and break the handles. Topological correction typically involves two steps, *i.e.*, (1) locating topologically defected regions and (2) correcting these topologically defected regions. Based on the priori knowledge, that each brain hemisphere has a simple spherical topology, several methods have been proposed to locate topologically-defected regions, e.g., finding cyclic graph loops [3] or overlapping surface meshes after spherical mapping [4,5]. Note, the second step is much challenging, because holes and handles are in the sense of anatomical correctness, but are hard to be distinguished by solely geometric information. Thus, several heuristics methods have been proposed for this issue. Among them, some methods are based on the minimal correction criterion, assuming that the change of voxels should be as small as possible [3,4]. For the complex cortical structure, this criterion might not be reliable enough. Many methods adopt *ad hoc* rules based on intensity images, achieving good performance on adult cortical surfaces [6,7], but are not very suitable for infant cortical surface. This is because infant MR images have extremely low tissue contrast and dynamically-changing image appearances in both T1w and T2w images along time, thus making the intensities less reliable and also resulting in much more complicated topological errors. To address these issues, a sparse representation based method has been proposed for correcting the topological defects on infant cortical surfaces [8]. This method does not need any predefined rules, and achieves good performance on topological defects correction on infant cortical surfaces. However, it relies on nonlinear image registration between the to-be-corrected image and a set of brain atlases, and thus is very time-consuming.

Advances in deep learning, e.g., U-Net [9,10], have shown competitive performance in medical image analysis. Inspired by this, we proposed an anatomically constrained U-Net method for topological correction of infant cortical surfaces. Specifically, in the training stage, we first locate topologically-defected regions by using a topology-preserving level set method [11]. Then, we construct the training dataset based on located topological-defected regions. Finally, we train the anatomically constrained U-Net. Different from the conventional U-Net, we *not only* train the network based on the ground truth, *but also* leverage anatomical prior of corresponding patches from a set of atlas images (free of topological defects). In the testing stage, we first locate the candidate voxels by topological-preserving level set method [11]. Then, we apply the trained anatomically constrained U-Net to infer the new labels of candidate voxels. To completely remove large topological errors, we gather the two steps in the testing stage into an iterative framework. Of note, our method only needs image registration in the training stage, not in the testing stage. To our knowledge, this is the *first work* on infant cortical topological correction using deep learning. Experimental results demonstrate the effectiveness of our method.

2   Method

To remove cortical topological defects, we leverage U-Net to reconstruct the image patches with errors and also incorporate anatomical prior into the model. For each patch, we collect its corresponding patches in a set of atlas images (free of topological defects) to help train U-Net.

2.1   Training Set Construction

Denote the tissue segmented images by $\mathbf{I}_{train} = \{\mathbf{I}_1, \mathbf{I}_2, .., \mathbf{I}_P\}$ with topological errors and their manually-corrected label maps (with experts) by $\mathbf{L}_{train} = \{\mathbf{L}_1, \mathbf{L}_2, .., \mathbf{L}_P\}$. Since the regions without topological errors have no contribution to the loss, we only extract the candidate voxels suffered from topological defects in training stage. Specifically, we locate the topologically defect regions by using a shrinking-wrapping topology-preserving level set method [11]. The converged volume of the level set evolution $\mathbf{V}_{LS}$ is a pure hole-filling process on the white matter volume ($\mathbf{V}_{WM}$). We extract candidate voxels with topological defects by a simple XOR operations ($\mathbf{V}_{CAN} = \mathbf{V}_{LS} \oplus \mathbf{V}_{WM}$). All holes are successfully fixed by the topology-preserving level set method, while all handles failed. Some candidate holes are caused by erroneous perforation of white matter (*i.e.*, real holes in anatomy.), while other are spin-off products of the erroneous connection of white matter (i.e., handles). Thus, we use a morphological dilation method to further enroll the neighboring candidate voxels in $\mathbf{V}_{CAN}$. In this way, the candidate set contains both holes and handles. Subsequently, for each candidate voxel v, we gather the tissue labels from v and its

$d \times d \times d$ neighbors. Thus we obtain a 3D patch $\mathbf{x}(v)$, encoding information of local anatomical structure. Each training patch has its corresponding label map (free of topological errors). We use $\mathbf{D} = \{\mathbf{x}_1, \mathbf{x}_2, .., \mathbf{x}_N | \mathbf{x}_i \in \mathbb{R}^{d \times d \times d}\}$ and $\mathbf{Y} = \{\mathbf{y}_1, \mathbf{y}_2, .., \mathbf{y}_N | \mathbf{y}_i \in \mathbb{R}^{d \times d \times d}\}$ to denote the training data and corresponding label maps, respectively. In addition, the atlases $\mathbf{A} = \{\mathbf{A}_1, \mathbf{A}_2, .., \mathbf{A}_K\}$ are non-linearly registered onto the tissue-segmented images by the diffeomorphic demons method [12]. For each atlas $\mathbf{A}_k$, we extract v's corresponding reference patch $\mathbf{p}^k(v)$ from its label map $\mathbf{L}_k^A$. Hence, we can construct the reference set $\mathbf{R} = \{\mathbf{r}_1, \mathbf{r}_2, .., \mathbf{r}_N\}$, where $\mathbf{r}_i = [\mathbf{p}^1(v), \mathbf{p}^2(v), .., \mathbf{p}^K(v)] \in \mathbb{R}^{d \times d \times d \times K}$, N and K represent the number of training data and atlases, respectively. The training dataset thus consists of $\mathbf{D}$, $\mathbf{Y}$ and $\mathbf{R}$.

2.2   Anatomically Constrained U-Net

The proposed anatomically constrained U-Net architecture is illustrated in Fig. 2. Specifically, the contracting path consists of the repeated two convolution layers and a max-pooling layer. We perform two convolutions operation with $3 \times 3 \times 3$ convolution kernels, with each convolution layer followed by batch normalization and rectified linear units. Then, a $2 \times 2 \times 2$ max-pooling operation with stride 2 is used for downsampling. The expansive path consists of the repeated one deconvolution layer, a concatenation with corresponding feature map from the contracting path and two convolutional layers. We perform deconvolution operation with $2 \times 2 \times 2$ convolution kernels, and convolution operation with $3 \times 3 \times 3$ with convolution kernels, with each convolution layer also followed by batch normalization and rectified linear units. At the final layer, a $1 \times 1 \times 1$ convolution followed by softmax non-linear units is used to output the probability maps $\mathbf{H} = \{\mathbf{h}_1, \mathbf{h}_2, .., \mathbf{h}_N | \mathbf{h}_i \in \mathbb{R}^{d \times d \times d \times C}\}$, where C is the number of tissue categories. Typically, each segmentation image has four labels *i.e.*, white matter (WM), gray matter (GM), cerebrospinal fluid (CSF) and background. Therefore, the output map has 4 channels, each corresponding to the probability of respective category.

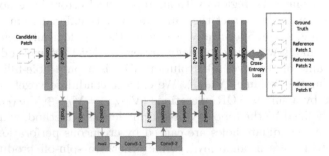

Fig. 2. The architecture of our proposed anatomically constrained U-Net. The purple, blue, green and red arrows represent the concatenation, convolution, max pooling and deconvolution respectively.

A patch with topological errors is reconstructed by our anatomically constrained U-Net. Therefore, we use the cross-entropy based reconstruction loss as the loss function. Meanwhile, we also leverage anatomical prior of corresponding patches from a set of atlas images (free of topological defects). Thus, the final loss function is defined by

$$L = -\frac{1}{N} \sum_{i=1}^{N} \sum_{j=1}^{d^3} \sum_{c=1}^{C} [\delta(y_{i,j} = c) \log h_{i,j,c} + \frac{\lambda}{K} \sum_{k}^{K} \delta(p_{i,j,k} = c) \log h_{i,j,c}] \quad (1)$$

where $\delta(a = b)$ is a Dirac function, which equal to 1 when $a = b$ and 0 otherwise. $h_{i,j,c}$ represents the probability of the j-th voxel in the i-th patch belonging to the c-category. The first term in the Eq. 1 is the reconstruction loss and the second term makes the network learn the anatomical information from the reference volumes. λ balances the loss from the ground truth and anatomical references.

2.3 Inferring the New Labels of Candidate Voxels

In the testing stage, giving a tissue-segmentation image $\mathbf{I}_{test}$, we first locate its candidate voxels with potential topological errors, similar to the process of training stage. Then we infer the probability maps for the candidate patches using the trained network. As each candidate voxel may be contained in multiple candidate patches, we calculate the probability of the voxel v *not only* based on the probability map that v is sitting the patch center, *but also* the probability maps that v in its neighboring patches. Thus, the probability of $l_v = c$ is calculated as follows:

$$p(l_v = c) = \frac{1}{V} \sum_{i}^{V} p(l_v = c|r_i) \quad (2)$$

where $p(l_v = c|r_i)$ is the voxel v's probability belonging to class c in the probability map of the patch center at voxel r_i. V is the number of candidate patches containing voxel v. Finally, we use the MAP criteria to obtain the new labels of candidate voxels.

Nevertheless, the infant cortical surfaces contain many large handles or holes, which are usually difficult to correct in one time. Hence, we further repeat the process of correction step to refine the correction results until convergence. Finally, we re-apply the topology preserving level set method to guarantee a spherical topology. The whole algorithm is summarized in Algorithm 1.

3 Experiments

3.1 Dataset and Experimental Settings

To validate our method, we adopted 55 infants brain MR images with the resolution of $1 \times 1 \times 1 \, \text{mm}^3$ at 6 months of age. The motivation is that brain MR images

---

Algorithm 1 Topological Correction Using Anatomically Constrained U-Net

---

Input: $\mathbf{I}_{train}$, $\mathbf{L}_{train}$, $\mathbf{A}$ and $\mathbf{I}_{test}$

Output: $\mathbf{I}_{out}$

Training:

1: Extract $\mathbf{V}_{CAN}$ from $\mathbf{I}_{train}$

2: Construct training set $\mathbf{D}$ and its label map set $\mathbf{Y}$ as well as reference label map set $\mathbf{R}$ from $\mathbf{I}_{train}$, $\mathbf{L}_{train}$ and $\mathbf{A}$ based on $\mathbf{V}_{CAN}$

3: Train the anatomically constrained U-Net

Testing:

1: Initialize the corrected image $\mathbf{I}_0 = \mathbf{I}_{test}$

2: **for** $t = 1:T$ **do**

3:     Extract $\mathbf{V}_t$ from $\mathbf{I}_{t-1}$

4:     Construct testing set $\mathbf{D}_t$ from $\mathbf{I}_{t-1}$ based on $\mathbf{V}_t$

5:     Infer the new labels of candidate voxels using the trained anatomically constrained U-Net

6:     Update $\mathbf{I}_t$ by replacing the old labels in $\mathbf{I}_{t-1}$

7: **end for**

8: **return** $\mathbf{I}_{out}$ by refining $\mathbf{I}_t$ with the topology-preserving level set method

---

of 6-month-olds exhibit the lowest tissue contrast and suffered the severest topological errors in tissue segmentation. Among 55 pairs of images with topological errors and their manually-corrected images, 10 subjects are randomly selected as atlas images, 15 subjects are randomly selected as the training images, and 30 subjects are used as the testing images. In the experiment, we fix patch size, atlas number and iteration number as $19 \times 19 \times 19$, 10 and 4, respectively. We set the learning rate and λ as 10^{-4} and 0.5, respectively.

We use successful rate (SR) to assess our method in anatomical consistency between the corrected surface and ground truth. SR is the topological defects that have been successfully corrected in proportion to the total topological defects. The successfully correct topological defects indicate that the holes are appropriately filled or handles are appropriately broken. Besides, we also use the Dice ratio (DR) and average surface distance (ASD) to measure the corrected performance. The DR and ASD are defined as follows:

$$DR = \frac{2 \times |W_1 \cap W_2|}{|W_1| + |W_2|} \qquad (3)$$

$$ASD = \frac{1}{2}\left(\frac{1}{n_1} \sum_{w_1 \in S(W_1)} d(w_1, S(W_2)) + \frac{1}{n_2} \sum_{w_2 \in S(W_2)} d(w_2, S(W_1))\right) \qquad (4)$$

where W_1 and W_2 denote the corrected white matter volumes by our proposed method and the manually corrected white matter volumes (i.e., ground truth), respectively. It is noteworthy that, when computing DR and ASD, we only use local regions enclosing the candidate voxels and their neighboring voxels, obtained by the dilation of the set of the candidate voxels. In Eq. 3, $|\cdot|$ calculates the number of voxels. In Eq. 4, $d(\cdot, \cdot)$ measures the Euclidean distance, and n_1 and n_2 are the numbers of vertices in surface $S(W_1)$ and surface $S(W_2)$, respectively.

3.2   Result

We compare our proposed anatomically constrained U-Net (ACU-Net) with the recent sparse representation based method [8], and show the results in Fig. 3 and Table 1. Meanwhile, we also compare with the conventional U-Net method without anatomical constraint. As can be seen, our proposed method achieves competitive results in anatomical consistency between the corrected surfaces and ground truth. The successful rates are 97.80% and 98.35% by U-Net and ACU-Net, respectively, in comparison with and 96.70% by Hao's method [8]. In addition, our proposed method also achieves the best result on Dice ratio and average surface distance. The Dice ratio is 98.83 ± 0.33% by ACU-Net, compared with 98.65 ± 0.79% by U-Net and 92.91 ± 1.60% and Hao's method, respectively. The average surface distance is 0.018 ± 0.006 mm, compared with 0.022 ± 0.014 mm by U-Net and 0.105 ± 0.025 mm and Hao's method, respectively. We also show the impact of the number of atlases in Table 1. As expected, increasing the number of atlases increases the correction performance. In Fig. 3, the red squares and blue squares are handles and holes, respectively, demonstrating superior performance of our proposed method. All these results suggest that our proposed method based on U-Net can effectively correct topological defects and achieve high anatomical accuracy. Also, incorporating anatomical information can further improve topological correction results by U-Net. Meanwhile, Hao's method needs non-linear image registration when inferring the new labels, which is very time-consuming. In comparison, our proposed method only needs registration in the training stage. Thus, our proposed method is much faster than Hao's method in practical application. Typically, the time consumed by our method is around 20 min, compared with 200 min by Hao's method.

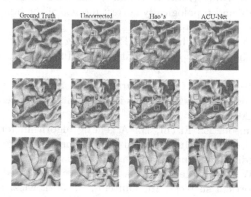

Fig. 3. Comparison with the state-of-the-art method.

Table 1. Quantitative comparison with other topological correction methods.

Method	SR	$DR(mean \pm std)$	$ASD(mean \pm std)$
Hao's [8]	96.70%	92.91 $\pm$ 1.60%	0.105 $\pm$ 0.025 mm
U-Net	97.80%	98.65 $\pm$ 0.79%	0.022 $\pm$ 0.014 mm
ACU-Net (5 atlases)	97.91%	98.75 $\pm$ 0.38%	0.020 $\pm$ 0.008 mm
ACU-Net (10 atlases)	**98.35%**	**98.83 $\pm$ 0.33%**	**0.018 $\pm$ 0.006 mm**

4   Conclusion

In this paper, we proposed an anatomically constrained U-Net for topological correction of infant cortical surfaces. Our main contributions are twofold. First, to the best of our knowledge, we are the first to leverage a convolutional neural network (CNN) method for topological correction, by incorporating it with a topology-preserving level set method. Second, we use the anatomical prior from a set of atlases to guide the network training, where incorporating more atlases can lead to better accuracy. Experimental results on 6-month infant brain images show excellent performance.

References

1. Li, G., et al.: Mapping region-specific longitudinal cortical surface expansion from birth to 2 years of age. Cereb. Cortex **23**(11), 2724–2733 (2012)
2. Paus, T., Collins, D., Evans, A., Leonard, G., Pike, B., Zijdenbos, A.: Maturation of white matter in the human brain: a review of magnetic resonance studies. Brain Res. Bull. **54**(3), 255–266 (2001)
3. Shattuck, D.W., Leahy, R.M.: Automated graph-based analysis and correction of cortical volume topology. IEEE TMI **20**(11), 1167–1177 (2001)
4. Fischl, B., Liu, A., Dale, A.M.: Automated manifold surgery: constructing geometrically accurate and topologically correct models of the human cerebral cortex. IEEE TMI **20**(1), 70–80 (2001)
5. Yotter, R.A., Dahnke, R., Thompson, P.M., Gaser, C.: Topological correction of brain surface meshes using spherical harmonics. Hum. Brain Mapp. **32**(7), 1109–1124 (2011)
6. Shi, Y., Lai, R., Toga, A.W.: Cortical surface reconstruction via unified reeb analysis of geometric and topological outliers in magnetic resonance images. IEEE TMI **32**(3), 511–530 (2013)
7. Ségonne, F., Grimson, E., Fischl, B.: A genetic algorithm for the topology correction of cortical surfaces. In: Biennial International Conference on Information Processing in Medical Imaging, Springer (2005) 393–405
8. Hao, S., Li, G., Wang, L., Meng, Y., Shen, D.: Learning-based topological correction for infant cortical surfaces. In: Ourselin, S., Joskowicz, L., Sabuncu, M.R., Unal, G., Wells, W. (eds.) MICCAI 2016. LNCS, vol. 9900, pp. 219–227. Springer, Cham (2016). https://doi.org/10.1007/978-3-319-46720-7_26

9. Ronneberger, O., Fischer, P., Brox, T.: U-Net: convolutional networks for biomedical image segmentation. In: Navab, N., Hornegger, J., Wells, W.M., Frangi, A.F. (eds.) MICCAI 2015. LNCS, vol. 9351, pp. 234–241. Springer, Cham (2015). https://doi.org/10.1007/978-3-319-24574-4_28
10. cCiccek, Ö., Abdulkadir, A., Lienkamp, S.S., Brox, T., Ronneberger, O.: 3D U-net: learning dense volumetric segmentation from sparse annotation. In: Ourselin, S., Joskowicz, L., Sabuncu, M.R., Unal, G., Wells, W. (eds.) MICCAI 2016. LNCS, vol. 9901, pp. 424–432. Springer, Cham (2016). https://doi.org/10.1007/978-3-319-46723-8_49
11. Han, X., Xu, C., Prince, J.L.: A topology preserving level set method for geometric deformable models. IEEE TPAMI **25**(6), 755–768 (2003)
12. Vercauteren, T., Pennec, X., Perchant, A., Ayache, N.: Diffeomorphic demons: efficient non-parametric image registration. NeuroImage **45**(1), S61–S72 (2009)

Self-taught Learning with Residual Sparse Autoencoders for HEp-2 Cell Staining Pattern Recognition

Xian-Hua Han[1]($\boxtimes$), JiandDe Sun[2], Lanfen Lin[3], and Yen-Wei Chen[4]

[1] Graduate School of Science and Technology for Innovation, Yamaguchi University, 1677-1 Yoshida, Yamaguchi City, Yamaguchi 753-8511, Japan
`hanxhua@yamaguchi-u.ac.jp`
[2] ShanDong Normal University, JianNan, ShanDong, China
[3] Zhejiang University, Hangzhou, China
[4] Ritsumeikan University, Kusatsu, Shiga, Japan

Abstract. Self-taught learning aims at obtaining compact and latent representations from data them-selves without previously manual labeling, which would be time-consuming and laborious. This study proposes a novel self-taught learning for more accurately reconstructing the raw data based on the sparse autoencoder. It is well known that autoencoder is able to learn latent features via setting the target values to be equal to the input data, and can be stacked for pursuing high-level feature learning. Motivated by the natural sparsity of data representation, sparsity has been imposed on the hidden layer responses of autoencoder for more effective feature learning. Although the conventional autoencoder-based feature learning aims at obtaining the latent representation via minimizing the approximation error of the input data, it is unavoidable to produce reconstruction residual error of the input data and thus some tiny structures are unable to be represented, which may be essential information for fine-grained image task such as medical image analysis. Even with the multiple-layer stacking for high-level feature pursuing in autoencoder-based learning strategy, the lost tiny structure in the former layers can not be recovered evermore. Therefore, this study proposes a residual sparse autoencoder for learning the latent feature representation of more tiny structures in the raw input data. With the unavoidably generated reconstruction residual error, we exploit another sparse autoencoder to pursuing the latent feature of the residual tiny structures and this self-taught learning process can continue until the representation residual error is enough small. We evaluate the proposed residual sparse autoencoding for self-taught learning the latent representations of HEp-2 cell image, and prove that promising performance for staining pattern recognition can be achieved compared with the conventional sparse autoencoder and the-state-of-the-art methods.

Keywords: Self-taught learning · Unsupervised feature learning
Latent representation · Residual sparse autoencoder · HEp2 cell
Staining patterns

© Springer Nature Switzerland AG 2018
Y. Shi et al. (Eds.): MLMI 2018, LNCS 11046, pp. 134–142, 2018.
https://doi.org/10.1007/978-3-030-00919-9_16

1 Introduction

Medical image analysis plays an important role for assisting medical experts to understand the internal organs of human and recognize characterization of different tissues. Unlike the frequently used generic images photoed in the real world where the features are often well-defined [1, 2] and are familiar to us, medical data is hard to be distinguishable and to define the characterization for the specific fine-grained tasks since the visibility even for very tiny structures is required for providing acceptable performance. Furthermore, contrast to the possible *enough* images with ground-truth provided for training generalized machine learning models in generic image vision applications, medical images are more difficult to collect especially for patient data with the abnormalities arising from disease, and the manually labels require substantially more specialist knowledge to define and is a time-consuming task, which strongly motivates the extensive research for development of automated methods with unlabeled data, generally called unsupervised learning.

Unsupervised learning ranging from the conventional methods such as principle component analysis, sparse coding, to neural network based method extracts hidden and compact features from unlabeled training data. Recently, the neural network based unsupervised approach has manifested the impressive performance for learning latent features in different vision applications [3–6], and mainly includes two categories: data distribution approximating model such as the restricted Boltzmann machine [3,4] and reconstruction error minimization strategy (Self-taught learning) such as aotoencoder [5,6]. RBM aims at estimating the entropy of candidate features consistent with the data to infer the hidden feature, and has been applied for wide vision problems. Autoencoder (AE) is able to learn latent features via setting the target values to be equal to the input data, and is formulated to minimizing the reconstruction error of the input data. Motivated by the natural sparsity of data representation, sparsity has been imposed on the hidden layer responses of AE for more effective feature learning, which called sparse autoencoder (SAE). Recent dedication on the neural network-based unsupervised learning is to stack several layers for building much deeper framework pursuing high-level latent features, and validated further performance improvement for several applications. In addition, the unsupervised learning can be used as a pretraining step for further supervised learning in deep networks. Thus for more effectively using the pre training knowledge, understanding unsupervised learning is of fundamental importance.

This study aims at exploring a novel unsupervised learning (self-taught learning) framework for medical image analysis. As we know that the target data in the medical image processing tasks usually are just a specific organ or a region of interests from different patients, which are generally called fine-grained task in generic image vision problem, and there exists only slight difference for distinguishing abnormality from normal tissue compared to the distinct difference of objects in generic vision problem. How to learn the latent and compact feature for medical data representation without lost of tiny structures, which are likely useful to the specific medical task, is essential issue for the fine-grained medical task. Although the conventional AE-based feature learning aims at obtaining the latent representation via minimizing the approximation error of the input data, it is unavoidable to produce reconstruction residual error of the input data and thus some tiny structures are unable to be represented, which may be essential information for fine-grained medical image task. Even with the multiple-layer stacking for high-level feature pursuing in AE-based learning strategy, the lost tiny structure in the former layers can not be recovered evermore. Therefore, this study proposes a residual SAE for learning the latent feature representation of more tiny structures in the raw input data. With the unavoidably generated reconstruction residual error, we exploit further SAE for pursuing the latent feature of the residual tiny structures and this self-taught learning process can continue until the representation residual error is enough small. We evaluate the proposed residual SAE for extracting the latent features of HEp-2 cell image [7], and visualize the activation maps of some sparse neurons for understanding the learned latent feature. In order to generate the same-dimensional features for the HEp-2 cell representation, we divided the activation maps of SAE into donut-shaped spatial regions, and aggregate the activations in one region as a mean value to form a representation vector of HEp-2 images. Experimental results for HEp-2 staining pattern recognition with the learned features by the proposed residual SAE can obtain promising performance compared with the conventional SAE and the state-of-the-art methods.

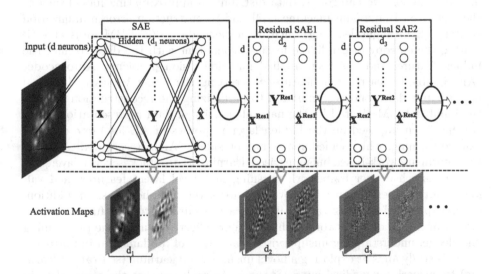

Fig. 1. The schematic concept of the proposed residual SAE. We stack several SAE to learn the latent feature of the unrecoverable residual in the former SAE until the reconstruction error are enough small.

2   Method

This study seeks to develop an automatic method for extraction latent feature with unlabeled images, and classifies staining patterns of HEp-2 cell IIF images. This section firstly describes the used dataset of the cell classification by Fluorescent Image Analysis, and then introduces the proposed residual SAE for learning latent and robust feature even for tiny structure representation. Finally, we analyze the activation maps of the residual SAE and propose a donut-shaped activation aggregation method for extracting the same dimensional feature vector of a HEp-2 cell image.

2.1   Material

We evaluate our self-taught learning method using the open ICIP2013 HEp-2 dataset [7] that includes two intensity types of HEp-2 cells, intermediate and positive, and the research purpose of the dataset is to recognize the staining pattern given the intensity types (intermediate or positive). The studied staining patterns primarily include six classes: Homogeneous, Speckled, Nucleolar, Centromere, Golgi and NuMem straining patterns. There are more than 10000 images with different sizes, each showing a single cell, which were obtained from 83 training IIF images by cropping the bounding box of the cell. Since AE-based network only accepts the same-length vector as the input, we divide the entire HEp-2 cell image into multiple $l \times l$ regions, and learn the latent feature for the local regions in HEp-2 cell image.

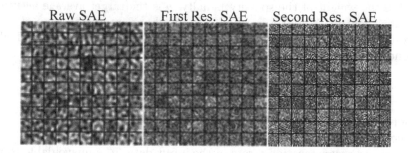

Fig. 2. The visualized weights in the raw SAE, the first- and second-level residual SAE.

2.2   Residual SAE for Self-taught Learning

Our proposed residual SAE mainly aims at learning the latent and compact features for more effectively representing tiny structures via self-taught learning procedure, which mainly based on the basic idea of autoencoder. An AE is a symmetrical neural network to learn the features by minimizing the reconstruction error between the input data at the encoding layer and its reconstruction at the decoding layer. Given a sample of input data $\mathbf{x} \in \mathbb{R}^{d \times 1}$, the encoding procedure is implemented by applying a linear mapping and a nonlinear activation function in the AE network:

$$y = sign(\mathbf{W}\mathbf{x} + \mathbf{b}_1), \tag{1}$$

where $\mathbf{W} \in \mathbb{R}^{d_o \times d}$ is a weight matrix with d_o features (d_o neurons in the encoding layers), $\mathbf{b}_1 \in \mathbb{R}^{d_o}$ is the encoding bias, and $sigm(\cdot)$ is the logistic sigmoid function. Decoding of the latent feature y in the encoding layer is performed using a separate decoding matrix:

$$\hat{\mathbf{x}} = \mathbf{V}^T y + \mathbf{b}_2, \tag{2}$$

where the decoding matrix is $\mathbf{V} \in \mathbb{R}^{d_o \times d}$ and $\mathbf{b}_2 \in \mathbb{R}^d$ is a decoding bias. Given training sample ensembles $\mathbf{X} = [\mathbf{x}_1, \mathbf{x}_2, \cdots, \mathbf{x}_N]$, the latent features $\mathbf{Y}$ in the data are learned by minimizing the reconstruction error of the likelihood function $L(\mathbf{X}, \hat{\mathbf{X}}) = \|\mathbf{X} - \hat{\mathbf{X}}\|^2 = \sum_i^N \|\mathbf{x}_i - \hat{\mathbf{x}}_i\|^2$, where $\hat{\mathbf{X}}$ are all the reconstructed data, and the parameters $\mathbf{W}, \mathbf{V}$ can be optimized via minimizing $L(\mathbf{X}, \hat{\mathbf{X}})$. Motivated by the natural sparsity of data representation, sparsity has been imposed to the target activation function, that is called as a sparse autoencoder (SAE) [5,6], for learning more effective feature, and the cost function in a SAE is formulated as:

$$< \mathbf{W}, \mathbf{V}, \mathbf{b} >= \underset{\mathbf{W}, \mathbf{V}, \mathbf{b}}{\operatorname{argmin}} \ L(\mathbf{X}, \hat{\mathbf{X}}) + \lambda \sum_{j=1}^{d_o} KL(\rho \parallel \hat{\rho}_j) \tag{3}$$

where λ is the weight of the sparsity penalty, ρ is the target average activation of the latent feature $\mathbf{Y}$ and $\hat{\rho}_j = \frac{1}{N} \sum_{i=1}^N y_{ji}$ is the average activation of $j - th$ input vector y_j over the N training data. $KL(\cdot)$ denotes the Kullback–Leibler divergence [5], and is given by:

$$KL(\rho \parallel \hat{\rho}_j) = \rho \log \frac{\rho}{\hat{\rho}_j} + (1 - \rho) \log \frac{1 - \rho}{1 - \hat{\rho}_j} \tag{4}$$

which provides the sparsity constraint on the latent features.

Although the AE and SAE aim at optimizing the parameters $< \mathbf{W}, \mathbf{V}, \mathbf{b} >$ via minimizing reconstruction errors of the input data, it is unavoidable to produce the residual error: $\mathbf{X}^{Res} = \mathbf{X} - \hat{\mathbf{X}}$, which cannot be recoverable evermore with further processing. The lost residual error may be discriminated for the target task especially fine-grained image processing, thus this study proposes to stack further SAE to encoder the residual error instead of the learned hidden feature in the conventional stacked SAE framework, and the cost function of the proposed residual SAE is formulated as:

$$< \mathbf{W}^{Res}, \mathbf{V}^{Res}, \mathbf{b}^{Res} >= \operatorname{argmin} \ L^{Res}(\mathbf{X}^{Res}, \mathbf{X}^{\hat{Res}}) + \lambda \sum_{j=1}^{d_o} KL(\rho^{Res} \parallel \hat{\rho}_j{}^{Res})$$

$$\tag{5}$$

where $\mathbf{W}^{Res}, \mathbf{V}^{Res}, \mathbf{b}^{Res}$ are the encoding weight matrix, decoding matrix and the encoding/decoding bias in the residual SAE. We can stack more residual layers for learning latent feature of the very tiny structures, and the global objective function can be formulated as:

$$< \theta, \theta^{Res1}, \theta^{Res2}, \cdots > = \mathrm{argmin} \beta_1 L(\mathbf{X}, \hat{\mathbf{X}}) + \beta_2 L^{Res1}(\mathbf{X}^{Res1}, \mathbf{X}^{\hat{Res1}})$$
$$+ \cdots + \lambda \sum KL(\rho, \rho^{Res1}, \cdots) \tag{6}$$

where $\theta = < \mathbf{W}, \mathbf{V}, \mathbf{b} >$, $\theta^{Res1} = < \mathbf{W}^{Res1}, \mathbf{V}^{Res1}, \mathbf{b}^{Res1} >$, $\theta^{Res2} = < \mathbf{W}^{Res2}, \mathbf{V}^{Res2}, \mathbf{b}^{Res2} >$ denote the optimized parameter in the raw SAE, the first- and second-level residual SAE, respectively. β_1, β_2 and β_3 are the weights of the reconstruction errors in different levels of residual SAEs. The activation values in the hidden layers of the SAE, residual SAE can be combined as the represented features of the input data. The schematic concept of the proposed residual SAE is shown in Fig. 1, where $d, d_1, d_2, \cdots$ are the neuron numbers of the input layer, the hidden layers in the raw SAE, the first- and second-level residual SAE. The visualized weights of the residual SAE are shown in Fig. 2, which manifest more detail structure in the later-level residual SAE,

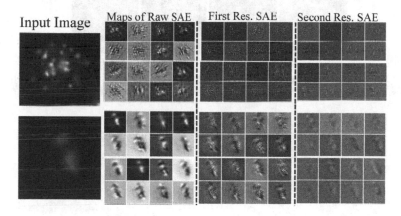

Fig. 3. Several activation maps of the hidden layers in three-level residual SAE for HEp-2 cell images.

2.3 The Aggregated Activation of the Residual SAE for Image Representation

As we mentioned that the input data in the raw SAE are the vectorized $l \times l$ local regions, which are sliding-extracted from the input image. We assume the neuron numbers of the hidden layers in the raw, the first- and second-level residual SAE are d_1, d_2 and d_3, respectively, we can obtain d_1, d_2 and d_3 activated values for each local region. Generally, given a $m \times n$ image, we can extract the $l \times l$ local regions for $(m - l) \times (n - l)$ centered pixels as the focused pixels, and thus the produced activation values of the hidden layer with d_k neurons in a (residual) SAE can be rearranged as d_k maps with size $(m - l) \times (n - l)$. The bottom row of Fig. 1 manifests the obtained activation maps for different level SAEs. We also provide several activation maps of the hidden layers in three-levels residual SAEs for HEp-2 cell images in Fig. 3, which manifests the detailed structures in the latter-level of residual SAE. Since the sizes of HEp-2 cell images are different, the activation maps in the residual SAE would accordingly change their sizes. For obtaining the same-length features for HEp-2 image representation, we divide each activation map into same number of regions, and averagely aggregate the activations in one region to form the final representation. Accompanying with the HEp-2 cell image, the cell region masks are also provided in this dataset, we apply morphological operators (dilation/erosion etc.) on cell mask image to form the center, middle and boundary regions for activation aggregation, as shown in Fig. 4. With the neuron numbers: d_1, d_2 and d_3 of the hidden layers in three-level residual SAE, a $(d_1 + d_2 + d_3) * 3$-dimensional feature vector can be generated for HEp-2 image representation.

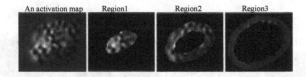

Fig. 4. The divided donut-shaped spatial regions for aggregating the activation value to form same-length feature vector as HEp-2 image representation.

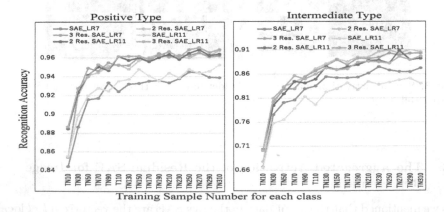

Fig. 5. The compared accuracy of HEp-e cell staining pattern recognition with raw/residual SAE, different local region sizes and training image numbers.

3   Experimental Results

Using HEp-2 cell images of two types of intensity (Intermediate and Positive), we validated the recognition performance by applying our proposed residual SAE and the conventional SAE. In our experiment, we randomly selected $Q(Q = 10, 30, \cdots, 310)$ cell images from each of the six patterns as training images, and the remainder are used as testing images for both Positive and Intermediate intensity types. The linear SVM was used as the classifier because of its effectiveness as compared with other classifiers, such as K-nearest neighbor, and its efficiency as compared with a nonlinear SVM, which requires much more time to classify a sample. The compared results with different training numbers and local region sizes $l = 7, 11$ (Denoted as LR7, LR11) are shown in Fig. 5, which manifests the proposed residual SAE can achieve much better performances than the conventional SAE.

Next, we compare the experimental results using our proposed residual SAE with the state-of-the-art methods [8–10] under the same experimental conditions for HEp-2 cell staining pattern recognition in Table 1, and show the promising performance can be obtained by our proposed method.

Table 1. The compared performance of our proposed Residual SAE and the state-of-the-art methods [8–10].

	GLRL [8]	SGLD [8]	Laws [8]	rSIFT [9]	MP [9]	FN [10]	Our
Positive	77.23	84.37	94.68	91.9	95.29	97.90	**98.45**
Intermediate	39.33	49.75	81.06	78	86.91	91.93	**92.24**

4   Conclusions

We have proposed a novel residual SAE network for self-taught learning the latent features of much tiny structure in the fine grained medical task. Instead of stacking the SAE for learning the high-level features from the output of the former SAE, we exploited residual SAE to model the residual reconstruction errors, which is vanished and cannot be recovered evermore in the former SAE, for learning the latent representation of more tiny structures. We have evaluated the proposed residual SAE for HEp-2 image representation, and proven that the promising performance for staining pattern recognition can be achieved.

References

1. Lowe, D.G.: Object recognition from local scale-invariant features. In: Proceedings of the International Conference on Computer Vision (ICCV1999), vol. 2, pp. 1150–1157 (1999)

2. Dalal, N., Triggs, B.: Histograms of oriented gradients for human detection. In: Proceedings of the International Conference on Computer Vision and Pattern Recognition (2005)
3. Sun, L., Shao, W., Zhang, D.Q.: High-order boltzmann machine-based unsupervised feature learning for multi-atlas segmentation. In: 2017 IEEE 14th International Symposium on Biomedical Imaging (ISBI 2017)
4. Zhao, Z.J., Xu, T.D., Dai, C.Y.: Classifying images using restricted Boltzmann machines and convolutional neural networks. In: Proceedings of SPIE 10420, Ninth International Conference on Digital Image Processing (ICDIP 2017), 104202U (21 July 2017)
5. Shin, H.-C., Orton, M.R., Collins, D.J., Doran, S.J., Leach, M.O.: Stacked autoencoders for unsupervised feature learning and multiple organ detection in a pilot study using 4D patient data. IEEE Trans. Pattern Anal. Mach. Intel. 35(8), 1930–1943 (2013)
6. Xu, J., et al.: Stacked Sparse Autoencoder (SSAE) for nuclei detection on breast cancer histopathology images. IEEE Trans. Med. Imaging 35, 119–130 (2015)
7. Foggia, P., Percannella, G., Soda, P., Vento, M.: Benchmarking hep-2 cells classification methods. IEEE Trans. Med. Imaging 32(10), 1878–1889 (2013)
8. Agrawal, P., Vatsa, M., Singh, R.: HEp-2 cell image classification: a comparative analysis. In: Wu, G., Zhang, D., Shen, D., Yan, P., Suzuki, K., Wang, F. (eds.) MLMI 2013. LNCS, vol. 8184, pp. 195–202. Springer, Cham (2013). https://doi.org/10.1007/978-3-319-02267-3_25
9. Manivannan, S., Li, W., Akbar, S., Wang, R., Zhang, J., McKenna, S.J.: An automated pattern recognition system for classifying indirect immunofluorescence images of hep-2 cells and specimens. Pattern Recognit. 15, 12–26 (2016)
10. Han, X.-H., Chen, Y.-W.: HEp-2 staining pattern recognition using stacked fisher network for encoding weber local descriptor. Pattern Recognit. 63, 542–550 (2017)

Semantic-Aware Generative Adversarial Nets for Unsupervised Domain Adaptation in Chest X-Ray Segmentation

Cheng Chen[1]([⊠]), Qi Dou[1], Hao Chen[1,2], and Pheng-Ann Heng[1]

[1] Dept. of Computer Science and Engineering, The Chinese University of Hong Kong, Hong Kong, China
cchen@cse.cuhk.edu.hk
[2] Imsight Medical Technology Co., Ltd., Shenzhen, China

Abstract. In spite of the compelling achievements that deep neural networks (DNNs) have made in medical image computing, these deep models often suffer from degraded performance when being applied to new test datasets with domain shift. In this paper, we present a novel unsupervised domain adaptation approach for segmentation tasks by designing semantic-aware generative adversarial networks (GANs). Specifically, we transform the test image into the appearance of source domain, with the semantic structural information being well preserved, which is achieved by imposing a nested adversarial learning in semantic label space. In this way, the segmentation DNN learned from the source domain is able to be directly generalized to the transformed test image, eliminating the need of training a new model for every new target dataset. Our domain adaptation procedure is unsupervised, without using any target domain labels. The adversarial learning of our network is guided by a GAN loss for mapping data distributions, a cycle-consistency loss for retaining pixel-level content, and a semantic-aware loss for enhancing structural information. We validated our method on two different chest X-ray public datasets for left/right lung segmentation. Experimental results show that the segmentation performance of our unsupervised approach is highly competitive with the upper bound of supervised transfer learning.

1 Introduction

Deep neural networks (DNNs) have achieved great success in automated medical image computing [4,11], attributing to their learned highly-representative features. However, due to domain shift, DNNs would suffer from performance degradation when being applied to new datasets, which are acquired with different protocols or collected from different clinical centers [6,9]. Actually, domain adaptation has been an important research topic in medical image computing and the traditional automated methods also encountered the same poor generalization problem. For example, Philipsen et al. [10] studied the influence of data

© Springer Nature Switzerland AG 2018
Y. Shi et al. (Eds.): MLMI 2018, LNCS 11046, pp. 143–151, 2018.
https://doi.org/10.1007/978-3-030-00919-9_17

distribution variations across chest radiography datasets on traditional segmentation methods based on k-nearest neighbor classification as well as active shape modeling.

To generalize DNNs trained on a *source domain* to a *target domain*, researches have been emerging for domain adaptation of deep learning models. A typical method is supervised transfer learning (STL), which fine-tunes the pre-trained source domain model with additional labeled target domain data. Remarkably, Ghafoorian *et al.* [6] studied on the number of fine-tuned layers to reduce the required amount of annotations for brain lesion segmentation across MRI datasets. However, the STL approaches still rely on extra labeled data, which is expensive or sometimes impractical to obtain.

Instead, unsupervised domain adaptation (UDA) is more appealing to generalize models in clinical practice. Early works have employed histogram matching to make test data resemble the intensity distribution of source domain data [15]. Recently, the generative adversarial networks (GANs) have made great achievements in generating realistic images and adversarial learning excels in mapping data distributions for domain adaptation [1,5,14]. In medical field, adversarial frameworks have been proposed to align feature embeddings between source and target data and presented promising results on cross-protocol brain lesion segmentation [9] and cross-modality cardiac segmentation [3]. Recent works adopted CycleGAN [16] as a data augmentation step to synthesize images from source domain to target domain, and used the pair of synthetic image and corresponding source label to train a segmentation model for target domain [2,7]. However, the synthetic images can be distorted on semantic structures, because the pure CycleGAN did not explicitly constrain the output of each single generator inside the cycle.

In this work, we propose a semantic-aware generative adversarial networks for unsupervised domain adaptation (named *SeUDA*) of medical image segmentation. Our method detaches the segmentation DNN from the domain adaptation process, and does not require any label from the test set. Given a test image, our *SeUDA* framework conducts image-to-image transformation to generate a source-like image which is directly forwarded to the established source DNN. To enhance the preservation of structural information during image transformation, we improve CycleGAN with a novel semantic-aware loss by embedding a nested adversarial learning in semantic label space. We validated our *SeUDA* on two different chest X-ray public datasets for lung segmentation. The performance of our unsupervised method exceeds the UDA baseline and is highly competitive with that of the supervised transfer learning. Last but not least, our transformed image results are visually observable, which sheds the light on the explicit intuition of our proposed method.

2   Method

Given the source domain images $x^s \in \mathcal{X}^s$ and the corresponding labels $y^s \in \mathcal{Y}$, we train a DNN model, denoted by f^s, which learns to segment the input images.

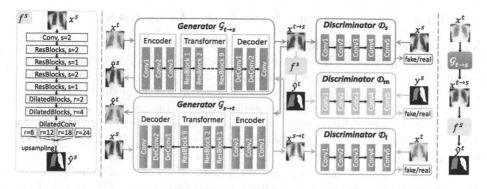

Fig. 1. The overview of our unsupervised domain adaptation framework. **Left**: the segmentation DNN learned on source domain; **Middle**: the *SeUDA* where the paired generator and discriminator are indicated with the same color, the blue/green arrows illustrate the data flows from original images (x^t/x^s) to transformed images $(x^{t\to s}/x^{s\to t})$ then back to reconstructed images $(\hat{x}^t/\hat{x}^s)$ in cycle-consistency loss, the orange part is the discriminator for the semantic-aware adversarial learning; **Right**: the inference process of *SeUDA* given a new target image for testing.

In UDA, we have unlabeled target images $x^t \in \mathcal{X}^t$ whose intensity distributions (or visual appearances) are not the same as the source domain data. Figure 1 presents an overview of our proposed *SeUDA* framework, which adapts the appearance of x^t to source image space $\mathcal{X}^s$, so that the established f^s can be directly generalized to the transformed image.

2.1 Segmentation Network Established on Source Domain

Our segmentation DNN model (referred as segmenter) is detached from the learning of our domain adaptation GANs. Compared with the integrated approaches, this advantage of an independent segmenter enables much more flexibility when designing a high-performance network architecture. In this regard, we establish a state-of-the-art segmentation network which makes complementary use of the residual connection, dilated convolution and multi-scale feature learning [11].

The backbone of our segmenter is modified ResNet-101. We replace the standard convolutional layers in the high-level residual blocks with the dilated convolutions. To leverage features with multi-scale receptive fields, we replace the last fully-connected layer with four parallel 3×3 dilated convolutional branches, with a dilation rate of $\{6, 12, 18, 24\}$, respectively. An upsampling layer is added in the end to produce dense predictions for the segmentation task. We start with 32 feature maps in the first layer and double the number of feature maps when the spatial size is halved or the dilation convolutions are utilized. The segmenter is optimized by minimizing the pixel-wise multi-class cross-entropy loss of the prediction $f^s(x^s)$ and ground truth y^s with standard stochastic gradient descent.

2.2   Image Transformation with Semantic-Aware GANs

After obtaining f^s which maps the source input space $\mathcal{X}^s$ to the semantic label space $\mathcal{Y}$, our goal is to make it generally applicable to new target datasets. Given that annotating medical data is quite expensive, we conduct the domain adaptation in an unsupervised manner. Specifically, we map the target images towards the source data space. The generated new image $x^{t\to s}$ appears to be drawn from $\mathcal{X}^s$ while the content and semantic structures remain unchanged. In this way, we can directly apply the well-established model f^s on $x^{t\to s}$ without re-training and get the segmentation result for x^t.

   To achieve this, we first construct a generator $\mathcal{G}_{t\to s}$ and a discriminator $\mathcal{D}_s$. The generator aims to produce realistic transformed image $x^{t\to s} = \mathcal{G}_{t\to s}(x^t)$. The discriminator competes with the generator by trying to distinguish between the fake generated data $x^{t\to s}$ and the real source data x^s. The GAN corresponds to a minimax two-player game and is optimized via the following objective:

$$\mathcal{L}_{\mathrm{GAN}}(\mathcal{G}_{t\to s}, \mathcal{D}_s) = \mathbb{E}_{x^s}[\log\mathcal{D}_s(x^s)] + \mathbb{E}_{x^t}[\log(1 - \mathcal{D}_s(\mathcal{G}_{t\to s}(x^t)))], \qquad (1)$$

where the discriminator tries to maximize this objective to correctly classify the $x^{t\to s}$ and x^s, while the generator tries to minimize $\log(1 - \mathcal{D}_s(\mathcal{G}_{t\to s}(x^t)))$ to learn the data distribution mapping from $\mathcal{X}^t$ to $\mathcal{X}^s$.

Cycle-consistency adversarial learning. For image transformation, the generated $x^{t\to s}$ should also preserve the detailed contents in the original x^t. Inspired by the CycleGAN [16] which sets the state-of-the-art for unpaired image-to-image transformation, we employ the cycle-consistency loss during the adversarial learning to maintain the contents with clinical clues of the target images.

   Inversely, we build a source-to-target generator $\mathcal{G}_{s\to t}$ and a target discriminator $\mathcal{D}_t$, so that the transformed image can be translated back to the original image. This pair of models are trained with a same-way GAN loss $\mathcal{L}_{\mathrm{GAN}}(\mathcal{G}_{s\to t}, \mathcal{D}_t)$ following the Eq. (1). In this regard, we derive the cycle-consistency loss which encourages $\mathcal{G}_{s\to t}(\mathcal{G}_{t\to s}(x^t)) \approx x^t$ and $\mathcal{G}_{t\to s}(\mathcal{G}_{s\to t}(x^s)) \approx x^s$ in the transformation:

$$\mathcal{L}_{\mathrm{cyc}}(\mathcal{G}_{t\to s}, \mathcal{G}_{s\to t}) = \mathbb{E}_{x^t}[||\mathcal{G}_{s\to t}(\mathcal{G}_{t\to s}(x^t)) - x^t||_1] + \mathbb{E}_{x^s}[||\mathcal{G}_{t\to s}(\mathcal{G}_{s\to t}(x^s)) - x^s||_1], \qquad (2)$$

where the L1-Norm is employed for reducing blurs in the generated images. This loss imposes the pixel-level penalty on the distance between the cyclic transformation result and the input image.

Semantic-aware adversarial learning. In our proposed *SeUDA*, we apply the established f^s to $x^{t\to s}$ which is obtained by inputting x^t to $\mathcal{G}_{t\to s}$. The image quality of $x^{t\to s}$ and the stability of $\mathcal{G}_{t\to s}$ are crucial for the effectiveness of our method. Therefore, besides the cycle-consistency loss which composes both generators and constraints the cyclic input-output consistency, we further try to explicitly enhance the intermediate transformation result $x^{t\to s}$. Specifically, for our segmentation domain adaptation task, we design a novel semantic-aware loss which aims to prevent the semantic distortion during the image transformation.

In our unsupervised learning scenario, we establish a nested adversarial learning module by adding another new discriminator $\mathcal{D}_m$ into the system. It distinguishes between the source domain ground truth lung mask y^s and the predicted lung mask $f^s(x^{t\to s})$ obtained by applying the segmenter on the source-like transformed image. Our underlying hypothesis is that the shape of anatomical structure is consistent across multi-center medical images. The prediction of $f^s(x^{t\to s})$ should follow the regular semantic structures of the lung to fool the $\mathcal{D}_m$, otherwise, the generator $\mathcal{G}_{t\to s}$ would be penalized by the semantic-aware loss:

$$\mathcal{L}_{\text{sem}}(\mathcal{G}_{t\to s}, \mathcal{D}_m) = \mathbb{E}_{y^s}[\log \mathcal{D}_m(y^s)] + \mathbb{E}_{x^t}[\log(1 - \mathcal{D}_m(f^s(\mathcal{G}_{t\to s}(x^t))))]. \quad (3)$$

This loss imposes an explicit constraint on the intermediate result of the cyclic transformation. Its gradients can assist the update of the generator $\mathcal{G}_{t\to s}$, which benefits the stability of the entire adversarial learning procedure.

2.3   Learning Procedure and Implementation Details

The configurations of the generators and discriminators follow the practice of [16]. Specifically, both generators have the same architecture consisting of an encoder (3 convolutions), a transformer (9 residual blocks) and a decoder (2 deconvolutions and 1 convolution). All the three discriminators process 70×70 patches and produce real/fake predictions via 3 stride-2 and 2 stride-1 convolutional layers. The overall objective for the generators and discriminators is as follows:

$$\mathcal{L}(\mathcal{G}_{s\to t}, \mathcal{G}_{t\to s}, \mathcal{D}_s, \mathcal{D}_t, \mathcal{D}_m) = \mathcal{L}_{GAN}(\mathcal{G}_{s\to t}, \mathcal{D}_t) + \alpha\mathcal{L}_{GAN}(\mathcal{G}_{t\to s}, \mathcal{D}_s) +$$
$$\beta\mathcal{L}_{\text{cyc}}(\mathcal{G}_{t\to s}, \mathcal{G}_{s\to t}) + \lambda\mathcal{L}_{\text{sem}}(\mathcal{G}_{t\to s}, \mathcal{D}_m), \quad (4)$$

where the $\{\alpha, \beta, \lambda\}$ denote trade-off hyper-parameters adjusting the importance of each component, which is empirically set to be $\{0.5, 10, 0.5\}$ in our experiments. The entire framework is optimized to obtain:

$$\mathcal{G}_{s\to t}^*, \mathcal{G}_{t\to s}^* = \arg\min_{\substack{\mathcal{G}_{s\to t} \\ \mathcal{G}_{t\to s}}} \max_{\mathcal{D}_s, \mathcal{D}_t, \mathcal{D}_m} \mathcal{L}(\mathcal{G}_{s\to t}, \mathcal{G}_{t\to s}, \mathcal{D}_s, \mathcal{D}_t, \mathcal{D}_m). \quad (5)$$

In our *SeUDA*, the generators $\{\mathcal{G}_{t\to s}, \mathcal{G}_{s\to t}\}$ and discriminators $\{\mathcal{D}_s, \mathcal{D}_t, \mathcal{D}_m\}$ are optimized altogether and updated successively. Note that the segmenter f^s is not updated in the process of image transformation. In practice, when training the generative adversarial networks, we followed the strategies of [16] for reducing model oscillation. Specifically, the negative log likelihood in $\mathcal{L}_{GAN}$ was replaced by a least-square loss to stabilize the training. The discriminator loss was calculated using one image from a collection of fifty previously generated images rather than the one produced in the latest training step. We used the Adam optimizer with an initial learning rate of 0.002, which was linearly decayed every 100 epochs. We implemented our proposed framework on the TensorFlow platform using an Nvidia Titan Xp GPU.

Table 1. Quantitative evaluation results of domain adaptation methods for both lung segmentations from chest X-ray images.

Methods	Right lung				Left lung			
	Dice	Recall	Precision	ASD	Dice	Recall	Precision	ASD
S-test	95.98	97.98	94.23	2.23	95.23	96.56	94.01	2.45
T-noDA	82.29	98.40	73.38	10.68	76.65	95.06	69.15	11.40
T-HistM [15]	90.05	92.96	88.05	5.72	91.03	94.35	88.45	4.66
T-FeatDA [9]	94.85	93.66	96.42	3.26	92.93	91.67	94.46	3.80
T-STL [6]	96.91	98.47	95.46	1.93	95.84	97.48	94.29	2.20
CyUDA	94.09	96.31	92.28	3.88	91.59	92.28	91.70	4.57
SeUDA	95.59	96.55	94.77	2.85	93.42	92.40	94.70	3.51

3   Experimental Results

Datasets and Evaluation Metrics. We validated our unsupervised domain adaptation method for lung segmentations using two public Chest X-ray datasets, i.e., the Montgomery set (138 cases) [8] and the JSRT set (247 cases) [13]. Both the datasets are typical X-ray scans collected in clinical practice, but their image distributions are quite different in terms of the disease type, intensity, and contrast (see the first and fourth column in Fig. 2(a)). The ground truth masks of left and right lungs are provided in both datasets. We randomly split each dataset into 7:1:2 for training, validation and test sets. All the images were resized to 512×512, and rescaled to $[0, 255]$. The prediction masks were post-processed with the largest connected-component selection and hole filling.

For evaluation metrics, we utilized four common segmentation measurements, i.e., the Dice coefficient ([%]), recall ([%]), precision ([%]) and average surface distance (ASD)([mm]). The first three metrics are measured based on the pixel-wise classification accuracy. The ASD assesses the model performance at boundaries and a lower value indicates better segmentation performance.

Experimental Settings. We employed the Montgomery set as source domain and the JSRT set as target domain. We first established the segmenter on source training data independently. Next, we test the segmenter under various settings: (1) testing on source domain (*S-test*); (2) directly testing on target data (*T-noDA*); (3) using histogram matching to adjust target images before testing (*T-HistM*); (4) aligning target features with the source domain as proposed in [9] (*T-FeatDA*); (5) fine-tuning the model on labeled target data before testing on JSRT (*T-STL*); In addition, we investigated the performance of our proposed domain adaptation method with and w/o the semantic-aware loss, i.e., *SeUDA* and *CyUDA*.

Comparison of Experimental Results Between Different Methods. As shown in Table 1, when directly applying the learned source domain segmenter

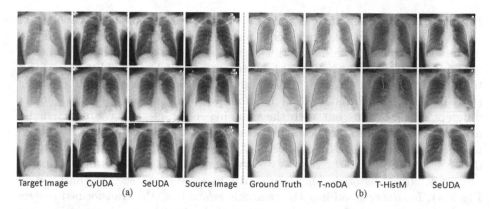

Target Image   CyUDA   SeUDA   Source Image | Ground Truth   T-noDA   T-HistM   SeUDA
(a)   (b)

Fig. 2. Typical results for the image transformation and lung segmentation. (a) Visualization of image transformation results, from left to right, are the target images in JSRT set, *CyUDA* transformation results, *SeUDA* transformation results, and the nearest neighbor of $x^{t \to s}$ got from source set; each row corresponds to one patient. (b) Comparison of segmentation results between the ground truth, *T-noDA*, *T-HistM*, and our proposed *SeUDA*; each row corresponds to one patient.

to target data (*T-noDA*), the model performance significantly degraded, indicating that domain shift would severely impede the generalization performance of DNNs. Specifically, the average Dice over both lungs dropped from 95.61% to 79.47%, and the average ASD increased from 2.34 to 11.04 mm.

With our proposed *SeUDA*, remarkable improvements have been achieved by applying the source segmenter on transformed target images. Compared with *T-noDA*, our *SeUDA* increased the average Dice by 15.04%. Meanwhile, the ASDs for both lungs were reduced significantly. Also, our method outperforms the UDA baseline histogram matching *T-HistM* with the average dice increased by 3.97% and average ASD decreased from 5.19 mm to 3.18 mm. Compared with the feature-level domain adaptation method *T-FeatDA*, our *SeUDA* can not only obtain higher segmentation performance, but also provide intuitive visualization of how the adaptation is achieved. Notably, the performance of our unsupervised *SeUDA* is even comparable to the upper bound of supervised *T-STL*. In Table 1, the gaps of Dice are marginal, i.e., 1.32% for right lung and 2.42% for left lung.

In Fig. 2(a), we can visualize typical transformed target images, demonstrating that *SeUDA* has successfully adapted the appearance of target data to look more similar to source images. In addition, the positions, contents, semantic structures and clinical clues are well preserved after transformation. In Fig. 2(b) we can observe that without domain adaptation, the predicted lung masks are quite cluttered. With histogram matching, appreciable improvements are obtained but the transformed images cannot mimic the source images very well. With our *SeUDA*, the lung areas are accurately segmented attributing to the successful target-to-source appearance transformation.

Effectiveness of Semantic-aware Loss. We investigated the contribution of our novel semantic-aware loss designed for segmentation domain adaptation. We implemented $CyUDA$ by removing the semantic-aware loss from the $SeUDA$. One notorious problem of GANs is that their training would be unstable and sensitive to initialization states [1,12]. In this study, we measured the standard deviation (std) of the $CyUDA$ and $SeUDA$ by running each model for 10 times under different initializations but with the same hyper-parameters. We observed significant lower variability on the segmentation performance across the 10 $SeUDA$ models than the 10 $CyUDA$ models, i.e., Dice std: 0.25% v.s. 2.03%, ASD std: 0.16 v.s. 1.19 mm. Qualitatively, we observe that the $CyUDA$ transformed images may suffer from distorted lung boundaries in some cases, see the third row in Fig. 2(a). In contrast, adding the semantic-aware loss, the transformed images consistently present a high quality. This reveals that the novel semantic-aware loss contributes to stabilize the image transformation process and prevent the distortion in structural contents, and hence contributes to boost the performance of segmentation domain adaptation.

4   Conclusion

This paper proposes a novel approach $SeUDA$ for unsupervised domain adaptation of medical image segmentation. The $SeUDA$ leverages GANs to transform the target images to resemble source images and generalize the source segmentation DNN directly on the transformed images. We design a novel objective which composes a GAN loss for mapping data distributions, a cycle-consistency loss to preserve the pixel-level content, and a semantic-aware loss to enhance the structural information. Our method is highly competitive with the supervised transfer learning on the task of lung segmentation in chest X-rays. Our proposed $SeUDA$ solution is general and can inspire more researches on domain adaptation problems in medical image computing.

Acknowledgments. The work described in this paper was supported by a grant from the Research Grants Council of the Hong Kong Special Administrative Region (Project no. GRF 14225616) and a grant from Hong Kong Innovation and Technology Commission (Project no. ITS/426/17FP).

References

1. Bousmalis, K., Silberman, N., Dohan, D., et al.: Unsupervised pixel-level domain adaptation with generative adversarial networks. In: CVPR. pp. 95–104 (2017)
2. Chartsias, A., Joyce, T., Dharmakumar, R., Tsaftaris, S.A.: Adversarial image synthesis for unpaired multi-modal cardiac data. In: Tsaftaris, S.A., Gooya, A., Frangi, A.F., Prince, J.L. (eds.) SASHIMI 2017. LNCS, vol. 10557, pp. 3–13. Springer, Cham (2017). https://doi.org/10.1007/978-3-319-68127-6_1
3. Dou, Q., Ouyang, C., Chen, C., Chen, H., Heng, P.: Unsupervised cross-modality domain adaptation of convnets for biomedical image segmentations with adversarial loss. In: IJCAI, pp. 691–697 (2018)

4. Dou, Q., et al.: Automated pulmonary nodule detection via 3d convnets with online sample filtering and hybrid-loss residual learning. In: MICCAI, pp. 630–638 (2017)
5. Ganin, Y., Ustinova, E., Ajakan, H.: Domain-adversarial training of neural networks. J. Mach. Learn. Res. **17**(1), 2096–2030 (2016)
6. Ghafoorian, M., et al.: Transfer learning for domain adaptation in MRI: application in brain lesion segmentation. In: Descoteaux, M., Maier-Hein, L., Franz, A., Jannin, P., Collins, D.L., Duchesne, S. (eds.) MICCAI 2017. LNCS, vol. 10435, pp. 516–524. Springer, Cham (2017). https://doi.org/10.1007/978-3-319-66179-7_59
7. Huo, Y., Xu, Z., Bao, S., et al.: Adversarial synthesis learning enables segmentation without target modality ground truth. arXiv preprint arXiv:1712.07695 (2017)
8. Jaeger, S.: Two public chest x-ray datasets for computer-aided screening of pulmonary diseases. Quant. Imaging Med. Surg. **4**(6), 475 (2014)
9. Kamnitsas, K., et al.: Unsupervised domain adaptation in brain lesion segmentation with adversarial networks. In: Niethammer, M., et al. (eds.) IPMI 2017. LNCS, vol. 10265, pp. 597–609. Springer, Cham (2017). https://doi.org/10.1007/978-3-319-59050-9_47
10. Philipsen, R.H., Maduskar, P., Hogeweg, L., Melendez, J., Sánchez, C.I., van Ginneken, B.: Localized energy-based normalization of medical images: application to chest radiography. IEEE Trans. Med. Imaging **34**(9), 1965–1975 (2015)
11. Ronneberger, O., Fischer, P., Brox, T.: U-Net: convolutional networks for biomedical image segmentation. In: Navab, N., Hornegger, J., Wells, W.M., Frangi, A.F. (eds.) MICCAI 2015. LNCS, vol. 9351, pp. 234–241. Springer, Cham (2015). https://doi.org/10.1007/978-3-319-24574-4_28
12. Salimans, T., Goodfellow, I., et al.: Improved techniques for training gans. Adv. Neural Inf. Process. Syst. 2234–2242 (2016)
13. Shiraishi, J., Katsuragawa, S., Ikezoe, J., Matsumoto, T., Kobayashi, T.: Development of a digital image database for chest radiographs with and without a lung nodule: receiver operating characteristic analysis of radiologists' detection of pulmonary nodules. Am. J. Roentgenol. **174**(1), 71–74 (2000)
14. Tzeng, E., Hoffman, J., Saenko, K., Darrell, T.: Adversarial discriminative domain adaptation. In: CVPR, pp. 2962–2971 (2017)
15. Wang, L.: Correction for variations in mri scanner sensitivity in brain studies with histogram matching. Magn. Reson. Med. **39**(2), 322–327 (1998)
16. Zhu, J., Park, T., Isola, P., Efros, A.A.: Unpaired image-to-image translation using cycle-consistent adversarial networks. In: ICCV, pp. 2242–2251 (2017)

Brain Status Prediction with Non-negative Projective Dictionary Learning

Mingli Zhang[1(✉)], Christian Desrosiers[2], Yuhong Guo[3], Caiming Zhang[4], Budhachandra Khundrakpam[1], and Alan Evans[1]

[1] Montreal Neurological Institute, McGill University, Montreal, Canada
mingli.zhang@mcgill.ca
[2] École de Technologie Supérieure, Montreal, Canada
[3] School of Computer Science, Carleton University, Ottawa, Canada
[4] Shandong Co-Innovation Center of Future Intelligent Computing, Yantai, China

Abstract. Study on brain status prediction has recently received increasing attention from the research community. In this paper, we propose to tackle brain status prediction by learning a discriminative representation of the data with a novel non-negative projective dictionary learning (NPDL) approach. The proposed approach performs class-wise projective dictionary learning, which uses an analysis dictionary to generate non-negative coding vectors from the data, and a synthesis dictionary to reconstruct the data. We formulate the learning problem as a constrained non-convex optimization problem and solve it via an alternating direction method of multipliers (ADMM). To investigate the effectiveness of the proposed approach on brain status prediction, we conduct experiments on two datasets, ADNI and NIH Study of Normal Brain Development repository, and report superior results over comparison methods.

1 Introduction

With the aging of the global population, age-related decline of cognitive functions and neurodegenerative disorders are becoming more prevalent. This leads to an important increase in health-related costs and constitutes a major burden on society. Brain degeneration is a complex process occurring progressively throughout life [2]. The high variability in this process also has a significant impact on human lifespan and the development of age-related diseases. Predicting brain status is therefore essential to identify subjects with higher risks of deterioration, estimate the progress of cognitive decline over time, and help to select optimal treatment.

Alzheimer's disease (AD) is the most common form of dementia, accounting for 60% to 80% of cases. Aging is the main risk factor for this neurodegenerative disease, the majority of patients being 65 years or older. However, in about 5%

© Springer Nature Switzerland AG 2018
Y. Shi et al. (Eds.): MLMI 2018, LNCS 11046, pp. 152–160, 2018.
https://doi.org/10.1007/978-3-030-00919-9_18

of cases, symptoms will occur before the age of 65 in what is known as early-onset Alzheimer's [13]. In the clinical context, an important task is to predict if a subject with mild cognitive impairment (MCI) will develop AD or not within a given period (e.g., 3 years) [11]. Discriminating between stable MCI (sMCI) and progressive MCI (pMCI) cases can help clinicians treat patients sooner so that potential disease-modifying therapies could be tested and applied.

Various studies in the literature have focused on predicting brain maturity (or *brain age*) [2,9] or MCI-to-AD conversion [3,10,11] using non-invasive neuroimaging techniques. Although large initiatives like Alzheimer's Disease Neuroimaging Initiative (ADNI) have led to significant improvements in recent years, the prediction of brain aging and AD progression remains challenging tasks.

This study proposes a novel approach called non-negative projective dictionary learning (NPDL) for brain status prediction. Based on the method of Gu et al. [6], our approach is similar to autoencoders [7] where input feature vectors are first encoded to a compact representation preserving semantic information and then reconstructed in a decoding step. In our approach, encoding and decoding steps are performed using two separate dictionaries: the analysis (or *projective*) dictionary and the synthesis dictionary. While autoencoders are an unsupervised feature learning technique, our approach also considers class labels to find class-specific dictionaries that can reconstruct accurately same-class examples but not those from other classes. The major contributions of this work are as follows:

- **Novel framework:** Our framework extends the dictionary pair learning (DPL) method of Gu et al. [6] in two important ways. While DPL applies simple norm constraints on the dictionary atoms, we also impose these atoms to be uncorrelated. In addition to helping avoid overfitting, this facilitates the visualization of features learned in the dictionary, as these features encode orthogonal components of the data. Moreover, unlike DPL, our framework also enforces non-negativity on the projected features. Our experiments show these strategies to improve classification accuracy compared to DPL.
- **Clinical applications:** We evaluate our NPDL framework using ADNI data [11] on the task of predicting MCI to AD conversion within three years, and show very competitive performance compared to recently proposed methods for this task. Our framework is also evaluated on longitudinal MRI data from the NIH Study of Normal Brain Development repository [4]. Results indicate our framework's ability to accurately predict the brain age of subjects from this dataset.

The rest of this paper is organized as follows. In Sect. 2, we present our NPDL model for class-wise projective dictionary learning. We describe how dictionaries can be obtained efficiently from training data using an alternating direction method of multipliers (ADMM) [1] and analyze the complexity and converge of the proposed training algorithm. Section 3 then evaluates our approach on the prediction of MCI-to-AD conversion and subject age. Finally, we conclude with a summary of main contributions and results.

2   The Proposed Approach

2.1   Non-negative Projective Dictionary Learning

We treat brain status prediction as a general classification problem over K classes. Let $\mathbf{X} = [\mathbf{X}_1, \cdots, \mathbf{X}_k, \cdots, \mathbf{X}_K]$ denote the data samples, where each $\mathbf{X}_k \in \mathbb{R}^{S \times N_k}$ represents the data samples belonging to the k-th class. We first propose to discriminatively model the data by performing separate projective dictionary learning on the subsamples from each different class. Specifically, we introduce an analysis dictionary $\mathbf{P}_k \in \mathbb{R}^{M \times S}$ and a synthesis dictionary $\mathbf{D}_k \in \mathbb{R}^{S \times M}$ for each class k, such that $\mathbf{P} = [\mathbf{P}_1, \cdots, \mathbf{P}_k, \cdots, \mathbf{P}_K]$ and $\mathbf{D} = [\mathbf{D}_1, \cdots, \mathbf{D}_k, \cdots, \mathbf{D}_K]$, and perform data modeling in the following class-specific dictionary pair learning framework:

$$\underset{\mathbf{P},\mathbf{D}}{\arg\min} \sum_{k=1}^{K} \|\mathbf{X}_k - \mathbf{D}_k\mathbf{P}_k\mathbf{X}_k\|_F^2 + \lambda\|\mathbf{P}_k\overline{\mathbf{X}}_k\|_F^2, \tag{1}$$

where $\|\cdot\|_F$ is the Frobenius norm and $\overline{\mathbf{X}}_k$ denotes the complementary data matrix of $\mathbf{X}_k$ in $\mathbf{X}$, i.e. $\overline{\mathbf{X}}_k = [\mathbf{X}_1, \cdots, \mathbf{X}_{k-1}, \mathbf{X}_{k+1}, \cdots, \mathbf{X}_K]$. In this framework, the regularization term $\|\mathbf{P}_k\overline{\mathbf{X}}_k\|_F^2$ is used to ensure class-specific dictionary learning by pushing $\mathbf{P}_k\mathbf{X}_j$ towards zero over data samples from any class j such that $j \neq k$. The analysis dictionary $\mathbf{P}_k$ projects the samples $\mathbf{X}_k$ into an encoding coefficient matrix $\mathbf{A}_k = \mathbf{P}_k\mathbf{X}_k$, which is then used to reconstruct $\mathbf{X}_k$ with the synthesis dictionary $\mathbf{D}_k$. Parameter $\lambda > 0$ controls the trade-off between the reconstruction accuracy and regularization terms.

To avoid overfitting, dictionary pair learning methods like [6] normally use a Frobenius norm regularization term over $\mathbf{D}_k$ or a Euclidean norm constraint over each column of this dictionary. Here, we aim to identify a compact synthesis dictionary $\mathbf{D}_k$ with uncorrelated dictionary basis vectors. Toward this goal, we impose an orthogonality constraint over the dictionary: $\mathbf{D}_k^\top\mathbf{D}_k = \mathbf{I}$. Moreover, we further assume the basis vectors of $\mathbf{D}_k$ model the representative latent components of $\mathbf{X}_k$. Hence, $\mathbf{X}_k$ can be taken as an additive combination of these components by enforcing the encoding coefficients $\mathbf{A}_k = \mathbf{P}_k\mathbf{X}_k$ to be non-negative. This leads to the following non-negative projective dictionary learning (NPDL) problem:

$$\underset{\mathbf{P},\mathbf{D}}{\arg\min} \sum_{k=1}^{K} \|\mathbf{X}_k - \mathbf{D}_k\mathbf{P}_k\mathbf{X}_k\|_F^2 + \lambda\|\mathbf{P}_k\overline{\mathbf{X}}_k\|_F^2$$

$$\text{s.t.} \quad \mathbf{D}_k^\top\mathbf{D}_k = \mathbf{I}, \quad \mathbf{P}_k\mathbf{X}_k \geq 0, \, k = 1, ..., K. \tag{2}$$

The next section presents an efficient optimization approach to learn dictionary sets $\mathbf{D}$ and $\mathbf{P}$ from training data.

2.2   Training Algorithm

The model in (2) is a non-convex optimization problem with both orthogonality and non-negativity constraints. We propose to solve it using an alternating direction method of multipliers (ADMM). Specifically, we introduce an explicit encoding coefficient matrix $\mathbf{A}_k$ with the equality constraint $\mathbf{A}_k = \mathbf{P}_k\mathbf{X}_k$ for each class k, and then incorporate such constraints into the objective with auxiliary variable matrices $\{\mathbf{Z}_k\}$. This leads to a minimization of the following augmented Lagrangian function:

$$\arg\min_{\mathbf{P},\mathbf{D},\mathbf{A}} \sum_{k=1}^{K} \|\mathbf{X}_k - \mathbf{D}_k\mathbf{P}_k\mathbf{X}_k\|_F^2 + \lambda\|\mathbf{P}_k\overline{\mathbf{X}}_k\|_F^2 + \mu\|\mathbf{A}_k - \mathbf{P}_k\mathbf{X}_k + \mathbf{Z}_k\|_F^2$$

$$\text{s.t. } \mathbf{D}_k^\top\mathbf{D}_k = \mathbf{I}, \quad \mathbf{A}_k \geq 0, \; k = 1, ..., K. \tag{3}$$

The ADMM algorithm then performs optimization in an iterative manner. In each iteration, it alternatively updates each variable matrix given the other variable matrices fixed, as follows.

Updating P: With fixed $\{\mathbf{D}, \mathbf{A}, \mathbf{Z}\}$, the minimization over each $\mathbf{P}_k$ is an unconstrained quadratic minimization problem:

$$\arg\min_{\mathbf{P}_k} \quad \|\mathbf{X}_k - \mathbf{D}_k\mathbf{P}_k\mathbf{X}_k\|_F^2 + \lambda\|\mathbf{P}_k\overline{\mathbf{X}}_k\|_F^2 + \mu\|\mathbf{P}_k\mathbf{X}_k - (\mathbf{A}_k + \mathbf{Z}_k)\|_F^2$$

which has the following closed-form solution:

$$\mathbf{P}_k = \left(\mathbf{D}_k^\top\mathbf{X}_k\mathbf{X}_k^\top + \mu(\mathbf{A}_k + \mathbf{Z}_k)\mathbf{X}_k^\top\right)\left((1+\mu)\mathbf{X}_k\mathbf{X}_k^\top + \lambda\overline{\mathbf{X}}_k\overline{\mathbf{X}}_k^\top + \gamma\mathbf{I}\right)^{-1} \tag{4}$$

where γ is a small constant used to increase invertibility. Following [6], we set this parameter to $\gamma = 10e^{-4}$.

Updating D: Given fixed $\{\mathbf{A}, \mathbf{P}, \mathbf{Z}\}$, the minimization over each $\mathbf{D}_k$ is an orthogonal constrained optimization problem:

$$\arg\min_{\mathbf{D}_k} \|\mathbf{X}_k - \mathbf{D}_k\mathbf{P}_k\mathbf{X}_k\|_F^2, \text{ s.t. } \mathbf{D}_k^\top\mathbf{D}_k = \mathbf{I}$$

which can be equivalently rewritten into

$$\arg\max_{\mathbf{D}_k} \text{tr}(\mathbf{D}_k^\top\mathbf{X}_k\mathbf{X}_k^\top\mathbf{P}_k^\top), \text{ s.t. } \mathbf{D}_k^\top\mathbf{D}_k = \mathbf{I}, \tag{5}$$

Let $\mathbf{U}\mathbf{\Sigma}\mathbf{V}^\top$ be the singular value decomposition (SVD) of $\mathbf{X}_k\mathbf{X}_k^\top\mathbf{P}_k^\top$. Then problem (5) has the following solution: $\mathbf{D}_k = \mathbf{U}\mathbf{V}^\top$.

Updating A: Given fixed $\{\mathbf{D}, \mathbf{P}, \mathbf{Z}\}$, we have a non-negative constrained minimization problem over each $\mathbf{A}_k$:

$$\arg\min_{\mathbf{A}_k} \|\mathbf{A}_k - (\mathbf{P}_k\mathbf{X}_k - \mathbf{Z}_k)\|_F^2, \text{ s.t. } \mathbf{A}_k \geq 0, \tag{6}$$

which has the following solution: $\mathbf{A}_k = \max(\mathbf{P}_k\mathbf{X}_k - \mathbf{Z}_k, 0)$.

Updating $\{\mathbf{Z}_k\}$: Finally, we update the dual variable $\mathbf{Z}_k$ following the standard ADMM algorithm: $\mathbf{Z}_k := \mathbf{Z}_k + (\mathbf{A}_k - \mathbf{P}_k\mathbf{X}_k)$.

2.3 Classification

Once learned, the dictionaries can be used to classify new samples by measuring the reconstruction error for each class. Let $\mathbf{x} \in \mathbb{R}^S$ be the feature vector of a sample to classify, we assign $\mathbf{x}$ to the class whose dictionary gives the lowest error:

$$k^* = \arg\min_k \|\mathbf{x} - \mathbf{D}_k\mathbf{P}_k\mathbf{x}\|_2. \tag{7}$$

Figure 1 shows an example of reconstruction residuals obtained with the same-class dictionary and with the dictionary of another class.

2.4 Complexity and Convergence

The computational complexity of the proposed dictionary learning framework is as follows. For updating dictionaries $\mathbf{P}_k$ with (4), since the matrix to invert is constant, its inverse can be computed only once in pre-processing. The complexity of this update step is therefore in $O\big(KM(S + \max_k\{N_k\})\big)$. Next, updating each $\mathbf{D}_k$ requires to calculate the SVD of $S \times M$ matrix $\mathbf{X}_k\mathbf{X}_k^\top\mathbf{P}_k^\top$. If the QR decomposition of $\mathbf{X}_k\mathbf{X}_k^\top$ is pre-computed, assuming that $M \leq S$, this step has a total complexity of $O(KM^3)$. Finally, updating all matrices $\mathbf{A}_k$ and $\mathbf{Z}_k$ can be done in $O(KM\max_k\{N_k\})$ operations.

While ADMM convergence analyses in the literature have mostly focused on convex problems, recent works have shown the convergence of this method for a broad set of non-convex problems [8]. The stability of ADMM has also been assessed empirically for various non-convex problems including biconvex formulations like the one in (2) [12]. An important factor for convergence is the choice of penalty parameter μ. In this work, we used a fixed value for μ as this strategy gave a good convergence in our experiments. However, an adaptive update scheme could also be employed to speed-up this convergence [1].

3   Experiments

The usefulness of our NPDL framework is assessed on the tasks of predicting the conversion of MCI subjects to AD and predicting brain age in developing subjects, using measures of cortical thickness. For both tasks, the following strategy was employed to tune parameters and measure performance. We first split available examples into a training set and validation set, the latter containing 10% of examples. The validation set was used to tune the regularization parameter λ and synthesis dictionary size M, and then discarded to avoid bias contamination in subsequent experiments. Afterwards, a 10-fold cross-validation is applied on the training set to measure performance in terms of prediction accuracy and area under the ROC curve (AUC). All experiments were performed in Matlab R2017b using a i7-6700K CPU with 16GB of RAM.

3.1   Prediction of MCI-to-AD Conversion

We first evaluate our framework with the pre-processed ADNI data used in [10,11]. In this experiment, cortical thickness measures obtained from a standard pipeline like CIVET[1] are aggregated with age and six cognitive scores: mini mental state examination (MMSE), clinical dementia rating-sum of boxes (CDR-SB), Rey's auditory verbal learning test (RAVLT), functional activities questionnaire (FAQ), and Alzheimer's disease assessment scale cognitive subset (AADAS-cog).

Table 1 compares the mean accuracy (ACC) and AUC obtained by our NPDL approach to that of recently proposed methods for MCI-to-AD prediction, all of which are based on random forest (RF) classifiers. We see that our approach outperforms all other methods, both in terms of accuracy and AUC. Compared to [11], our approach yields improvements of about 3% in accuracy and 1% in AUC. This difference is statistically significant with p-value < 0.05 in a one-sided t-test.

Table 1. Classification results of pMCI vs sMCI with the ADNI subset in [11].

Method	Data	pMCI/sMCI	Conv. time (months)	ACC	AUC
RF [10]	MRI, age, cog. scores	164/100	0–36	82%	90%
RF [11]	MRI, age, cog. scores	164/100	0–36	84%	92%
Ours	MRI, age, cog. scores	164/100	0–36	**87%**	**93%**

3.2   Prediction of Brain Age

We also demonstrate our approach's ability to predict the brain age of children and adolescents ranging from 5 to 22 years old, based only on cortical thickness measures. For this experiment, we used data from NIH-funded MRI Study of Normal Brain Development (hereafter, NIHPD, for NIH pediatric database) [4], using the same MRI acquisition protocol and cortical thickness measurements as [9]. This dataset contains 678 longitudinal scans from 308 subjects (172 females/136 males) with the following characteristics: average age 12.9 ± 3.8, full scale intelligence quotient FSIQ 111.7 ± 12.1, performance intelligence quotient (PIQ) 110.6 ± 12.7, verbal intelligence quotient (VIQ) 110.3 ± 12.9. Subjects were separated into female and male individuals, and then further divided in five age groups ([5]): preschool childhood (5−7 years), late childhood (8−11 years), early adolescence (12−16 years), middle adolescence (16−18 years), and late adolescence (19−22 years). The classification task is to predict the age group of a new subject.

---

[1] http://www.bic.mni.mcgill.ca/ServicesSoftware/CIVET.

Table 2. The Accuracy (ACC) on the database of NIHPD.

Method	ACC (male)	ACC (female)	Time (ms)
RF [11]	75.1%	74.7%	8.6
DPL [6]	86.3%	85.7%	0.3
Ours (w/o non-neg.)	87.5%	84.9%	0.4
Ours (with non-neg.)	**88.9%**	**87.6%**	0.4

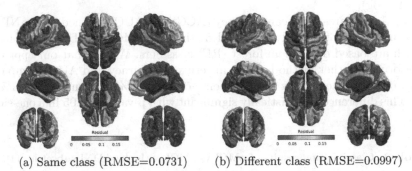

    (a) Same class (RMSE=0.0731)   (b) Different class (RMSE=0.0997)

Fig. 1. Example of reconstruction residuals obtained for a late-adolescent subject using (a) the same-class dictionary, and (b) the dictionary of a different class.

The mean prediction accuracy for male/female subjects and the runtime (in seconds) of our approach is given in Table 2. As comparison baseline, we also report the performance of the random forest method presented in [11] and of the dictionary pair learning (DPL) algorithm [6]. Furthermore, to measure the impact of non-negativity, we also give the accuracy obtained without this constraint. We note that DPL is equivalent to removing both non-negativity and orthogonality constraints from our NPDL model. Results show our method to be superior to the RF method of [11], in terms of both accuracy and efficiency. With respect to DPL, our approach improves accuracy by 2% to 3%, demonstrating the advantage of imposing orthogonality and non-negativity constraints in the dictionary learning model. Once again, these differences are statistically significant with p-value < 0.05. The benefit of having non-negative encoding coefficients is further supported by the improvement over using our model without these constraints.

Figure 1 shows an example or reconstruction residuals, i.e. $|\mathbf{x} - \mathbf{DPx}|$, obtained for a late-adolescent subject using the same class dictionary (*left*) and the dictionary of a different class (*right*). As expected, using the same-class dictionary leads to smaller residual values, with a global RMSE of 0.0731 compared to 0.0997. Moreover, to visualize features learned by our model, Fig. 2 plots the values of two atoms (i.e., columns of $\mathbf{D}$) for the dictionary of the late-adolescent class. We observe that these atoms encode information with very different spatial distribution.

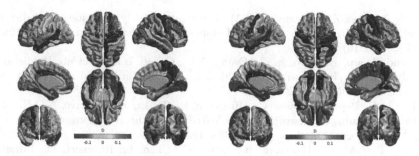

Fig. 2. Examples of dictionary atoms corresponding to the late-adolescent class.

4   Conclusion

We proposed a novel non-negative projective dictionary learning approach for predicting brain status. This approach extends conventional methods for learning discriminative dictionaries by imposing both orthogonality and non-negativity constraints. An efficient algorithm based on ADMM was presented to learn the dictionaries from training data. Experiments on the tasks of predicting the conversion from MCI to AD and predicting brain age showed the advantages of our approach compared to recent methods for these tasks. Future work includes a deeper analysis of learned features, to link these features with known results in the literature.

Acknowledgments. This work is supported by HBHL FRQ/CCC Axis X-C (Funding No. 246117), Canada, NSFC Joint Fund with Zhejiang Integration of Informatization and Industrialization under Key Project (U1609218), China.

References

1. Boyd, S., Parikh, N., Chu, E., Peleato, B., Eckstein, J.: Distributed optimization and statistical learning via the alternating direction method of multipliers. Found. Trends®. Mach. Learn. **3**(1), 1–122 (2011)
2. Cole, J.H., Franke, K.: Predicting age using neuroimaging: innovative brain ageing biomarkers. Trends Neurosci. **40**, 681–690 (2017)
3. Eskildsen, S.F., Coupé, P., Fonov, V.S., Pruessner, J.C., Collins, D.L., Initiative, A.D.N.: Structural imaging biomarkers of Alzheimer's disease: predicting disease progression. Neurobiol. Aging **36**, S23–S31 (2015)
4. Evans, A.C., Group, B.D.C., et al.: The NIH MRI study of normal brain development. Neuroimage **30**(1), 184–202 (2006)
5. Franke, K., Luders, E., May, A., Wilke, M., Gaser, C.: Brain maturation: predicting individual BrainAGE in children and adolescents using structural MRI. Neuroimage **63**(3), 1305–1312 (2012)
6. Gu, S., Zhang, L., Zuo, W., Feng, X.: Projective dictionary pair learning for pattern classification. Adv. Neural Inf. Process. Syst. 793–801 (2014)
7. Hinton, G.E., Salakhutdinov, R.R.: Reducing the dimensionality of data with neural networks. Science **313**(5786), 504–507 (2006)

8. Hong, M., Luo, Z.Q., Razaviyayn, M.: Convergence analysis of alternating direction method of multipliers for a family of nonconvex problems. SIAM J. Optim. **26**(1), 337–364 (2016)
9. Khundrakpam, B.S., Tohka, J., Evans, A.C., Group, B.D.C., et al.: Prediction of brain maturity based on cortical thickness at different spatial resolutions. Neuroimage **111**, 350–359 (2015)
10. Moradi, E., Pepe, A., Gaser, C., Huttunen, H., Tohka, J., Initiative, A.D.N., et al.: Machine learning framework for early MRI-based Alzheimer's conversion prediction in MCI subjects. Neuroimage **104**, 398–412 (2015)
11. Tong, T., Gao, Q., Guerrero, R., Ledig, C., Chen, L., Rueckert, D., Initiative, A.D.N.: A novel grading biomarker for the prediction of conversion from mild cognitive impairment to Alzheimer's disease. IEEE Trans. Biomed. Eng. **64**(1), 155–165 (2017)
12. Xu, Z., De, S., Figueiredo, M., Studer, C., Goldstein, T.: An empirical study of admm for nonconvex problems. arXiv preprint arXiv:1612.03349 (2016)
13. Zhu, X.C., et al.: Rate of early onset alzheimers disease: a systematic review and meta-analysis. Ann. Trans. Med. **3**(3) (2015)

Classification of Pancreatic Cystic Neoplasms Based on Multimodality Images

Weixiang Chen[1,2,3], Hongchen Ji[4], Jianjiang Feng[1,2,3(✉)], Rong Liu[4(✉)],
Yi Yu[1], Ruiquan Zhou[4], and Jie Zhou[1,2,3]

[1] Department of Automation, Tsinghua University, Beijing, China
jfeng@tsinghua.edu.cn
[2] State Key Lab of Intelligent Technologies and Systems, Tsinghua University,
Beijing, China
[3] Beijing National Research Center for Information Science and Technology,
Beijing, China
[4] Department of Hepatobiliary and Pancreatic Surgical Oncology, Chinese PLA
General Hospital and Chinese PLA Medical School, Beijing, China
liurong301@126.com

Abstract. Classification of pancreatic cystic neoplasms (PCN) into subclasses is crucial since their treatments are different. However, accurate
classification is very difficult even for radiologists, due to similar appearance and shape. We propose a network called PCN-Net which makes
use of T1/T2 MRI of abdomen by its three stages design. The first and
second stages are trained on T1 and T2 separately for detection and
inter-modality registration. After a Z-Continuity Filter and modalities
fusion, the third stage predict the results with registered image pairs.
On a database of 48 patients, our method can predict with slice level
accuracy of 80.0% and patient level accuracy of 92.3%, which are much
better than other baseline methods.

1 Introduction

Pancreatic Cystic Neoplasms (PCN) represent for approximately 10%–15% of
primary cystic masses of the pancreas [5]. Mucinous Cystic Neoplasms (MCN),
Intraductal Papillary Mucinous Neoplasm (IPMN) and Serous Cystic Neoplasms
(SCN) are three main kinds of PCN, and they represent separately for 45%, 25%
and 30% [3]. Different subclasses of PCN have quite different malignant poten-
tials where IPMN and MCN have a high malignant potential, while SCN is
largely benign lesion. Hence, accurate classification based on noninvasive imaging (CT, MRI) is very desirable. However, reported classification accuracy of
radiologists is quite low, 53.9% for CT and 59.6% for MRI [9]. As a result, diagnosis of PCN, especially distinction between MCN and SCN, via medical images
remains a challenge for both clinicians and researchers.

W. Chen and H. Ji—contributed equally to this work.

© Springer Nature Switzerland AG 2018
Y. Shi et al. (Eds.): MLMI 2018, LNCS 11046, pp. 161–169, 2018.
https://doi.org/10.1007/978-3-030-00919-9_19

CAD publications focused on diagnosis of pancreatic disease appeared just in recent years. It is a challenging problem because pancreas is a small organ hiding deeply in abdomen and pancreatic diseases have many subclasses. Previous publications about pancreas mainly focused on pancreas segmentation [2,11,15] and pancreatic cysts segmentation [14]. In more recent years, [4] proposed methods to identify IPMN via T2 MRIs, [8] used shape of pancreas segmentation to identify Pancreatic Ductal Adenocarcinoma (PDAC), which is another type of pancreatic disease. Distinction between MCN and SCN is much more challenging, and has not been studied to the best of our knowledge.

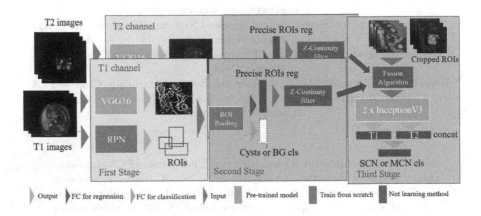

Fig. 1. Framework of our proposed method.

In this paper, we proposed a detection and classification network called PCN-Net for MCN and SCN using two modalities of MRI, which are T2 and T1 weighted MRIs since they are routinely captured in hospitals. For detection, instead of using pancreas to cyst localization like [14], we proposed a modified Faster-RCNN [10] to detect cysts in both modalities. Together with detection, approximate registration between modalities is done. After modality fusion method, we used deep networks for classification. We yield an accuracy of 80.0% at slice level and 92.3% at patient level on dataset collected by clinicians in cooperation hospital. The contributions of this paper include:

1. Propose a three-stage modified Faster-RCNN for multimodality cysts detection and classification.
2. Propose the first deep learning algorithm for on MCN and SCN detection and identification.
3. Yield good accuracy in diagnosis of MCN and SCN.

2 Methodology

2.1 Framework of PCN-Net

Our proposed PCN-Net extends the Faster-RCNN from two stages to three stages, as Fig. 1 shows. The first stage is used for feature extraction and region proposal. The second stage is used to compute accurate bounding boxes and the third stage is used for classification. First two stages compute separately for two modalities. After a carefully designed Z-Continuity filter and fusion procedure, features of two modalities are merged together into image pairs. Finally the image pairs are used for identification in the third stage.

2.2 First Stage: Feature Extraction and Region Proposal

We use VGG16 [12] with weights trained on ImageNet [12] as our feature extraction network. MRI images are rescaled to $h \times 600 \times 3$ by repeating 3 times to match number of channels (in order to use pretrained weights). The shorter side is rescaled to 600 and h represents the rescaled longer side (block ratio of length to width).

RPN of the proposed method will firstly sample the the feature maps extracted from former part with a 3×3 kernel. Because the cyst is usually small comparing to the whole image, our method propose 1024 regions of interest per image to make sure some of them capture the cyst. In addition, cysts vary in size and shape, so we design 25 kinds of anchors with scales of $4, 8, 16, 24, 32$ pixels and ratios of $0.5, 0.75, 1, 1.5, 2$. After RPN, more than 20,000 Region Of Interests (ROI) are proposed and a Non Maximum Suppression (NMS) procedure is used to decrease the number.

2.3 Second Stage: Intra-modality Localization and Inter-modality Registration

The second stage of PCN-Net aims to precisely detect cysts via ROIs. In this stage, both MCN and SCN are labeled as the same class, cyst, because results of separately detecting two kinds of neoplasms are worse than detecting them together (see Sect. 3.3). For every ROI from the first stage, ROI-pooling is done and two fully-connected layers are set to learn the precise offsets of bounding box from input positions.

The first and the second layers are trained together and their loss function for an image is defined as follow:

$$
\begin{aligned}
L_{Ti} &= L_{rpn} + L_{head} \\
&= \frac{1}{N_1} \sum_i \mathrm{CE}_{rpn}(P_i^*, T_{cls}) + \frac{1}{N_2} \sum_i \mathrm{SL1}_{rpn}(Pos_i^*, T_{pos}) + \\
&\quad \frac{1}{N_3} \sum_i \mathrm{CE}_{head}(P_i, T_{cls}) + \frac{1}{N_3} \sum_i \mathrm{SL1}_{head}(Pos_i, T_{pos})
\end{aligned}
\tag{1}
$$

in which L_{Ti} means loss functions for T1 or T2 modalities, CE means cross-entropy loss for two classes (cyst and background) and SL1 means smooth L1 distance between two positions. N_1 denotes the num of boxes provided for RPN (which is 1024); N_2 denotes the boxes to regress in RPN, which only computes for the cysts regions; N_3 denotes the number of input ROIs for the second stage.

Because offsets, sizes and resolutions of two modalities are different, inter modality registration is important before modality combination. If our second stage can produce reliable bounding boxes, the detection in two modalities can be regarded as a registration procedure. After feature maps of two modalities are separately extracted, NMS and **Z-Continuity Filter (ZCF)** are used to make sure the outputs of both modalities are precise and the registration is reliable. Our experiments prove our assumption and show that our method can detect cysts with a high recall, which is shown in Sect. 3.3.

Z-Continuity Filter is a ROI filter based on spatial continuity in Z-axis, which is illustrated in Fig. 2. Based on our statistics, all the cysts appear within a certain range in an abdomen MRI volume. For T1 MRI, if we compute the relative index to the whole volume's height, cysts in all cases appear from about 22% to 75% and for T2 the range is from 26% to 95%. We firstly remove all slices beyond the ranges. Then, discontinuous boxes whose offsets to boxes of two adjacent slices are too large are removed; when no box is detected and two adjacent slices have output boxes in almost the same position, an interpolated box will be added.

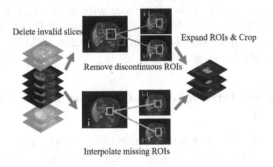

Fig. 2. Z-Continuity Filter

2.4   Third Stage: Modality Fusion and Classification

This part is trained alone and the classification backbone is InceptionV3 [13]. As Fig. 3 shows, multimodality image pairs are input to the network and their bottlenecks are concatenated for prediction. The two modalities are arranged to pairs using a simple fusion algorithm. Loss function for this part is cross entropy:

$$L = \frac{1}{N} \sum_{i=1}^{N} (q_i \log(p_i) + (1 - q_i) \log(1 - p_i)) \tag{2}$$

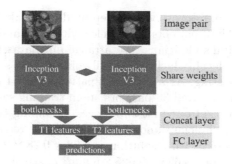

Fig. 3. Modality fusion and classification

where N is batch size; q denotes the one-hot binary codes of groundtruth (MCN or SCN); p denotes the codes of predictions. We use model pretrained on ImageNet and finetuned on OCT2017 [6]. OCT2017 dataset are composed of 100 thousands of OCT images which is another kind of medical images. Weights of networks before the bottleneck are fixed for transfer learning.

Our InceptionV3 network can identify image pairs with MCN or SCN. After procedure on all image pairs is done, we use a simple voting algorithm to get patient level classification. All the results are voted with weights (which are the confidence degrees in classification).

Fusion algorithm: After ZCF, every slice of image must have no more than one ROI. We arrange all slices with a ROI into a volume (simply jump the blank slices when testing) with their Z-axis index. Then we resample the modality with fewer slices to increase the number of slices. As a result, images of two modalities have the same number for every patient. For training set, we use groundtruth bounding box to replace detected ROIs. We then expand every sides of ROIs for 50 pixels in X-Y plane, and crop ROIs and resize them into 299×299 pixels. Reasons for such a expansion is that the raw width of ROIs are about 30–50 pixels and thus 299 pixels is too large for them. An even more important reason is that the annotated bounding boxes enclose the cysts for detection. Without ROI expansion, much of information around cysts will be abandoned, which is important for diagnosis.

3   Experiment

3.1   Dataset and Annotation

Our dataset has been collected in cooperation hospital from December 2015 to December 2017. There are 52 preoperative T1 MRI volumes data and 68 preoperative T2 MRI volumes data from 48 different patients and all of them are abdomen MRIs. All patients have been diagnosed as either SCN or MCN in the department of pathology using surgical specimens (36 SCNs and 12 MCNs) and all have both T1 and T2 modalities. Some patients have more than one volume for a modality. In fusion procedure, the volumes of a patient for the modality with fewer volumes will be used repeatedly to make sure all T1 and T2 volumes are in pair. All of patients are labeled with clinical diagnosis offered by the cooperative hospital's clinicians. We arrange our dataset into training and testing set in patients level, which means all volumes of a same patient appear either in training or testing. As a result, 13 patients with 4 MCNs and 9 SCNs are divided into testing set and 35 patients are in training set with 8 MCNs and 27 SCNs. In order to train our first two stages, bounding boxes for MCN and SCN are annotated by clinicians and radiologists in our research team.

T1 MRIs are captured with resolution of $0.78 \times 0.78 \times 2.5$ mm^3 and T2 are with $0.74 \times 0.74 \times 4.8$ mm^3, $0.625 \times 0.625 \times 6$ mm^3 or $0.625 \times 0.625 \times 8$ mm^3. So for most situations, PCNs only appear in 3 to 8 slices, which is the reason for using 2D method instead of 3D. The numbers of 2D slices with PCNs for T1 and T2 are separately 533 and 476. Training set for the first two stages is augmented by rotation and translation, and the augmented set has about 60,000 slices. Training set for the third stage is augmented only for MCN cases to balance the numbers of two classes. After resampling and augmentation 483 multi-modality image pairs are used in training.

3.2 Implementation Details

We implement our method with Tensorflow [1]. Both two parts of training are optimized by [7] with initial learning rate 10^{-4}. Training for first and second stages on T1 and T2 separately takes 30,000 and 25,000 iterations with batch size 1 image. Training for the third stages takes 4000 iterations with batch size 256. Training for two detection nets takes 16 h and for InceptionV3 takes 25 min. Test process takes about 0.5 s for a 2D image pair, and about 16 s for whole volumes of two modalities for a patients.

3.3 Result and Comparisons

ROI Detection The ROI detection results are shown in Table 1. A box with Dice's coefficient larger than 0.5 will be regarded as an accurate match. Boxes with confidence larger than 0.6 is kept. "Reg 2 classes" means detection with annotation of MCN and SCN (the proposed method regresses with 1 class, cyst).

Table 1. ROI detection results of T1/T2 (%).

Metric	Without ZCF	With ZCF	Reg 2 classes
Precision	41.7/36.9	58.9/59.8	50.9/43.2
Recall	74.5/71.1	87.3/88.9	57.2/36.9

The result shows that our proposed ZCF can increase both precision and recall. In addition, the experiment shows that detecting SCN and MCN together

Table 2. Classification results (%) at slice level.

Method	ROIs	All Acc	SCN Acc.	MCN Acc.
SVM T1/T2	GT	66.7/73.5	81.0/87.9/	29.0/34.6
KNN k=8 T1/T2	GT	61.6/78.1	73.4/90.8/	21.5/29.5
Proposed Cls T1/T2/fusion	GT	80.6/68.5/88.7	80.1/88.0/90.8	83.3/28.6/82.1
Faster-RCNN T1/T2	detection	57.3/60.3	59.6/72.7	12.3/6.8
Proposed method T1/T2/fusion	detection	73.4/74.4/80.0	77.7/86.5/89.1	61.0/44.1/56.0

is better than detecting them as two types. The low precision will influence slice level classification, but is not serious for patient level classification.

Classification at slice level Since we have not found related PCN classification algorithm published, results from single modality and some traditional methods are used as baselines. We use accuracy as our metric, which means both the cysts areas and the classifications are correct. The result is shown in Table 2. The notations are described as follow:

- **SVM**: Use a Support Vector Machine (SVM) to classify on T1/T2 modality with groundtruth bounding boxes. Boxes are resized to 64 × 64.
- **KNN**: Utilize a K-Nearest Neighbor (KNN) to classify on T1/T2 modality groundtruth boxes. Boxes are resized to 64 × 64.
- **Proposed Cls**: Utilize proposed classification method on T1/T2/multimodality with groundtruth boxes.
- **Faster-RCNN**: Utilize Faster-RCNN [10] on T1/T2 modality.
- **Proposed method**: Utilize proposed method on T1/T2/multimodality.

The results of proposed multimodality method prove that T1 and T2 images have complementary information. By combining them the proposed classification method with manual or automatic detection procedure both perform better than using two modalities alone. In addition, by comparing results of Faster-RCNN and our proposed network for single modality, we can conclude that our three-stage method might help classification procedure work better. Traditional methods (like SVM and KNN) can hardly overcome the data imbalance. The accuracy of the smaller class, MCN is both low for KNN and SVM. When using groundtruth boxes for localization and inter modality registration, our accuracies are very high for this difficult diagnosis problem, significantly higher than reported accuracies of radiologists (although datasets are different) in [9]. The main shortcoming of our detection procedure is that many false positive boxes are present even after ZCF, which will be addressed by patient level fusion.

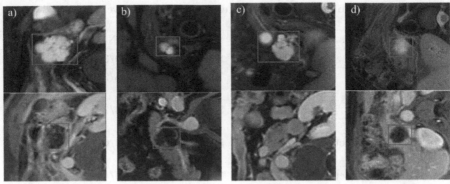

(a) Big and round SCN with unclear sub-cavity walls.

(b) Round SCN reacts weakly in T2.

(c) SCN with a round sub-cavity in T2; false detection in T1.

(d) Small MCN with unclear boundary.

Fig. 4. Some cases classified incorrectly in either T1 or T2 but correctly in multimodality. UP: T2 images. Below: T1 images. Every column is an image pair.

Table 3. Classification results (%) at patient level.

Method	Proposed multimodality	Proposed T1	Proposed T2	Decision level fusion
Acc	92.3	84.6	84.6	84.6

Diagnosis at patient level We do the experiments to combine all predictions of images pairs for a patient, and then use a simple voting algorithm to get the patient level diagnosis. The result are shown in Table 3. Decision level fusion means fusing two modalities after classification by voting their classification results. The proposed multimodality method performs much better since fusion at earlier level can capture more complementary information.

Though many false positive boxes influence slice level classification, it can hardly influence patient level diagnosis. Our classification procedure is trained on ground-truth boxes, so the classification confidence degree is a good metric to identify whether the testing inputs are false positive detections or not. When voting for patient level results, the false positive detections will have lower weights, thus the diagnosis result is not affected by them. Figure 4 shows some cases diagnosed wrong in single modality but correctly in multimodality.

4   Discussion and Conclusion

In this paper, we proposed PCN-Net for detection and identification of SCN and MCN. We modified Faster-RCNN and combined two kinds of modalities, T1 and T2 weighted MRI. A carefully designed Z-Continuity Filter and fusion procedure are added. The identification accuracy is as high as 80.0% and the diagnostic performance is 92.3% (which in fact is just one failure case in all 13 cases).

A limitation of the current study is the relatively small dataset. Limited by the small amount of data, we only train and test our method on samples of MCN and SCN, two major types of PCN. However, our method can be extended to other subclasses of PCN. Collecting more data of different subclasses of PCN is one of our future works. Although the Z-Continuity Filter performs well in keeping continuity and increasing recall rate, it still has some false positive cases, which will be addressed in future.

Acknowledgments. This work is supported by the National Natural Science Foundation of China under Grant 61622207.

References

1. Abadi, M., Agarwal, A., Barham, P., Brevdo, E., et al.: TensorFlow: large-scale machine learning on heterogeneous systems. arXiv:1603.04467 (2016). Software available from https://tensorflow.org
2. Cai, J., Lu, L., Xing, F., Yang, L.: Pancreas segmentation in CT and MRI images via domain specific network designing and recurrent neural contextual learning. arXiv:1803.11303 (2018)
3. del Castillo C, F., Warshaw, A.L.: Cystic tumors of the pancreas. Surg. Clin. North Am. **75**(5), 1001–16 (1995)
4. Hussein, S., Chuquicusma, M.M., Kandel, P., Bolan, C.W., Wallace, M.B., Bagci, U.: Supervised and unsupervised tumor characterization in the deep learning era. arXiv:1801.03230 (2018)
5. Hutchins, G.F., Draganov, P.V.: Cystic neoplasms of the pancreas: a diagnostic challenge. World J. Gastroenterol. **15**(1), 48 (2009)
6. Kermany, D.S., et al.: Identifying medical diagnoses and treatable diseases by image-based deep learning. Cell **172**(5), 1122–1131 (2018)
7. Kingma, D., Ba, J.: Adam: a method for stochastic optimization. Computer Science (2014)
8. Liu, F., Xie, L., Xia, Y., Fishman, E.K., Yuille, A.L.: Joint shape representation and classification for detecting PDAC. arXiv:1804.10684 (2018)
9. Lu, X., Zhang, S., Ma, C., Peng, C., Lv, Y., Zou, X.: The diagnostic value of eus in pancreatic cystic neoplasms compared with CT and MRI. Endosc. Ultrasound **4**(4), 324–329 (2015)
10. Ren, S., He, K., Girshick, R., Sun, J.: Faster R-CNN: towards real-time object detection with region proposal networks. In: NIPS, pp. 91–99 (2015)
11. Roth, H., et al.: Towards dense volumetric pancreas segmentation in CT using 3D fully convolutional networks. arXiv:1706.07346 (2017)
12. Russakovsky, O., et al.: ImageNet large scale visual recognition challenge. IJCV **115**(3), 211–252 (2015)
13. Szegedy, C., Vanhoucke, V., Ioffe, S., Shlens, J., Wojna, Z.: Rethinking the inception architecture for computer vision. Computer Science, pp. 2818–2826 (2015)
14. Zhou, Y., Xie, L., Fishman, E.K., Yuille, A.L.: Deep supervision for pancreatic cyst segmentation in abdominal CT scans. In: MICCAI, pp. 222–230 (2017)
15. Zhou, Y., Xie, L., Shen, W., Wang, Y., Fishman, E.K., Yuille, A.L.: A fixed-point model for pancreas segmentation in abdominal CT scans. In: MICCAI, pp. 693–701 (2017)

Retinal Blood Vessel Segmentation Using a Fully Convolutional Network – Transfer Learning from Patch- to Image-Level

Taibou Birgui Sekou[1,3]([✉]), Moncef Hidane[1,3], Julien Olivier[1,3],
and Hubert Cardot[2,3]

[1] Institut National des Sciences Appliquées Centre Val de Loire, Blois, France
[2] Université de Tours, Tours, France
[3] LIFAT EA 6300, Tours, France
taibou.birgui_sekou@insa-cvl.fr

Abstract. Fully convolutional networks (FCNs) are well known to provide state-of-the-art results in various medical image segmentation tasks. However, these models usually need a tremendous number of training samples to achieve good performances. Unfortunately, this requirement is often difficult to satisfy in the medical imaging field, due to the scarcity of labeled images. As a consequence, the common tricks for FCNs' training go from data augmentation and transfer learning to patch-based segmentation. In the latter, the segmentation of an image involves patch extraction, patch segmentation, then patch aggregation. This paper presents a framework that takes advantage of all these tricks by starting with a patch-level segmentation which is then extended to the image level by transfer learning. The proposed framework follows two main steps. Given a image database $\mathcal{D}$, a first network $\mathcal{N}_P$ is designed and trained using patches extracted from $\mathcal{D}$. Then, $\mathcal{N}_P$ is used to pre-train a FCN $\mathcal{N}_I$ to be trained on the full sized images of $\mathcal{D}$. Experimental results are presented on the task of retinal blood vessel segmentation using the well known publicly available DRIVE database.

Keywords: Retinal blood vessel segmentation · Fully convolutional neural networks · Transfer learning

1 Introduction

The human vascular system is an important risk biomarker in a large number of diseases. In particular, retinal blood vessels serve as a cue to diagnose diabetic retinopathy, age-related macular degeneration and glaucoma. As the eye shares neural and vascular similarities with the brain, its vascularization also offers a direct window to cerebral pathology.

Manual delineation of blood vessels from images by ophthalmologists is a tedious task. It is also subject to inter- and intra-operator variability. To alleviate this difficulty, an intensive body of work has concentrated on developing

© Springer Nature Switzerland AG 2018
Y. Shi et al. (Eds.): MLMI 2018, LNCS 11046, pp. 170–178, 2018.
https://doi.org/10.1007/978-3-030-00919-9_20

automatic retinal blood vessel segmentation (RBVS) techniques. Fraz *et al.* [1] presented a review and a taxonomy of the proposed methods in the field, up to 2012. A recent reviews is presented in [2].

State-of-the-art methods for RBVS are supervised and mainly based on deep learning. They associate a label to each pixel in the image, indicating whether it belongs to a vessel or to the background.

In [3], each pixel is labeled using a (preprocessed) surrounding $m \times m$ patch (a small neighborhood centered around it). The classification is performed using a freely designed deep convolutional neural network. The authors also presented an interesting variation of their method where they framed the segmentation task as a structured inference problem. This leads to a deep neural network that predicts the class assignments for all pixels in a small window, of size $s \times s$ (with $s < m$), located inside the input patch. The same idea of structured prediction is employed in [4] to train a FCN using patches extracted from the training images. In [6,7], patch-based methods are proposed using discriminative dictionary learning techniques for RBVS.

In general, working at the patch level eases the possibility of learning arbitrarily designed deep networks since from few images one can extract millions of (overlapping) patches. However, a patch aggregation step, which may be time consuming, is needed to obtain the segmentation of an entire image. Moreover, a patch based segmentation labels a pixel using a restrained view and does not take advantage of the extra information located in other parts of the image. Instead, it is also possible to work at the image level, that is learning on complete images and segmenting each test image in one forward pass across the network.

On the task of RBVS, Mo et al. [8] proposed a VGG-like [12] network and included an additional contextual information in the network by aggregating the segmentation of different layers. The proposed model working at the image level, they performed a data augmentation technique to boost the database size. Still, the size of their training set was very small compared to the number of parameters in their network. Thus, the authors initialize their network using pre-trained weights from ImageNet.

Transfer learning from VGG, or other architectures, might lead to good performance but diminishes the degree for freedom when designing new networks since the transfered parts of the network must remain unchanged. This reduces the field of exploration and research.

This paper introduces a transfer learning based framework to train arbitrarily designed FCNs even on relatively small sized databases. The framework is tested on the task of RBVS using an example of freely designed FCN. The proposed framework consists of two steps. Given a database $\mathcal{D}$. In the first step, a fully convolutional network $\mathcal{N}_P$ is designed and trained using patches extracted from the training images of $\mathcal{D}$. The second step consists in re-using the weights of $\mathcal{N}_P$ to pre-train a FCN $\mathcal{N}_I$ which takes as inputs the full sized images of $\mathcal{D}$. Full size image segmentation means that an image is segmented in one forward pass, which is more practical in the medical field than aggregating extracted patches. In this manner, one can train various network architectures first at the patch level then transfer the weights to segment images in one forward pass. We experimentally show that our network outputs outstanding results on the well known publicly available DRIVE dataset.

The overview of the paper is as follows. Section 2 presents our framework and the proposed network in terms of its architecture. In Sect. 3, we present all the experimental aspects of the work including the dataset, the training set generation and the results along with a discussion. Section 4 sums up the paper and introduces possible future work.

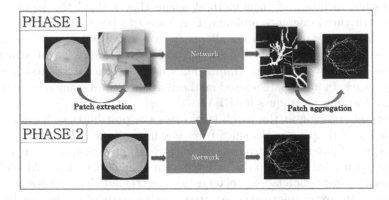

Fig. 1. The proposed framework. Phase 1: The network is fed with patches extracted from the original images. Phase 2: The network is fine-tuned with the full sized images.

2 Proposed Model

This section presents the core components of our proposition: the different steps of the framework and the network.

2.1 Fully Convolutional Networks and Transfer Learning

Deep neural networks generally consist of multiple layers of different type and purpose. The convolution or the fully connected layers aim at learning efficient patterns in the training set. The patterns are either discriminative (e.g. classification tasks) or generative (e.g. generative models). Layers that perform pooling, non-linearity or batch-normalization inject more robustness in the model and provide a way for the network (i) to be more invariant to some change in the input, and (ii) to have better generalization power. A detailed presentation of common layers of a deep network is presented in [11].

The proposed framework is mainly based on fully convolutional networks [13] which are particular deep neural networks that do not include fully connected layers. As a consequence, the spatial and structural information of the input can be preserved throughout the network. A FCN, by construction, only imposes its inputs to share the same number of dimensions and channels. For example, a FCN trained on an input of shape $10 \times 10 \times 3$ to output a shape 5×5 can, theoretically, be applied on an input of shape $20 \times 20 \times 3$ to output 10×10. On the task of medical image segmentation, to train FCNs, one usually makes use of a transfer learning technique. Transfer learning consists in reusing some weights of a network $\mathcal{N}_s$ trained on a source database $\mathcal{D}_s$ as a starting point for a network $\mathcal{N}_t$ to be trained on a target database $\mathcal{D}_t$ [14].

In the following, the proposed framework is introduced. It makes use of (i) the FCNs shape preservation between the input and output, and (ii) the transfer learning from patch- to image-level.

2.2   The Proposed Framework

As aforementioned, RBVS is a major phase in the diagnostic system. It needs to be as fast and accurate as possible. And, this applies to all medical image segmentation tasks. To guarantee a fast segmentation time, we need to segment each image at once instead of working at the patch level.

On the other hand, the number of images makes the training phase highly challenging, thus the need for a good starting point. On RBVS tasks, Mo et al. [8] initialized their network with pre-trained weights learned on a large-scale natural image dataset (ImageNet).

In this paper, we introduce another pre-training possibility. We propose to initialize the network with weights learned from the patches of the same dataset. The proposed framework consists of two phases as depicted on Fig. 1.

Phase 1 (patch level) In this phase, we first create a patch training set $\mathcal{D}_P$ by extracting a large number of patches from the training images. Then, a fully convolutional network $\mathcal{N}_P$ is freely designed and fed with samples of $\mathcal{D}_P$. Given a patch of shape $m \times n$ the network $\mathcal{N}_P$ will output its segmentation map of the same shape. Hence, at this level, one need to aggregate patches of different location to segment an entire image (*see* First row of Fig. 1).

Phase 2 (image level) At this stage, we already have a network that outputs good results at the patch level. The goal is to have similar performance but at the image level. To do so, we first design a network $\mathcal{N}_I$ that takes as an input an entire image and produces its overall segmentation mask. Suppose, the images are of shape $h \times w$, then the only difference between a patch and an image is the number of pixel, their number of dimension and channel being the same. As aforementioned, FCNs can process inputs of similar shapes regardless of their number of pixels. Our transfer learning consists in reusing all the weights of $\mathcal{N}_P$ in $\mathcal{N}_I$. In other words, the only difference between $\mathcal{N}_P$ and $\mathcal{N}_I$ is the size of their inputs. The network $\mathcal{N}_I$ can the be trained using the full sized images of $\mathcal{D}$. This training process can be seen as a fine-tuning of $\mathcal{N}_P$ at the image level.

In the following, the patch level network refers to $\mathcal{N}_P$ while the one fine-tuned at the image level refers to $\mathcal{N}_I$.

174   T. Birgui Sekou et al.

2.3   Neural Network Architecture

In this work, we present a fully convolutional auto-encoder-like network depicted
on Fig. 2. The encoder phase (first eleven layers) extracts high-level abstract
patterns. From these underlying structures, the decoder phase tries to recover
the segmentation of an input.

The network consists of convolution and deconvolution layers. The down-
samplings are performed with convolution of stride 2. And, to recover the initial
input size, the deconvolution layers which apply transposed convolutions with
a certain stride, are used. All convolutions are followed by a ReLU activation
except the last one which uses a Sigmoid to output a class probability for each
pixel of the input. The network may have the same look as other well know architectures but has less weights and less down-sampling levels. This architecture has
been experimentally selected and performs better than very deep and complex
propositions of the literature on the task of retinal blood vessel segmentation.

A classical cross-entropy, which is based on the distance between probability
distribution, is used as loss function.

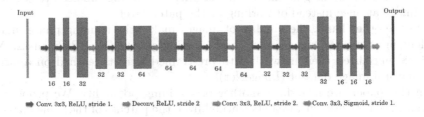

Fig. 2. Network architecture.

3   Experiments

We applied the proposed method on the task of RBVS. The evaluation is performed on the publicly available DRIVE dataset. This section presents practical details about the training including the normalizations and the patches
extraction procedure. Afterwards, our numerical and some qualitative results
are exposed and discussed.

The DRIVE[1] (Digital Retinal Images for Vessel Extraction) [15] contains
RGB fundus image of size $585 \times 564 \times 3$. The mask image delineating the field of
view (FoV) of each image is also provided. The DRIVE dataset is divided into
two sets of 20 images: the training and testing sets.

---

[1] http://www.isi.uu.nl/Research/Databases/DRIVE/.

3.1   Data Preparation and Network Training

We applied three operations on each image before any procedure: (1) gray-scale conversion, (2) gamma correction (with gamma set to 1.7), and (3) Contrast Limited Adaptive Histogram Equalization (CLAHE). The database is boosted by adding for each image its vertically and horizontally flipped version.

At the patch level, to avoid storing the entire patch dataset, their are extracted on the fly. That is, at each epoch and for each image, we extract randomly 3200 patches of shape 32×32, where half of them are centered on a vessel pixel and the other half are centered on a background pixel.

At the image level, if needed, we concatenate a zero matrix to an image to ensure an output with the same size. In other words, if the input image is of size (584×565) we zero-pad the second dimension to obtain (584×568) so that the down-sampling by 4 in the network will be straightforward.

The network is implemented using the Keras library. The training is carried out on a GPU Nvidia GeForce GTX 1080 Ti, with 64 batch size when using patches and 1 at the image level. The *adadelta* [16] learning algorithm is adopted. We performed 15 epochs at the patch level and 300 at the image level.

3.2   Results

The proposed model is compared to the most recent and state-of-the-art methods using the Area Under the ROC Curve (**AUC**) metric. The latter is a commonly used metric for RBVS. The AUC score is an important metric in the sense that it aggregates metrics of various threshold. Let TP, TN, FP, and FN respectively denote the number of true positive, true negative, false positive, and false negative. We computed with a 0.5 threshold the sensitivity $\textbf{Sens} = \frac{TP}{TP+FN}$, the specificity $\textbf{Spec} = \frac{TN}{TN+FP}$ and the accuracy $\textbf{Acc} = \frac{TP+TN}{TP+TN+FP+FN}$.

Our numerical results are presented on Table 1 and are discussed in the next section. On Table 1, *Proposed-patches* are the results obtained with the network trained only on patches and *Proposed-images* are the results achieved when the network is fine-tuned at the image level. The line *Images-nopretrain* is added to present the results at the image level without pretraining from the patches, obtained after convergence on a validation set (300 epochs).

Figure 3 illustrates some qualitative results of the proposed method.

3.3   Discussion

Firstly, note that, the comparison of RBVS methods is rather biased in the sense that the field of view usually differ from one method to another. For example, the results in [3] are computed on an eroded version of the field of view. Thus, we focused on reaching competitive results and proposing an interesting training procedure that can be generalized to any medical image segmentation task.

The numerical results show that our metrics are state-of-the-art on the DRIVE dataset. On the one hand, we reach the results in [3] when working at the patch level. That is, the network is efficiently trained at the patch level

Table 1. Results on the DRIVE database.

Methods	AUC	Spec	Sens	Acc
Proposed-patches	**98.01**	**98.37**	76.65	**95.58**
Proposed-images	97.87	97.82	79.90	95.52
Images-nopretrain	97.01	98.27	72.91	95.02
Birgui S. et al. [7] (JDCL)**	–	96.32	**80.60**	94.93
Dasgupta et al. [4]*	97.44	98.01	76.91	95.33
Javidi et al. [6]**	–	97.02	72.01	94.50
Liskowski et al. [3]*	97.90	98.07	78.11	95.35
Mo et al. [8]*	97.82	97.80	77.79	95.21
Vega et al. [5]*	–	96.00	74.44	94.12
Zhang et al. [9]	96.36	97.25	77.43	94.76

*deep learning — **dictionary learning

in the Phase 1 of the proposed framework. On the other hand, at the image level, our transfer learning from the patch level outperforms the one from the VGG proposed in [8]. Moreover, we notice that, at least with this network, at the image level it is better to work with transfer learning than without (*see* Proposed-images and Images- nopretrain on the Table 1).

Using the framework, One can also see that the results obtained at the image level are rather close to the ones from the patch level. When trained at the patch level, the network is constrained to be precise in a small window (*i.e.* the patch). While at the image level, the constraint window becomes much larger and the network may miss some fine details. A loss function that consider the output's size or the classes' balance may improve the metrics at the image level.

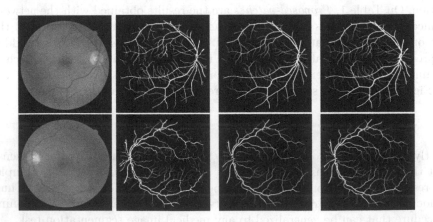

Fig. 3. Qualitative results. From left to right: RGB original image, ground-truth, segmentation at patch level, segmentation after fine-tuning at image level.

4 Summary and Perspectives

We proposed a fully convolutional network training framework and applied it on the task of retinal blood vessel segmentation. First, The framework is employed to train a freely designed FCN using patches extracted from the training images. Then, to meet the real-time necessity of the medical field, we fine-tuned the network using the full size images.

The training at the patch level being the first step, future work may include more ways to improve the latter such as data augmentation and preprocessing. Furthermore, we plan to examined the results on various networks such as residual networks and on other medical image modalities. Moreover, detailed studies of the patch and image levels and their correlation are left for future work.

References

1. Fraz, M.M., et al.: Blood vessel segmentation methodologies in retinal images a survey. Comput. Methods Prog. Biomed. **108**(1), 407–433 (2012)
2. Srinidhi, C.L., Aparna, P., Rajan, J.: Recent advancements in retinal vessel segmentation. J. Med. Syst. **41**(4), 70:1–70:22 (2017)
3. Liskowski, P.: Segmenting retinal blood vessels with deep neural networks. IEEE Trans. Med. Imaging **35**(11), 2369–2380 (2016)
4. Dasgupta, A., Singh, S.: A fully convolutional neural network based structured prediction approach towards the retinal vessel segmentation. In: ISBI, IEEE, pp. 248–251 (2017)
5. Roberto, V., et al.: Retinal vessel extraction using lattice neural networks with dendritic processing. Comput. Biol. Med. **58**, 20–30 (2015)
6. Javidi, M.: Vessel segmentation and microaneurysm detection using discriminative dictionary learning and sparse representation. Comput. Methods Prog. Biomed. **139**, 93–108 (2017)
7. Sekou, B.T., Hidane, M., Olivier, J., Cardot, H.: Segmentation of retinal blood vessels using dictionary learning techniques. In: Cardoso, M.J. (ed.) FIFI/OMIA -2017. LNCS, vol. 10554, pp. 83–91. Springer, Cham (2017). https://doi.org/10.1007/978-3-319-67561-9_9
8. Mo, J., Zhang, L.: Multi-level deep supervised networks for retinal vessel segmentation. Int. J. Comput. Assist. Radiol. Surg. **12**(12), 2181–2193 (2017)
9. Zhang, J., et al.: Robust retinal vessel segmentation via locally adaptive derivative frames in orientation scores. IEEE Trans. Med. Imaging **35**(12), 2631–2644 (2016)
10. Ronneberger, O., Fischer, P., Brox, T.: U-Net: convolutional networks for biomedical image segmentation. In: Navab, N., Hornegger, J., Wells, W.M., Frangi, A.F. (eds.) MICCAI 2015. LNCS, vol. 9351, pp. 234–241. Springer, Cham (2015). https://doi.org/10.1007/978-3-319-24574-4_28
11. Ian, G., Yoshua, B.: Deep learning (adaptive computation and machine learning). MIT Press, Cambridge (2016)
12. Simonyan, K., Zisserman, A.: Very deep convolutional networks for large-scale image recognition, CoRR, vol. abs/1409.1556 (2014)
13. Shelhamer, E., Long, J., Darrell, T.: Fully convolutional networks for semantic segmentation. IEEE Trans. Pattern Anal. Mach. Intell. **39**(4), 640–651 (2017)

14. Yosinski, J., Clune, J., Bengio, Y., Lipson, H.: How transferable are features in deep neural networks? Adv. Neural Inf. Process. Syst. 27 (2014)
15. Staal, J., et al.: Ridge-based vessel segmentation in color images of the retina. IEEE Trans. Med. Imaging **23**(4), 501–509 (2004)
16. Zeiler, M.D.: ADADELTA: An adaptive learning rate method, CoRR, vol. abs/1212.5701 (2012)

Combining Deep Learning and Active Contours Opens The Way to Robust, Automated Analysis of Brain Cytoarchitectonics

Konstantin Thierbach[1], Pierre-Louis Bazin[1,2], Walter de Back[5],
Filippos Gavriilidis[1], Evgeniya Kirilina[1,3], Carsten Jäger[1], Markus Morawski[4],
Stefan Geyer[1], Nikolaus Weiskopf[1], and Nico Scherf[1(✉)]

[1] Max Planck Institute for Human Cognitive and Brain Sciences, Leipzig, Germany
nscherf@cbs.mpg.de
[2] University of Amsterdam, Amsterdam, The Netherlands
[3] Center for Cognitive Neuroscience Berlin, Free University Berlin, Berlin, Germany
[4] Paul Flechsig Institute of Brain Research, University of Leipzig, Leipzig, Germany
[5] Institute for Medical Informatics and Biometry, TU Dresden, Dresden, Germany

Abstract. Deep learning has thoroughly changed the field of image analysis yielding impressive results whenever enough annotated data can be gathered. While partial annotation can be very fast, manual segmentation of 3D biological structures is tedious and error-prone. Additionally, high-level shape concepts such as topology or boundary smoothness are hard if not impossible to encode in Feedforward Neural Networks. Here we present a modular strategy for the accurate segmentation of neural cell bodies from light-sheet microscopy combining mixed-scale convolutional neural networks and topology-preserving geometric deformable models. We show that the network can be trained efficiently from simple cell centroid annotations, and that the final segmentation provides accurate cell detection and smooth segmentations that do not introduce further cell splitting or merging.

Keywords: Histology · Image segmentation · Cell detection
Deep learning · Convolutional neural networks · Active contours

1 Introduction

Systematic studies of the cortical cytoarchitecture are indispensable to understand the functional organization of the human brain. Classical works based on qualitative description of cell counts and shapes in physical 2D sections of the human cortex revealed functional areas and segregation in the brain [2,4,15].

The research leading to these results has received funding from the European Research Council under the European Union's Seventh Framework Programme (FP7/2007-2013)/ERC grant agreement no. 616905.

© Springer Nature Switzerland AG 2018
Y. Shi et al. (Eds.): MLMI 2018, LNCS 11046, pp. 179–187, 2018.
https://doi.org/10.1007/978-3-030-00919-9_21

These brain parcellations are currently updated and refined using automated image analysis [18]. Even 3D imaging of post mortem brain tissue at microstructural resolution are within reach using recent light sheet fluorescence microscopy (LSFM) [7] and tissue clearing protocols [3]. Combined with advanced image analysis these techniques enable studying cortical cellular organisation in the human brain with unsurpassed precision. To reach this goal we need robust computational analysis relying on minimal manual annotations, facing the following challenges:

- Clearing of aged, unperfused human tissue is imperfect, and optical distortions due to scattering and refraction remain. This leads to varying background intensities across the image and shading artifacts.
- The penetration of antibody stains and thus contrast is uneven across the sample. The tissue degenerates with longer post-mortem times. These effects increase the already high variability of neural shape and appearance across the cortical samples (Fig. 1a).
- The resolution is lower along the optical axis in the 3D stack. Additional imperfection in depth focusing and sample movement create artifacts through the depth of the stack (Fig. 1b).
- Cell density varies locally, leading to false segmentation of cells into clusters.

Machine Learning methods improved the analysis of microscopy data [13]. Deep Learning, in particular Convolutional Neural Networks (CNNs), can address challenging problems in biomedical imaging because they learn multilevel internal representations of the data [9,13]. These, typically supervised, methods require a lot of annotated data: For cell segmentation pixel-accurate masks have to be supplied [12]. Manually annotating data for training is often prohibitive in biomedical applications where data are specialized, scarce and expert knowledge is required. Abstract concepts at the object level (Gestalt principles such as continuation, closure [8], or object topology) are hard to learn with CNNs. Additional annotation of the border region between adjacent cells is needed to reduce false merging of neighboring cells [12]. Human vision exploits high level concepts using top-down processing [8] which is not represented in feedforward architectures.

Active Contour methods have been designed to embody high level concepts of object shapes. They can guarantee the smoothness of contours and a consistent topology [1]: features that improve cell segmentation in challenging conditions and prevent splitting and merging of contours during segmentation. But active contour methods require an initialization with the number and approximate position of objects in the image. Robust initial localization of cells is hard to define a priori and should be learned from data. This is where Deep Learning has a clear advantage: CNNs can be trained to robustly predict cell positions in images using only sparse centroid annotations [16].

In this work we combine the complementary strengths of CNNs and topology-aware active contours into a robust workflow to detect and segment cells that delivers high quality results and most importantly, requires only minimal

annotations (sparse annotations of approximate cell centers are enough).[1]
Additionally, our approach works with 2D and 3D microscopy data. Here, we
demonstrate and validate the method using 2D slices from a 3D microscopy
image volume obtained of cleared post mortem human brain blocks and as a
proof of concept we show that our methods easily extends to full 3D processing.

2   Methodology

2.1   Sample Preparation

Blocks from a human post mortem brain (temporal lobe cortex, male, 54 yr.,
post-mortem interval 96 h) have been provided by the Brain Banking Centre
Leipzig of the German Brain-Net. The entire procedure of case recruitment,
acquisition of the patient's personal data, the protocols and the informed consent
forms, performing the autopsy, and handling the autoptic material have been
approved by the local ethics committee. For details on tissue preparation and
clearing see [10].

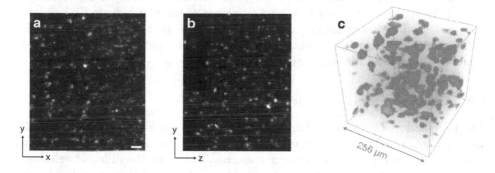

Fig. 1. Example of image data. An xy (a) and yz (b) slice of a $1080 \times 1280 \times 1000 \, \mu$m
subvolume (scale bar 100 μm). (c) Direct volume rendering of cuboid volume randomly
sampled from the image stack.

2.2   Image Data

A commercial light-sheet fluorescence microscope (LaVision BioTec, Bielefeld,
Germany) was used to image the cleared specimen. The microscope was equipped
with 10x CLARITY-objective (Olympus XLPLN10XSVMP, numerical aperture
(NA) 0.6, working distance (WD) 8 mm; Zeiss Clr Plan-Apochromat, NA 0.5,
WD 3.7 mm) and operated with 630 nm excitation wavelength and band-pass 680

---

[1] Related ideas integrating deep learning and level set formulations have been proposed
by [14] or [6]. In contrast to our approach based on sparse centroid annotations these
methods require pixel-accurate object masks for training.

nm emission filter. Samples were stained with a fluorescent monoclonal antibody against human neuronal protein HuC/HuD (a specific marker for neuronal cell bodies). The acquisition covered a 1.1 mm × 1.3 mm × 2.5 mm volume resulting in a stack of 2601 16-bit TIFF images (2560 × 2160 pixels, 0.51 μm lateral resolution) using a 1 μm step size.

For the 2D analysis workflow we took 19 slices at regular intervals from the entire stack. We used 15 images for training and validation and kept 4 images as a test set. The images for the test set were used for final assessment of segmentation and detection performance only. A single image typically contains around 300 cells (Fig. 1). To analyze 2D segmentation accuracy, an expert created reference cell masks on the 2D test images. The masks were independently checked and corrected by a second expert.

For the 3D analysis pipeline we first resampled the image stack to an isotropic resolution of 1 μm. One expert manually annotated cell centroids for a subregion of the size 2304 × 256 × 280 (z, x, y), which we subsequently used for the training and validation of the CNN for cell localization. We additionally annotated cell centroids in three separate regions of size 256 × 256 × 256, which served as a test set to measure the performance of our method. As manually segmenting cells in 3D is very laborious and error-prone we only annotated 2D reference cell masks in regularly spaced xy, and yz planes of the test images. To validate the agreement between annotated masks and segmentation we computed the segmentation entirely in 3D but exported the results only in those 2D planes that have been used for annotation.

2.3   Cell Segmentation Workflow

The proposed method is based on a Fully Convolutional Neural Network for cell localization and a topology-preserving multi-contour segmentation [1] to control smoothness and topology of the segmentation. To handle the different cell sizes we use the recently proposed Mixed-scale Dense (MS-D) architecture by [11] to robustly predict masks of cell centroid regions in 2D and 3D. The basic concept is as follows: **Training:** Pairs of image stacks (annotated centroids convolved by a spherical kernel and raw data) are fed into MS-D network. The network is trained to directly segment a spherical region of radius 3 around the annotated cell centroid. **Prediction:** MS-D predicts probability maps of cell positions from the raw image. These centroid probabilities are thresholded and used to initialize the active contour segmentation that segments the cells from the raw images. The workflow is schematically depicted for the general 3D case in Fig. 2.

Cell Localization For the 2D cell localization we used the MS-D architecture, with a *width* of 8 (multi-scale feature channels), a *depth* of 8 and a kernel size of 3 × 3 (see [11] for details). As the loss function we used the $1 - F_\beta$ score on the binary pixel labels between reference and prediction. This score combines precision (p) and recall (c) as $F_\beta = (1 + \beta^2) * \frac{p*r}{(\beta^2*p)+r}$. We set $\beta = 0.7$, putting more emphasize on precision of the predicted cell centroid regions. For

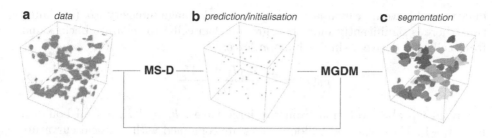

Fig. 2. Schematic overview of method in 3D. We train a MS-D network on manually labeled cell centroids. The predicted cell positions are used as initialization and topology prior for the multi-object geometric deformable model (MGDM).

optimization we used stochastic gradient descent with an adaptive learning rate (ADADELTA) [17]. We trained the network on randomly sampled image sections of size 256×256 pixels and the annotated centroids, convolved with a spherical kernel of radius 3. We used a batch size of 8 and applied data augmentation to the training samples in form of image rotation up to $90°$. To derive cell centroids from the MS-D predictions, we thresholded the predictions at 70% probability level.

Extension to 3D. For the 3D images we used a 5×8 (width×depth) MS-D to fit into the GPU memory, with all 2D convolutional layers replaced by 3D convolutions with corresponding kernel size of $3 \times 3 \times 3$.

We trained the network, with a batch size of 1 and without augmentation. As input we used pairs of randomly sampled image sections of size $96 \times 96 \times 96$ pixels and the annotated centroids, convolved with a 3D spherical kernel of radius 3. Predictions were thresholded at 70% probability level.

Multi-object Geometric Deformable Model Once cell centroids have been detected, the final segmentation is handled by a Multi-object Geometric Deformable Model (MGDM), an extension of the classical Deformable Geometric Model which ensures fast segmentation of an arbitrarily large number of cells while enforcing topological constraints between them [1]. The deformable model can be driven by any number of active contour forces. For simplicity, we only include balloon forces derived from the microscopy images and curvature regularisation, as follows.

For each detected cell c, we first find the maximum intensity M_c of the microscopy image inside the non-zero probability region around each detected centroid. We set the MGDM balloon forces to decrease linearly with the distance to M_c:

$$F_c(x) = \frac{M_c - |I(x) - M_c|}{M_c}. \tag{1}$$

where $I(x)$ is the image intensity. Because fluorescence intensity varies between cells, this calibration ensures that each cell is within its detection range. For the background b, we first estimate the mean overall image intensity M_b (assuming that there is significantly more background than cells) to separate background from cells and derive a similar balloon force:

$$F_b(x) = \frac{M_b - (I(x) - M_b)}{M_b} \tag{2}$$

To avoid unstable evolution from too large forces, F_c and F_b are all bounded in $[+1, -1]$. These specific balloon forces are combined with classical curvature regularisation forces in the MGDM evolution equation, with ϕ_c, ϕ_b the signed distance function level sets defining the implicit curve evolution and κ_c, κ_b the corresponding level set mean curvature for cells c and background b:

$$\frac{\partial \phi_c}{\partial t} = (w_\kappa \kappa_c + w_c F_c)|\nabla \phi_c|, \qquad \frac{\partial \phi_b}{\partial t} = (w_\kappa \kappa_b + w_b F_b)|\nabla \phi_b| \tag{3}$$

We used the same parameters for all 2D and 3D studies and fixed the weights for curvature regularisation to $w_\kappa = 0.6$, and the balloon forces to $w_c = w_b = 0.3$. The evolution was run for 200 iterations.

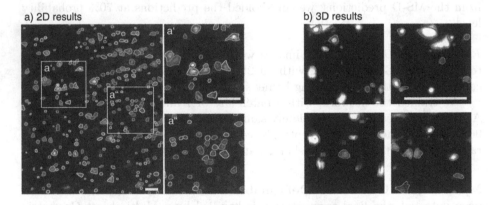

Fig. 3. Segmentation result. (a) An image from the 2D test set showing (randomly colored) outlines of segmented cell masks, subregions were magnified for better visibility. (b) Example planes from the 3D test set showing the outlines of annotated reference masks (red) and segmentation results (blue). (All scale bars 100 µm.)

3   Results

2D Cell Localization and Segmentation. To assess cell localization accuracy, we compared the MS-D net prediction to the manually annotated reference centroids and computed precision, recall, and the combined F1-score for the annotated images. Examples of final segmentation masks on the test set are shown in Fig. 3a. The segmentation performed well across regions with varying cell appearance and density. The cell localization step produced a few fusion and splitting errors, particularly in regions where small, dim cells were concentrated (Fig. 3a"). Quantitative results were aggregated over all four test images and summarized in Table 1. The proposed method improved cell detection and segmentation accuracy. We used the fastER segmentation [5] as a reference baseline because it produces state-of-the art results on par with deep learning methods such as [12] and can be trained with few annotations.[2] We further compare our results to a simple baseline using adaptive thresholding.

Table 1. Comparison of segmentation across test set. Best results shown in bold.

Method	Precision	Recall	F1-score	JI (median)
Ours	**0.895**	**0.942**	**0.918**	**0.672**
Adapt. threshold	0.255	0.855	0.393	0.634
FastER	0.834	0.917	0.874	0.521

3D Cell Localization and Segmentation. Examples of segmentation results on a test sample are shown in Fig. 2c and on 2D sub-slices in Fig. 3b (blue contours). Over the three test stacks our method achieved a good performance in 3D with a cell localization precision of 0.81, a recall of 0.873 resulting in an F1-score of 0.84 and a median Jaccard index of 0.732 for segmentation. The MGDM segmentation tended to result in slightly larger 3D masks compared to the manual reference as illustrated in Fig. 3b showing the annotated outlines in red and the segmentation result in blue.

4 Conclusions

As a proof of concept we present a hybrid strategy to segment neural cells combining a mixed-scale neural network and a topology-preserving geometric deformable model. Our method robustly detects and segments cell bodies in light-sheet microscopy images of cleared post mortem human brain tissue. High-quality results were obtained despite large variations in cell shape and intensity, anisotropic resolution and challenging imaging artifacts. Our method works for 2D and 3D images and only requires sparse centroid annotations for training. This is a crucial prerequisite for large-scale histological analysis of desired quality as fully annotated cell segmentations are tedious and error-prone in 3D.

While there exist many different options for multi-label segmentation given the initial detected cell centroids, such as watersheds or graph cuts, we chose multi-object geometric deformable models for their ability to constrain the cell boundary curvature and enforce topological relationships while allowing for a

---

[2] Note that fastER is limited to 2D images only.

flexible design of the segmentation cost function based on local rather than global intensity variations. Thus, the method can be adapted to alternative clearing, staining and imaging protocols.

As a next step we will systematically optimize the neural network architecture, the loss function, and the forces of the MGDM segmentation. Finally, the entire segmentation pipeline could also be trained end-to-end by directly learning the MGDM output using a semi-supervised approach.[3]

References

1. Bogovic, J.A., Prince, J.L., Bazin, P.L.: A multiple object geometric deformable model for image segmentation. Comput. Vis. Image Underst. **117**(2), 145–157 (2013)
2. Brodmann, K.: Vergleichende Lokalisationslehre der Grosshirnrinde in ihren Prinzipien dargestellt auf Grund des Zellenbaues. Barth (1909)
3. Chung, K., Deisseroth, K.: CLARITY for mapping the nervous system. Nat. Methods **10**(6), 508–513 (2013)
4. von Economo, C.F., Koskinas, G.N.: Die cytoarchitektonik der hirnrinde des erwachsenen menschen. J. Springer (1925)
5. Hilsenbeck, O., Schwarzfischer, M., Loeffler, D., Dimopoulos, S., Hastreiter, S., Marr, C., Theis, F.J., Schroeder, T.: fastER: a user-friendly tool for ultrafast and robust cell segmentation in large-scale microscopy. Bioinformatics (2017)
6. Hu, P., Shuai, B., Liu, J., Wang, G.: Deep level sets for salient object detection. In: 2017 IEEE Conference on Computer Vision and Pattern Recognition (CVPR), pp. 540–549. IEEE Computer Society (2017)
7. Huisken, J., Swoger, J., Del Bene, F., Wittbrodt, J., Stelzer, E.H.K.: Optical sectioning deep inside live embryos by selective plane illumination microscopy. Science **305**(5686), 1007–1009 (2004)
8. Kandel, E.R., Schwartz, J.H., Jessell, T.M., Siegelbaum, S.A., Hudspeth, A.J.: Others: Principles of Neural Science, vol. 4. McGraw-hill, New York (2000)
9. LeCun, Y., Bengio, Y., Hinton, G.: Deep learning. Nature **521**(7553), 436–444 (2015)
10. Morawski, M., et al.: Developing 3D microscopy with CLARITY on human brain tissue: towards a tool for informing and validating MRI-based histology. Neuroimage (2017)
11. Pelt, D.M., Sethian, J.A.: A mixed-scale dense convolutional neural network for image analysis. Proc. Natl. Acad. Sci. U.S.A. 115(2), 254–259 (2018)
12. Ronneberger, O., Fischer, P., Brox, T.: U-Net: convolutional networks for biomedical image segmentation. In: Navab, N., Hornegger, J., Wells, W.M., Frangi, A.F. (eds.) MICCAI 2015. LNCS, vol. 9351, pp. 234–241. Springer, Cham (2015). https://doi.org/10.1007/978-3-319-24574-4_28
13. Shen, D., Wu, G., Suk, H.I.: Deep learning in medical image analysis. Annu. Rev. Biomed. Eng. (2017)

---

[3] This would also speed up the entire pipeline as MGDM segmentation is the computationally more expensive part taking about 5 min for a 256^3 volume, while prediction with the MS-D net is about 10 times faster.

14. Tang, M., Valipour, S., Zhang, Z., Cobzas, D., Jagersand, M.: A deep level set method for image segmentation. In: Cardoso, M.J., et al. (eds.) DLMIA/ML-CDS -2017. LNCS, vol. 10553, pp. 126–134. Springer, Cham (2017). https://doi.org/10. 1007/978-3-319-67558-9_15
15. Vogt, C., Vogt, O.: Allgemeine ergebnisse unserer hirnforschung I-IV. J. Psychol. Neurol. (Lpz.) 25, Erg. heft 1, 279–462 (1919)
16. Xie, W., Noble, J.A., Zisserman, A.: Microscopy cell counting and detection with fully convolutional regression networks. Comput. Methods Biomech. Biomed. Eng. Imaging Vis. 1–10 (2016)
17. Zeiler, M.D.: Adadelta: an adaptive learning rate method. CoRR arXiv:abs/1212.5701 (2012)
18. Zilles, K., Schleicher, A., Palomero-Gallagher, N., Amunts, K.: Quantitative analysis of cyto-and receptor architecture of the human brain. Brain Mapping: The Methods (Second Edition), pp. 573–602. Elsevier, New York (2002)

Latent3DU-net: Multi-level Latent Shape Space Constrained 3D U-net for Automatic Segmentation of the Proximal Femur from Radial MRI of the Hip

Guodong Zeng[1], Qian Wang[2], Till Lerch[3], Florian Schmaranzer[3],
Moritz Tannast[3], Klaus Siebenrock[3], and Guoyan Zheng[1(✉)]

[1] Institute of Surgical Technology and Biomechanics, University of Bern,
Bern, Switzerland
guoyan.zheng@istb.unibe.ch
[2] School of Biomedical Engineering, Shanghai Jiao Tong University,
Shanghai, China
[3] Department of Orthopaedic Surgery, Inselspital,
University of Bern, Bern, Switzerland

Abstract. Radial 2D MRI scans of the hip are routinely used for the diagnosis of the cam-type of femoroacetabular impingement (FAI) and of avascular necrosis (AVN) of the femoral head, which are considered causes of hip joint osteoarthritis in young and active patients. However, for computer assisted planning of surgical treatment, it is highly desired to have 3D models of the proximal femur. In this paper, we propose a novel volumetric convolutional neural network (CNN) based framework to fully automatically extract 3D models of the proximal femur from sparsely hip radial slices. Our framework starts with a spatial transform to interpolate sparse 2D radial MR images to a densely sampled 3D volume data. Automated segmentation of the interpolated 3D volume data is very challenging due to the poor image quality and the interpolation artifact. To tackle these challenges, we introduce a multi-level latent shape space constrained 3D U-net, referred as *Latent3DU-net*, to incorporate prior shape knowledge into voxelwise semantic segmentation of the interpolated 3D volume. Comprehensive results obtained from 25 patient data demonstrated the effectiveness of the proposed framework.

1 Introduction

Femoroacetabular Impingement (FAI) and avascular necrosis (AVN) of the femoral head are known causes of osteoarthritis of the hip joint in young and active patients. Depending on clinical and imaging findings, two types of impingement are distinguished: pincer impingement is the acetabular cause of FAI and is characterized by focal or general over-coverage of the femoral head. Cam impingement is the femoral cause of FAI and is due to aspherical portion of the femoral-neck junction [1]. On the other hand, in AVN the blood flow to

© Springer Nature Switzerland AG 2018
Y. Shi et al. (Eds.): MLMI 2018, LNCS 11046, pp. 188–196, 2018.
https://doi.org/10.1007/978-3-030-00919-9_22

the femoral head is interrupted, which can progressively lead to the collapse of the hip. A lot of joint-preserving treatments have been developed in an attempt to slow or reverse its progression, as it usually affects young patients [2]. MRI has been recognized as an important assisting tool for the diagnosis and the assessment of FAI and AVN as, in addition to the non-ionizing nature, MRI can capture the vascular status of the femoral head. Moreover, MR scanners typically have the capability to directly scan planes of arbitrary orientation. A radiologist can take advantage of this in order to acquire planes perpendicular to the curvature of the acetabulum. Such a scanning protocol is often referred to as radial imaging of the hip. The appeal of using radial scans over 3D MRI for image-assisted diagnosis is its motion insensitivity and reduced scanning time, as a typical radial scan of the hip consists of much fewer slices. Radial scans around the femoral neck axis are increasingly recognized as an important tool for morphological assessment of FAI.

To enhance surgeon's ability to assess the presence, location, and severity of impingement as well as to plan hip preservation surgery, computer-assisted diagnosis and planning systems have been developed [3]. In such a system, it is highly desired to have 3D models of the proximal femur, better derived from the radial MR images of the hip to avoid extra logistic efforts and cost.

The topic of automated MR image segmentation of the hip joint has been addressed by a few studies which relied on atlas-based segmentation [4], active shape models [5] and statistical shape models [6]. Recently, with the advance of deep convolutional neural network (CNN) based techniques, deep CNN-based methods, especially those based on fully convolutional networks (FCN), are introduced for segmentation of 3D volumetric data [7–9]. Despite impressive results achieved by these methods, they all assume that densely sampled 3D volumetric data are available. To the best of our knowledge, no 3D segmentation method has been proposed for segmenting the proximal femur that relies solely on sparse radial slices, though there exists work on segmentation of other organs such as the cardiac left ventricle from radial images [10]. The method introduced in [10] depends on a matching of 3D-active shape model to sparse, arbitrarily oriented image data. The initialization of the matching is done manually. After that, the matching is driven by feature points detected using fuzzy inference.

In this paper, we propose a novel volumetric FCN-based framework to fully automatically extract 3D models of the proximal femur from sparse radial MR images of the hip. More specifically, we first perform a spatial transform to interpolate the sparse radial slices to a densely sampled volumetric data. Automated segmentation of the proximal femur from such a 3D volumetric data is challenging due to the poor image quality and the interpolation artifacts. To solve these challenges, we introduce a multi-level latent shape constrained 3D U-net, referred as *Latent3DU-net*, to incorporate prior shape knowledge into a voxelwise semantic segmentation of the proximal femur from the interpolated 3D volume.

2   Methods

Figure 1 illustrate the proposed framework, which mainly consists of two steps, i.e., spatial transform and Latent3DU-net-based segmentation of the proximal femur. Below the details about each step will be presented.

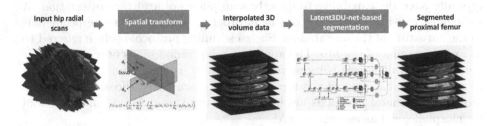

Fig. 1. A schematic illustration of the proposed framework, which mainly consists of two steps, i.e, spatial transform and Latent3DU-net-based 3D segmentation.

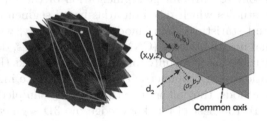

Fig. 2. A schematic illustration of how to do spatial transform.

2.1   Spatial Transform

The purpose of spatial transform is to interpolate the sparse hip radial slices to a densely sampled 3D volume data, which is done as follows. First, we compute the common axis of the radial scan by computing the intersections of all radial imaging planes. Around this axis, we then define a volume data sampling space. In order to fill the space with image data, we conduct an intensity interpolation as shown in Fig. 2. More specifically, for a point with coordinate (x, y, z) in the sampling space, we first determine the two radial planes which have the shortest distances to this point, as shown in Fig. 2-left, and denote these two plane as the ith plane and the jth plane, respectively. Assuming that the distances from this point to the two planes are d_1 and d_2, respectively, and further assuming that projections of this point onto these two planes have image coordinates of (a_1, b_1) and (a_2, b_2), respectively, we can compute the intensity value $f(x, y, z)$ at point (x, y, z) via interpolation. Although there exist many different interpolation methods, empirically we find that a distance inversely weighted interpolation as follows is enough for our purpose.

$$f(x, y, z) = (\frac{1}{d_1} + \frac{1}{d_2})^{-1} \cdot (\frac{1}{d_1} \cdot g_i(a_1, b_1) + \frac{1}{d_2} \cdot g_j(a_2, b_2)) \qquad (1)$$

where $g_i(a_1, b_1)$ and $g_j(a_2, b_2)$ denotes the image intensity values of the two image point (a_1, b_1) and (a_2, b_2), respectively.

Figure 3 shows several slices extracted from an interpolated 3D volume data.

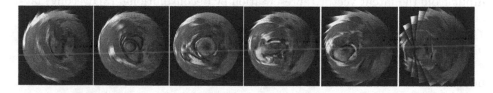

Fig. 3. Slices extracted from an interpolated 3D volume data.

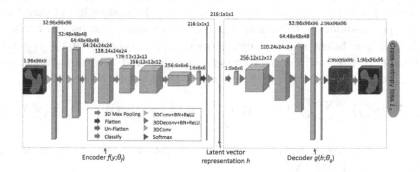

Fig. 4. Fully convolutional denoising auto-encoder for volumetric representation.

2.2 Segmentation of the Proximal Femur

It is useful to incorporate prior shape knowledge into image segmentation algorithms to obtain more accurate and plausible results. As summarized in a recent survey paper on deep learning in medical image analysis [11], most of the classification and regression models utilize a pixel-level loss function such as cross-entropy or Dice loss. Prior knowledge is usually incorporated in a post-processing step. Recently, based on the TL networks of [12], Oktay et al. [13] proposed anatomically constrained neural networks to incorporate anatomical prior knowledge into CNNs. In this paper, inspired by the fully convolutional denoising auto-encoder of [14], we propose a fully convolutional volumetric auto-encoder that learns volumetric representation from noisy data. The learned volumetric representation can then be treated as a denoised generative vector representation of anatomical knowledge in a latent space. We further propose a multi-level latent shape constrained 3D U-net, referred as *Latent3DU-net*, for accurate segmentation of the proximal femur from the interpolated volume data.

Fully convolutional denoising auto-encoder. Figure 4 shows the architecture of the fully convolutional denoising auto-encoder to learn an end-to-end, voxel-to-voxel mapping. The left half of our network can be seen as an encoder stage that results in a condensed representation (indicated by "latent vector representation"). In the second stage (right half), the network reconstructs back the input from the latent vector representation by deconvolutional (3DDeconv) layers. The network is trained using cross-entropy loss. After training, the encoder $f(y; \theta_f)$ can be used to map a noisy volumetric label to a vector representation h in the latent space.

Latent3DU-net. Figure 5 illustrates the architecture of the Latent3DU-net. It is an extension of 3D U-net [7] with multi-level deep supervision. We further leverage multi-level Euclidean losses calculated at the latent space to enforce the prediction to follow the learnt shape/label distributions. More specifically, let W be the weights of main network and $\{w^c\}$ be the weights of classifiers. Then the cross-entropy loss function of a classier is: $L_{ce}^c(\chi; W, w^c) = \sum_{x_i \in \chi} - \log p(y_i = t(x_i)|x_i; W, w^c)$, where χ represents the training samples; y_i is the ground truth label; $p(y_i = t(x_i)|x_i; W, w^c)$ is the probability of target class label $t(x_i)$ corresponding to sample $x_i \in \chi$. Additionally, as shown in Fig. 5, the Euclidean loss at latent space of a classifier is: $L_{he}^c = \|f(\phi(x)^c; \theta_f) - f(y; \theta_f)\|_2^2$, where $\phi(x)^c$ is the prediction of the cth classifier and y is the ground truth segmentation. Then the total loss function of the Latent3DU-net is:

$$L(\chi, W, \{w^c\}) = \sum_c (\alpha^c L_{ce}^c(\chi, W, w^c) + \lambda^c L_{he}^c) + \gamma(\psi(W) + \sum_c \psi(w^c)) \quad (2)$$

where $\psi()$ is the regularization term (L_2 norm in our experiment) with hyper parameter γ, $\{\alpha^c\}$ and $\{\lambda^c\}$.

For both fully convolutional denoising auto-encoder as shown in Fig. 4 and Latent3DU-net as shown in Fig. 5. All convolutional layers use kernel size of $3 \times 3 \times 3$ and strides of 1 and all max pooling layers use kernel size of $2 \times 2 \times 2$ and strides of 2. In the convolutional and deconvolutional layers of our networks, batch normalization (BN) [15] and rectified linear units (ReLU) [16] are adopted to speed up the training and to enhance the gradient back-propagation.

3   Experiments and Results

3.1   Dataset and Preprocessing

We evaluated the proposed framework on a dataset consisting of MR gadolinium-enhanced radial scans of 25 patients with symptomatic FAI or AVN. No 3D MR data was available for these patients. The intra-slice spacing of these radial scans is 0.28 mm and the size of the images is either 448×448 or 512×512. There are 14 radial slices in each radial scan. A reference, manual segmentation of every slice of the radial scans was also provided. From the 2D manual segmentation of each radial scan, we used the method introduced by Carr et al. [17] to reconstruct a smooth 3D surface model of the proximal femur. We then conducted spatial transform for all radial scans. After that, we also converted the reconstructed 3D surface models of the proximal femur into dense binary volumetric labels. As there was no 3D MR scan available for these patients, we took the corresponding dense binary volumetric labels as the ground truth segmentation.

All the interpolated volume data and the corresponding binary volumetric labels were rescaled to a size of $96 \times 96 \times 96$ due to memory restrictions. To enlarge the training samples and to mitigate possible over-fitting problem, random noise was injected: random value between $(-3, 3)$ was added to each voxel. Finally, each training sample was normalized as zero mean and unit variance before fed into the network. A standard 5-fold cross-validation study was performed to evaluate the performance of the proposed framework.

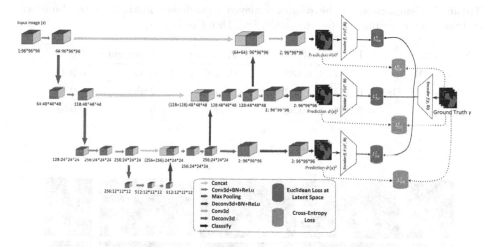

Fig. 5. Illustration of the architecture of Latent3DU-net.

3.2 Training

We trained our networks from scratch. The training was done in two stages. In the first stage, the fully convolutional denoising auto-encoder was trained for 5,000 iterations. After that, we trained the Latent3DU-net for another 5,000 iterations. All weights were initialized from a Gaussian distribution ($\mu = 0, \sigma = 0.01$) and were updated by the stochastic gradient descent(SGD) algorithm (momentum $= 0.9$, weight decay $= 0.005$). For each stage of the training, the initial learning rate was initialized as 1×10^{-3} and halved by every 1,500 times.

3.3 Testing and Evaluation

In the inference phase, only the prediction $\phi(x)^0$ of the 0th classifier was used to generate the segmentation result. After that, the segmentation was rescaled back to the original size. Implemented with Python using TensorFlow framework on a workstation with a 3.6GHz Intel(R) i7 CPU and a GTX 1080 Ti graphics card with 11GB GPU memory, on average it took Latent3DU-net about 10 s to finish one test case while the spatial transform took another 30 s.

The segmented results were compared with the associated ground truth segmentation. For each test case, we evaluated the distance between the surface models extracted from different segmentation as well as the volume overlap measurements including Dice overlap coefficient, precision and recall.

For further comparison, we implemented the 3D U-net with multi-level deep supervision (we referred it as "3DU-net-MLDS") as introduced in [9], which reported state-of-the-art results when applied to segmentation of the proximal femur from 3D MR images, and a 3D U-net [7].

Table 1. Comparison of the results achieved by different methods. HD: Hausdorff distance; ASD: average surface distance; DC: Dice Coefficient.

Methods	DC	HD (mm)	ASD (mm)	Precision	Recall
Latent3DU-net	0.954	6.18	0.74	0.958	0.950
3DU-net-MLDS	0.943	12.07	0.83	0.959	0.929
3DU-net	0.941	10.36	0.92	0.943	0.940

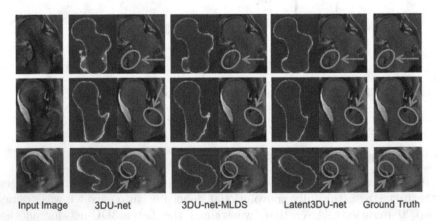

Input Image   3DU-net   3DU-net-MLDS   Latent3DU-net   Ground Truth

Fig. 6. Qualitative comparison of different methods. Data cropped for visualization purpose. For each method, the probability maps and the segmentation results are displayed. Green circles highlight the differences of different methods.

3.4   Results

Table 1 shows the segmentation results achieved by different methods. On average, our method achieved a mean ASD of 0.74 mm, a mean HD of 6.18 mm, a mean DC of 0.954, a mean precision of 0.958 and a mean recall of 0.95. When evaluated on the same dataset, the method introduced in [9] achieved a mean ASD of 0.83 mm, a mean HD of 12.07 mm, and a mean DC of 0.943 while 3D U-net achieved a mean ASD of 0.92 mm, a mean HD of 10.36 mm, and a mean DC of 0.941. Pairwise T-test on the DC measurements demonstrated that the difference between our method and the method introduced in [9] is statistically significant (p-value < 0.01). Figure 6 shows a qualitative comparison of the results achieved by these three methods.

4   Conclusions

In this paper, we presented a deep CNN-based framework to fully automatically extract a 3D model of the proximal femur from sparse hip radial slices. To the best of our knowledge, this is probably the first study addressing such a problem using deep learning. We compared the results achieved by our method to those achieved by a state-of-the-art methods. The experimental results clearly demonstrated the effectiveness of incorporating the latent space constraint for accurate segmentation of the proximal femur.

Acknowledgments. This study was partially supported by the Swiss National Science Foundation via project 205321_163224/1.

References

1. Leunig, M., Beaule, P., Ganz, R.: The concept of femoroacetabular impingement: current status and future perspectives. Clin. Orthop. Relat. Res. **467**, 616–622 (2009)
2. Chughtai, M., Piuzzi, N.: An evidence-based guide to the treatment of osteonecrosis of the femoral head. Bone Joint J. **99**(10), 1267–1279 (2017)
3. Tannast, M., Kubiak-Langer, M.: Noninvasive three-dimensional assessment of femoroacetabular impingement. J. Orthop. Res. **25**(1), 122–131 (2007)
4. Xia, Y., Fripp, J.: Automated bone segmentation from large field of view 3d MR images of the hip joint. Phys. Med. Biol. **58**(20), 7375–7390 (2013)
5. Arezoomand, S., Lee, W.: A 3d active model framework for segmentation of proximal femur in MR images. Int. J. CARS **10**(1), 55–66 (2015)
6. Chandra, S.S., Xia, Y., et al.: Focused shape models for hip joint segmentation in 3d magnetic resonance images. Med. Image Anal. **18**(3), 567–578 (2014)
7. Çiçek, Ö., Abdulkadir, A., Lienkamp, S.S., Brox, T., Ronneberger, O.: 3D U-net: learning dense volumetric segmentation from sparse annotation. In: Ourselin, S., Joskowicz, L., Sabuncu, M.R., Unal, G., Wells, W. (eds.) MICCAI 2016. LNCS, vol. 9901, pp. 424–432. Springer, Cham (2016). https://doi.org/10.1007/978-3-319-46723-8_49

8. Dou, Q., Yu, L.: 3d deeply supervised network for automated segmentation of volumetric medical images. Med. Image Anal. **41**, 40–54 (2017)
9. Zeng, G., Yang, X., Li, J., Yu, L., Heng, P.-A., Zheng, G.: 3D U-net with multi-level deep supervision: fully automatic segmentation of proximal femur in 3D MR images. In: Wang, Q., Shi, Y., Suk, H.-I., Suzuki, K. (eds.) MLMI 2017. LNCS, vol. 10541, pp. 274–282. Springer, Cham (2017). https://doi.org/10.1007/978-3-319-67389-9_32
10. Van Assen, H., Danilouchkine, M.: Spasm: a 3d-ASM for segmentation of sparse and arbitrarily oriented cardiac MRI data. Med. Image Anal. **10**(2), 286–303 (2006)
11. Litjens, G., Kooi, T.: A survey on deep learning in medical image analysis. Med. Image Anal. **42**, 60–88 (2017)
12. Girdhar, R., Fouhey, D.F., Rodriguez, M., Gupta, A.: Learning a predictable and generative vector representation for objects. In: Leibe, B., Matas, J., Sebe, N., Welling, M. (eds.) ECCV 2016. LNCS, vol. 9910, pp. 484–499. Springer, Cham (2016). https://doi.org/10.1007/978-3-319-46466-4_29
13. Oktay, O., Kamnisas, K.: Anotomically constrained neural networks (ACNN): application to cardiac image enhancement and segmentation. IEEE Trans. Med. Imaging **37**(2), 384–395 (2018)
14. Sharma, A., Grau, O., Fritz, M.: VConv-DAE: deep volumetric shape learning without object labels. In: Hua, G., Jégou, H. (eds.) ECCV 2016. LNCS, vol. 9915, pp. 236–250. Springer, Cham (2016). https://doi.org/10.1007/978-3-319-49409-8_20
15. Ioffe, S., Szegedy, C.: Batch normalization: accelerating deep network training by reducing internal covariate shift. Proc. ICML 448–456 (2015)
16. Krizhevsky, A., Ilya, S., Hinton, G.: Imagenet classification with deep convolutional neural networks. Proc. NIPS 1097–1105 (2012)
17. Carr, J., Beatson, R., et al.: Reconstruction and representation of 3d objects with radial basis functions. Computer Graphics (2001) 67–76

Adversarial Image Registration with Application for MR and TRUS Image Fusion

Pingkun Yan[1]([✉]), Sheng Xu[2], Ardeshir R. Rastinehad[3], and Brad J. Wood[2]

[1] Department of Biomedical Engineering, Rensselaer Polytechnic Institute,
Troy, NY 12180, USA
yanp2@rpi.edu
[2] National Institutes of Health, Center for Interventional Oncology,
Radiology and Imaging Sciences, Bethesda, MD 20892, USA
[3] Icahn School of Medicine at Mount Sinai, New York City, NY 10029, USA

Abstract. Robust and accurate alignment of multimodal medical images is a very challenging task, which however is very useful for many clinical applications. For example, magnetic resonance (MR) and transrectal ultrasound (TRUS) image registration is a critical component in MR-TRUS fusion guided prostate interventions. However, due to the huge difference between the image appearances and the large variation in image correspondence, MR-TRUS image registration is a very challenging problem. In this paper, an adversarial image registration (AIR) framework is proposed. By training two deep neural networks simultaneously, one being a generator and the other being a discriminator, we can obtain not only a network for image registration, but also a metric network which can help evaluate the quality of image registration. The developed AIR-net is then evaluated using clinical datasets acquired through image-fusion guided prostate biopsy procedures and promising results are demonstrated.

1 Introduction

Prostate cancer is one of the leading causes of cancer death among men in the western world. The fusion of magnetic resonance (MR) and transrectal ultrasound (TRUS) images, benefited by the good sensitivity and specificity of multiparametric MR (mpMR) on identifying suspicious prostate cancer regions, has been demonstrated improving the biopsy yield by as much as 30% [1]. For a fusion system to work effectively, accurate registration of different imaging modalities is critical. However, multi-modality image registration is a very challenging task, as it is hard to define a robust image similarity metric [2]. The registration of MR and TRUS is more difficult due to the noisy appearance of ultrasound images and the inhomogeneous imaging resolutions between MR and TRUS.

With the rapid advancement of deep learning technology in the past several years, a number of new image registration methods based on deep learning have

© Springer Nature Switzerland AG 2018
Y. Shi et al. (Eds.): MLMI 2018, LNCS 11046, pp. 197–204, 2018.
https://doi.org/10.1007/978-3-030-00919-9_23

been proposed, which gained better performance compared to the traditional methods. The early deep learning based image registration methods still follow the classical framework of iteratively optimizing over certain similarity metric through updating the transformation. Deep learning was initially only used for acquiring a better similarity metric. For example, Cheng et al. [3] used a multi-layer perceptron network to learn the correspondence between a pair of images. Simonovsky et al. [4] developed a convolutional neural network (CNN) based similarity learning network and embedded it into an image registration framework for multi-modal image alignment. Compared with the traditional manually defined similarity measures like mutual information, deep learning similarity metric uses huge number of automatically extracted features to achieve better performance. Its output value can also provide a good sense of the registration quality due to the pre-defined value range.

With more powerful CNN being designed to extract more representative image features, Miao et al. [5] proposed a CNN based method to directly estimate the transformation parameters instead of using an iterative process. Therefore, the registration can be performed very fast and efficient. De Vos et al. [6] further developed an end-to-end unsupervised registration method, which however is limited to same modality image registration. Recently, Hu et al. [7] proposed a label-driven registration method by using CNN to evaluate not only image pairs but also the object label pairs for MR-TRUS image registration. Cao et al. [8] developed a deep learning method for inter-modality image registration without using ground truth but supervised by intra-modality similarity. However, such methods lack a direct feedback of registration quality, which can be important for image-fusion guided interventions.

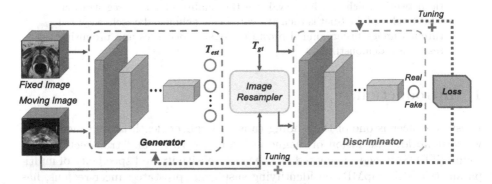

Fig. 1. Overall structure of the proposed AIR-net registration framework.

Inspired by the previous works, in this paper, we propose a multi-modality image registration method based on the generative adversarial network (GAN) framework [9] with simultaneously trained CNNs for transformation parameter estimation and registration quality evaluation. The proposed adversarial image registration network (AIR-net) consists of two sub-networks, registration generator and registration discriminator, which are trained in the adversarial fashion. An overview of the proposed AIR-net is shown in Fig. 1.

In the proposed method, the registration generator network (**G**) directly estimates transformation parameters between the input image pair. The image resampler then uses either the estimated transformation T_{est} or the ground truth transformation T_{gt} to interpolate the input moving image to get a new resampled moving image. The registration discriminator (**D**) tries to tell if its input image pair is aligned using transformation T_{est} or T_{gt}. As the training goes on, both **G** and **D** are iteratively updated. The feedback of **D** will be used to improve **G**, so that eventually **G** will be well trained to generate transformations close to T_{gt} to pass the test of **D**.

Our work in this paper has two major contributions. First, the proposed AIR-net not only estimates transformation parameters directly with an efficient feed-forward pass of G-network but also evaluates the quality of the estimated registration with the D-network, which makes it very suitable for applications like image-guided intervention. Second, the AIR-net is trained in an end-to-end fashion, where both **G** and **D** become available once the training is completed. Our experimental results demonstrate the effectiveness of the proposed approach.

The rest of this paper is organized as follows. Section 2 gives details of the proposed AIR-net. The network training and experimental results are presented in Sect. 3. Finally, Sect. 4 draws conclusions.

2 Adversarial Image Registration (AIR)

2.1 Generator and Discriminator Networks

In our work, the G- and D-networks are designed using CNNs due to their strong capability for image feature extraction and compact representation. The MR and TRUS volumes in our work are 3D data. However, to build deep CNNs to effectively deal with the complex nature of this challenging multi-modality image registration problem, we consider each 3D volume as multi-channel 2D image. In this way, much deeper neural networks can be trained on a single GPU with limited memory compared with using 3D CNNs. We also experimented with 3D CNNs with shallower structures, and our results showed that deeper 2D CNNs indeed performed better.

The structure of the designed G-network is as follows. It first starts with a dilated convolutional layer, aka atrous convolution, to enlarge the perceptive field. The layer has 128 filters with dilation of 2. All the convolutional filters in the designed networks are in the size of 3×3, if not explicitly noted. Each convolutional layer is followed by a rectified linear unit (ReLU) layer as activation. The first convolutional layer is followed by two more convolutional layers with 128 filters and stride of 2 to reduce the output tensor size. After that, a residual block containing 3 convolutional layers with residual connections as in [10] is used to have both high- and low-level features. The number of filters remains to be 128. We then used a 1×1 convolutional layer to decrease the number of filters from 128 to 8, in order to reduce the number of parameters. Two fully connected layers are then used to get the final output. The first fully connected layer has 256 hidden units, while the number of the units for the second one is equal to the transformation parameters, e.g. 6 for 3D rigid transformation and 12 for 3D affine transformation. There is no activation function for the output layer of G-network. The D-network has almost identical structure as the G-network, except that the last fully connected layer has only one output unit with Sigmoid activation function, which is for evaluating the performance of registration.

The input to the networks is in the form of "two-channel" images, which are obtained by concatenating the MR and TRUS image pair. The choice is made based on the extensive experiments performed in [11], where CNN was used to compare image patches from natural images. We believe that the conclusion also applies to medical image registration, as confirmed by the work of Simonovsky et al. [4].

2.2 Adversarial Training

The designed networks can then be trained in the adversarial fashion. However, as it is known that the original GAN [9] can be tricky to train due to the unstable loss, the improved version of Wasserstein GAN (WGAN) by Arjovsky et al. [12] is adopted in our work. To make the network quickly converge to generate good image registrations, perturbed transformations are also used to compute part of the loss so the networks can recognize poor registrations. Let I_f and I_m denote the fixed image and the moving image, respectively, corresponding to MR image and TRUS image in this application. Assume that I_m has been properly registered to I_f by using the ground truth transformation. Then the discriminator loss $\mathcal{L}(D)$ is defined as

$$\mathcal{L}(D) = -\mathbb{E}_{T \sim p_{gt}(T)}[D(I_f, I_m)] + \mathbb{E}_{T \sim p_z(T)}[D(I_f, T(I_m)], \tag{1}$$

where $\mathbb{E}_{T \sim p_{gt}(T)}[D(I_f, I_m)]$ denotes the error expectation of the discriminator given a well aligned MR-TRUS image pair and $\mathbb{E}_{T \sim p_z(T)}[D(I_f, T(I_m)]$ defines the error expectation of the discriminator given a randomly perturbed transformation. The generator loss $\mathcal{L}(G)$ is defined as

$$\mathcal{L}(G) = \mathbb{E}_{T \sim p_z(T)}[1 - D(I_f, T_{est}(T(I_m))) + \alpha \|T_{est} - T^{-1}\|^2], \tag{2}$$

where T_{est} is the registration transform generated by the generator $G(I_f, T(I_m))$ and $\|T_{est} - T^{-1}\|^2$ is the Euclidean distance between the estimated transformation and the randomly created transformation. The latter is weighted by a positive weighting parameter α.

For WGAN, after each round of training, the parameters of the D-network needs to be clipped for stability. The clipping parameter was set to be 0.01 in our work. The G-network is trained once the D-network is updated twice, i.e. the parameter of critic is set to be 2. It is worth noting that although we used the square of difference between the transformation parameters as part of the generator loss, the AIR-net can still be trained without it. The training process just takes longer and the parameters need to be tuned carefully.

3   Experiments

The presented method is implemented in Python based on the PyTorch deep learning library [13]. To realize an end-to-end training of the network with resampling component in between of the two networks, the technique of spatial transform network proposed by Jaderberg et al. [14] is used.

3.1   Materials and Training

In our work, a total 763 sets of data have been used for experiments, with 679 from the National Institutes of Health and the other 84 from the Mount Sinai Hospital. The data were acquired from MR-TRUS fusion-guided prostate cancer biopsy procedures using FDA approved UroNav device (In Vivo, FL, USA). Each case contains a T2-weighted MR volume, a 3D TRUS volume reconstructed from 2D ultrasound sweep of the prostate under electro-magnetic tracking. Each MR volume has $512 \times 512 \times 26$ voxels with the resolution of $0.3\,mm \times 0.3\,mm \times 3\,mm$. The ultrasound volumes have varying sizes and resolutions, which are determined by the ultrasound scanning parameters used during the procedure. The data were randomly split into training and validation sets with a ratio of 5:1, resulting in 636 cases for training and 127 cases for validation.

The MR and TRUS volumes are sampled into the size of 256×256 multi-channel images. The perturbed transformation parameters are in the following ranges: rotation is in $[-25,25]$ degrees and translation is in $[-5,5]\,mm$.

The developed network is trained and tested on a workstation equipped with a NVIDIA Titan Xp GPU. It take about 8 hours for the network to get trained on our dataset. When testing on an image pair, it runs very fast, using less than $100\,ms$ for estimating a transformation. We then can use both the generator and discriminator networks efficiently to iteratively update the image registration until it converges.

3.2   Experimental Results

With the trained networks, performance evaluation was then carried out. For each evaluation case, an initial transformation was randomly created in the same way as the training data by perturbing the ground truth transformation. The target registration error (TRE) and the discriminator scores (D-Scores) are then computed on the initial registration. The initial poorly aligned image pairs are input into the G-network for registration and a new set of transformation parameters are generated. The TRUS volume is then resampled by using the new registration and put together with the MR volume to form a new pair. TRE of the new registration will be computed and the new pair will also be fed into the D-network for scoring.

In our current experiment, we limit the randomly generated transformation to be in 2D, i.e. only rotation and translations in the axial view with 3 degrees of freedom. We are extending the method to more general scenarios. Figure 2 first shows some example registration results. It can be seen that starting from

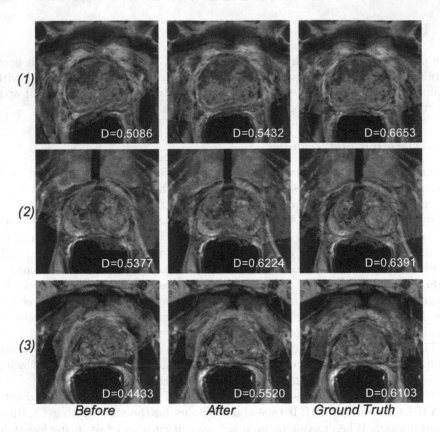

Fig. 2. Example registration results from 3 different cases. MR images are shown in gray level and corresponding TRUS images are superimposed in pseudo color. The columns from left to right are as follows. *Left*: Images aligned under a randomly generated transform before registration; *Middle*: Images aligned using the generated transformation after registration; *Right*: Images aligned using the manually performed registration by experts, which is considered as ground truth. The discriminator score for each pair of aligned images is shown in yellow at the lower right corner of the image.

some randomly perturbed registrations, the developed method was able to put the images back into alignment and get very close to the ground truth registration. The improved image alignment is also reflected by the D-Scores. As the registration quality improves, the D-scores also increase. This suggests that both the generator and discriminator networks are working effectively.

The registration performance of the developed AIR-net was then quantitatively evaluated and the results are given in Fig. 3. The evaluation was performed using both TRE and D-Scores given by the D-network, respectively. It can be seen from Fig. 3(a) that the TRE dropped significantly ($p < 0.01$) after registration, with mean TRE being decreased to 3.48 mm from 6.11 mm. in the same time, the D-scores are significantly ($p < 0.01$) improved after image registration,

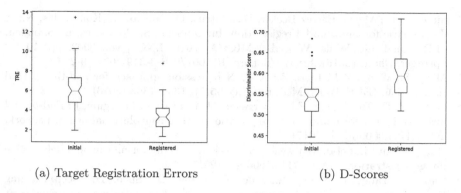

| (a) Target Registration Errors | (b) D-Scores |

Fig. 3. Evaluation of the AIR-net based image registration performance measured by TRE and D-Scores.

which shows very good correlation with TRE. Therefore, the results demonstrate that the G-network is able to generate improved registration with significantly smaller registration error and the D-network is able to tell good registration from poor registration.

4   Conclusions

In this paper, a new multi-modality image registration method of AIR-net based on the GAN framework is presented. To the best of our knowledge, this is the first work using GAN for multi-modality medical image registration. The proposed method provides not only a registration estimator, but also a quality evaluator in the same time, which can be used for quality check to detect potential registration failure. Being a major contribution of this work, it can be very useful in clinical practice to warn physicians about potential problems in image-fusion guided procedures. More evaluation will be performed in our future work against other state-of-the-art methods on registration performance.

Acknowledgment. The authors would like to thank NVIDIA Corporation for the donation of the Titan Xp GPU used for this research.

References

1. Siddiqui, M.M., et al.: Comparison of MR/ultrasound fusion-guided biopsy with ultrasound-guided biopsy for the diagnosis of prostate cancer. JAMA **313**(4), 390–397 (2015)
2. Cao, X., Gao, Y., Yang, J., Wu, G., Shen, D.: Learning-based multimodal image registration for prostate cancer radiation therapy. In: Ourselin, S., Joskowicz, L., Sabuncu, M.R., Unal, G., Wells, W. (eds.) MICCAI 2016. LNCS, vol. 9902, pp. 1–9. Springer, Cham (2016). https://doi.org/10.1007/978-3-319-46726-9_1
3. Cheng, X., Zhang, L., Zheng, Y.: Deep similarity learning for multimodal medical images. Comput. Methods Biomech. Biomed. Eng. Imaging Vis. 1–5 (2016)

4. Simonovsky, M., Gutiérrez-Becker, B., Mateus, D., Navab, N., Komodakis, N.: A deep metric for multimodal registration. In: Ourselin, S., Joskowicz, L., Sabuncu, M.R., Unal, G., Wells, W. (eds.) MICCAI 2016. LNCS, vol. 9902, pp. 10–18. Springer, Cham (2016). https://doi.org/10.1007/978-3-319-46726-9_2

5. Miao, S., Wang, Z.J., Liao, R.: A CNN regression approach for real-time 2d/3d registration. IEEE Trans. Med. Imaging 35(5), 1352–1363 (2016)

6. de Vos, B.D., Berendsen, F.F., Viergever, M.A., Staring, M., Igum, I.: End-to-end unsupervised deformable image registration with a convolutional neural network. arXiv:1704.06065 [cs] (2017)

7. Hu, Y., et al.: Label-driven weakly-supervised learning for multimodal deformable image registration. arXiv:1711.01666 [cs] (2017)

8. Cao, X., Yang, J., Wang, L., Xue, Z., Wang, Q., Shen, D.: Deep learning based inter-modality image registration supervised by intra-modality similarity. arXiv:1804.10735 [cs] (2018)

9. Goodfellow, I.J., et al.: Generative adversarial networks. arXiv:1406.2661 [cs, stat] (2014)

10. He, K., Zhang, X., Ren, S., Sun, J.: Deep residual learning for image recognition. In: 2016 IEEE Conference on Computer Vision and Pattern Recognition (CVPR), 770–778 (2016)

11. Zagoruyko, S., Komodakis, N.: Learning to compare image patches via convolutional neural networks. CoRR abs/ arXiv:1504.03641 (2015)

12. Arjovsky, M., Chintala, S., Bottou, L.: Wasserstein GAN. arXiv:1701.07875 [cs, stat] (2017)

13. Paszke, A., et al.: Automatic differentiation in pytorch. In: NIPS 2017 Workshop Autodiff (2017)

14. Jaderberg, M., Simonyan, K., Zisserman, A., Kavukcuoglu, K.: Spatial transformer networks. arXiv:1506.02025 [cs] (2015)

Reproducible White Matter Tract Segmentation Using 3D U-Net on a Large-scale DTI Dataset

Bo Li[1,2(✉)], Marius de Groot[2], Meike W. Vernooij[2], M. Arfan Ikram[2], Wiro J. Niessen[2,3], and Esther E. Bron[2]

[1] Northeastern University, Shenyang, China
[2] Erasmus MC, Rotterdam, The Netherlands
{b.li,e.bron}@erasmusmc.nl
[3] Delft University of Technology, Delft, the Netherlands

Abstract. Tract-specific diffusion measures, as derived from brain diffusion MRI, have been linked to white matter tract structural integrity and neurodegeneration. As a consequence, there is a large interest in the automatic segmentation of white matter tract in diffusion tensor MRI data. Methods based on the tractography are popular for white matter tract segmentation. However, because of the limited consistency and long processing time, such methods may not be suitable for clinical practice. We therefore developed a novel convolutional neural network based method to directly segment white matter tract trained on a low-resolution dataset of 9149 DTI images. The method is optimized on input, loss function and network architecture selections. We evaluated both segmentation accuracy and reproducibility, and reproducibility of determining tract-specific diffusion measures. The reproducibility of the method is higher than that of the reference standard and the determined diffusion measures are consistent. Therefore, we expect our method to be applicable in clinical practice and in longitudinal analysis of white matter microstructure.

Keywords: White Matter · Tract · Low resolution · DTI
Diffusion measurements · Segmentation · Convolution neural network
3D

1 Introduction

White matter (WM) tracts are the neural fibers enabling communication among brain regions. The changes in which have increasingly been associated with cognitive dysfunction and neurodegeneration. For improving understanding of neurodegenerative process and the study of pathogenesis triggered by abnormal changes, a quantitative description of WM tract is essential. Therefore, a precise segmentation method used for quantifying WM tract is needed [1].

© Springer Nature Switzerland AG 2018
Y. Shi et al. (Eds.): MLMI 2018, LNCS 11046, pp. 205–213, 2018.
https://doi.org/10.1007/978-3-030-00919-9_24

Tract segmentation is typically performed by tractography followed by a filtering step based on the prior information. After tractography reconstruction, millions of possible pathways are filtered into specific tract either via tract-specific thresholds [2], anatomical atlas based mask [3,4] or neighboring anatomical labels based prior probability [5]. However, these steps result in accumulating intermediate errors, multiple environment settings and limited consistency due to the property of tractography and, therefore, limit their application in clinical practice.

The U-Net architecture [6] has shown good performances in several segmentation tasks. Based on 3D U-Net, the newer V-Net [7] made further improvements by introducing residual function, strided convolution and convolution transpose operations. Recently a U-Net based WM tract segmentation method [8] showed competitive results to tractography-based methods. Model in [8] was trained on a high resolution dataset of only 20 subjects. In this paper we develop a method based on a large dataset of lower resolution data, and evaluate the potential of the method in this setting.

This work presents a novel deep learning method for direct segmentation of white matter tract. Our method was evaluated on the tasks of FMI and CST segmentation and determining diffusion measures. We will evaluate whether this method is reproducible and can be used to provide more insight into the role of WM microstructure in neurodegeneration.

2   Methods

2.1   Model

We built our model based on the 3D U-Net architecture. We added batch normalization after each convolution layer and replaced Relu activation function with PRelu. The used convolution layers are 3D with a kernel size of $3 \times 3 \times 3$.

As input to the model, voxel-wise diffusion tensor elements were used. The input was fed in random batches during each training iteration to increase the robustness. Its batch generation was "on-the-fly" paralleled to the training process for efficiency. The method outputs a binary segmentation of a specific tract.

2.2   Dataset

The method was developed based on the dataset of Rotterdam Study, an ongoing, population based cohort study [9]. After quality assessment, 9149 MRI scans from 4983 non-demented subjects were available for this work. Scans were performed at 1.5 Tesla. The diffusion weighted images (DWIs) were acquired with a maximum b-value of $1000\,s/mm^2$ in 25 gradient directions. Voxel size was resampled from $2.2 \times 3.3 \times 3.5\,mm^3$ to $1\,mm^3$.

We assign these scans into an optimization set (D1), a validation set (D2) and a reproducibility set (D3). Their sizes are as follows: $D1a_{train}$ 864 subjects, $D1a_{test}$ 218 subjects, size is same for $D1b_{train}$ and $D1b_{test}$ but with different subjects; $D2_{train}$ 7162 scans (including D1), $D2_{validate}$ 200 subjects and $D2_{test}$ 1036 subjects; $D3_{test}$ 80 subjects. The subjects (mean age of 69.7 years) in $D3_{test}$ had been scanned twice (mean interval of 19.3 days). A separate cohort was used for $D2_{validate}$ and $D2_{test}$ to ensure this is completely independent from $D2_{train}$. Additionally, all $D3_{test}$ related scans, which are their other rounds of scan, were excluded from D2 for the purpose of reproducibility evaluation.

2.3 Preprocessing

DWIs were corrected motion and eddy currents by co-registering all diffusion weighted volumes to the $b = 0$ volume with Elastix [10]. Diffusion tensors were estimated with ExploreDTI [11]. Diffusion measures, such as fractional anisotropy (FA) and mean diffusivity (MD), were computed based on the estimated tensors.

The diffusion tensor imaging (DTI) was used because this was the most suitable model for low-resolution DWIs. To evaluate location and structure information, with FLIRT [12] we registered the MNI_152 template and T1 weighted image (T1) to DTI space where most features were computed. Tissue masks including WM and gray matter (GM) were applied on all features. Due to the large image size and computation limitation of 3D convolution, we computed the region of interest (ROI) as input based on tract bounding boxes. The ROI sizes are $96 \times 64 \times 64$ (FMI) and $64 \times 96 \times 128$ (CST).

2.4 Reference Standard

As reference standard we used a clinical-accepted method [2], which consists of probabilistic tractography and tract-specific thresholds. Manual annotation can not be obtained as WM tracts are not visible on imaging and the semi-manual annotation on tractography images is also unrealistic for such a large dataset.

The method was evaluated on FMI and CST tract, since they are significantly related to aging [2], anatomically distinctive and have different degrees of difficulty for segmentation [8].

2.5 Evaluation Metrics

Segmentation accuracy was quantified by the Dice coefficient (DC). Binary segmentations were created from the probabilistic output by thresholding by 0.5.

To evaluate reproducibility, tract-specific metrics were compared between our method and the reference standard. Median FA and MD were individually computed inside the segmented tract, then averaged over $D3_{test}$. We computed the R^2 value of ordinary least squares (OLS) regression for measures in both scans. Cohen's kappa (K), which measures inter-rater agreement, was computed by rigidly aligning the FA image of rescan to the space of the first scan. We used t-test to compare K and paired scan-rescan differences of FA, MD and volumes with those of the reference standard, and used paired t-test to compare whether the measures determined by our method are consistent in both scans.

3   Experiments

The experiments were ran on one node of Cartesius, Dutch national supercomputer, with the Intel E5-2450 v2 CPU and NVidia Tesla K40m GPU.

3.1   Method Optimization Experiments

We optimized the method using the FMI tract on three key elements: (1) input, (2) the loss function and tract weight, and (3) network architecture. Experiments (1) and (3) were performed on $D1a$ and $D1b$, trained with default parameters of optimizers; experiment (2) was performed on $D2$. The following paragraphs will describe these optimization experiments.

We trained the V-Net based model with eleven different inputs. Nadam optimizer [13] and weighted inner product [14] loss function (L_{wip}) were used. The choice of input is based on DC and computation consumption. Since there are 25 diffusion weighted volumes in our raw DWIs and the number of volumes increases with resolution, e.g. 270 volumes in 7T scanner, it's an essential step to choose a concentrated and generalized input that works on different scanners. We considered diffusion tensor, FA, MD, location and T1 for training the model. we experimented to find the efficient input to avoid overlapping information and to reduce our high computation load due to the 3D convolution and large dataset.

To compare the L_{wip} and weighted cross entropy (L_{wce}) loss function, we trained two V-Net based models using

$$L_{wip} = -\frac{1}{N}\sum_{i=1}^{N} W * r_i * p_i + (1 - r_i) * (1 - p_i) \tag{1}$$

and

$$L_{wce} = -\frac{1}{N}\sum_{i=1}^{N} W * r_i * log(p_i) + (1 - r_i) * log(1 - p_i), \tag{2}$$

where $r_i \to \{0,1\}$ is the reference standard, $p_i \to \{0,1\}$ is the binarized prediction, N is the voxel number of the input and $W = [1,3,5,10,100]$ is the weight of tract. Due to the great frequency imbalance between classes, we evaluated different weights (W) for FMI segmentation, ranging from 1 to the mean frequency ratio of non-tract relative to tract, i.e. 100. Models were trained using Adam optimizer with an initial learning rate of 0.1, which was automatically reduced by 50% once the validation loss stopped improving for 10 epochs.

Similarly, to investigate if the newer V-Net architecture performs better than 3D U-Net in WM tract segmentation, two separate models were trained using diffusion tensor input and L_{wip}. Furthermore, to avoid the chance that one gradient descent algorithm works better for a particular back-propagation pathway, we doubled the number of experiments using Adam [15] and Nadam optimizer.

3.2   Validation Experiments

The optimized method was trained for FMI and CST tract on $D2_{train}$ to evaluate accuracy ($D2_{test}$) and reproducibility ($D3_{test}$). For $D3_{test}$, because of the short time interval between two scans (i.e. 19.3 days on average), tract segmentations and diffusion metrics are expected to be identical. We computed the paired scan-rescan differences, mean, standard deviation, R^2 value for FA, MD and volumes inside the segmented tracts in both scans and the Cohen's kappa to evaluate reproducibility of both segmentation and determining diffusion measures.

4   Results

4.1   Method Optimization Results

Figure 1 (left) presents the test DC of FMI for different combinations of input images. The figure shows that all combinations gave similar performances. Therefore, we used the simplest and most computation-efficient input, i.e. tensor only.

The performance when varying the loss function (L_{wip} and L_{wce}) and tract weight is provided in Fig. 2. L_{wip} in combination with $W = 3$ gave the best result. Both loss functions had instable performance when $W > 5$, especially L_{wce}. Based on the comparison, we used L_{wip} ($W = 3$) in the remainder of the experiments.

Since Fig. 1 (right) shows that the 3D U-Net architecture in combination with the Adam optimizer yielded a better performance than the other methods using either a V-Net architecture or the Nadam optimizer, we will adopt this combination in our method.

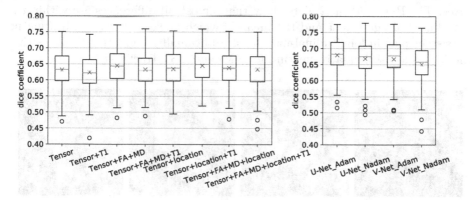

Fig. 1. Test dice coefficient of FMI for different: (left). Input images. The "Location" is an image of voxel-wise coordinates on MNI_152 template; (right). Architecture and optimizer.

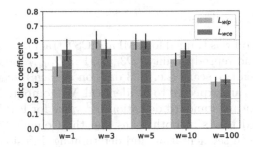

Fig. 2. Test dice coefficient of FMI using L_{wip} and L_{wce} loss function. W indicates the weight of tract.

4.2 Validation Results

Figure 3 provides a visualization of our segmentation result. It overlaps with the reference standard in (a) and (c) for FMI and right CST, respectively. The mean test DC of FMI is 0.66 (SD 0.06), that of CST is 0.77 (SD 0.03).

Figure 3(b)(d) provide its overlaps with segmented rescan, which was registered by rigidly aligning the FA images. Table 1 gives the reproducibility statistics. Typically, a $K > 0.60$ indicates "substantial" agreement between raters, and a $K > 0.80$ for "almost perfect" [16]. Our mean K for FMI longitudinal-segmentations achieved 0.74 and 0.80 for CST. The R^2 and K show that our method has better reproducibility than reference. Moreover, there was no difference in our longitudinal-measures (FA, MD, volume, paired t-test, $p > .1$). Our mean FA and MD are consistent with that of the reference. These results show that our method is applicable in longitudinal analysis of WM microstructure.

Figure 4 provides subject-wise reproducibility in determining diffusion measures. The Bland-Altman plots show that almost all differences are within the 95% limits of agreement and the mean of which is close to zero, indicating no consistent bias in longitudinal-measures. Additionally, Fig. 4 (right) shows that the MD is a discriminative feature for FMI and CST tract.

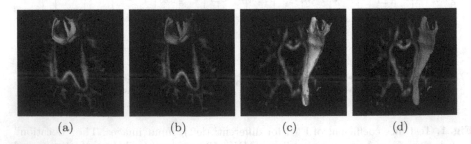

| (a) | (b) | (c) | (d) |

Fig. 3. Visualization of segmentation results: (a) FMI (blue) and reference (yellow), $DC = 0.67$; (b) FMI of the first scan and rescan (green), $K = 0.79$; (c) right CST (pink) and reference, $DC = 0.76$; (d) right CST of the first scan and rescan, $K = 0.84$.

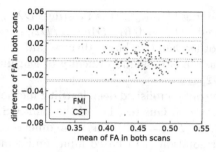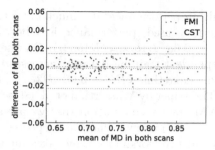

Fig. 4. The Bland-Altman plots. Difference (y-axis) and mean (x-axis) of diffusion measures (left) FA, (right) MD inside the segmented FMI and CST tract in both scans.

Table 1. Tract-specific reproducibility statistics. MD x $10^{-3}mm^2/s$. The "ref" indicates reference standard; "prop" indicates proposed method; SD standard deviation; "diff (SD)" indicates averaged absolute-differences between both scans; "mean (SD)" indicates mean value over all scans; R^2 is the R^2 value of OLS regression for measures in both scans; "Vol" indicates tract volume in ml; "K" indicates the Cohen's kappa; * significantly $(99\% - CI)$ improved from the reference, t-test, $p < .01$.

	FA			MD			Vol			K
	diff	mean	R^2	diff	mean	R^2	diff	mean	R^2	
FMI										
ref	.012 (.009)	.44 (.04)	.89	.0082 (.007)	.79 (.04)	.93	.26 (.21)	3.3 (.53)	.66	.64 (.02)
prop	.011 (.008)	.44 (.05)	.91	.0089 (.007)	.79 (.04)	93	.23 (.16)	3.8 (.58)	.79	.74* (.01)
CST										
ref	.011 (.008)	.46 (.03)	.83	.0053 (.005)	.70 (.03)	.92	.64 (.50)	6.1 (.93)	.39	.72 (.04)
prop	.009 (.003)	.46 (.03)	.84	.0052 (.004)	.69 (.03)	.93	.41*(.26)	6.5 (.69)	.52	.80* (.07)

5   Discussion

We developed and evaluated a novel deep learning method for direct WM tract segmentation. The method was trained and applied on a large set of low resolution DTI images and showed very good reproducibility. Therefore it can be applied to longitudinal imaging studies to investigate the process of neurodegeneration in WM microstructure as can be assessed with diffusion MRI.

Strengths of this study are the large size of dataset, which is representative of clinical variation, and the reproducibility validation in both segmentation and determining diffusion measures. Reproducibility is an essential indicator of a method that can be applied in clinical practice to ensure reliable and reproducible results. Moreover, comparing with the tractography-based methods, our direct method enables to segment a 3D tract in 0.5 s, and therefore avoid the processing time and storage space of tractography for researchers who only focus on the analysis of diffusion measures.

Based on the results of FMI segmentation we concluded that both the dependency of train and test datasets and their respective sizes are important for the resulting performance. If a much older training ($D1b_{train}$) than testing ($D2_{test}$) dataset is used, performance is suboptimal ($DC = 0.61$, $D1b_{train}/D2_{test}$ vs. $DC = 0.68$, $D1b_{train}/D1b_{test}$). On the other hand, a large, diverse and test-independent training dataset increases the robustness and difficulty of learning at the same time ($DC = 0.66$, $D2_{train}/D2_{test}$).

The paper by Wasserthal et al. [8] is the only published deep learning method of WM tract segmentation that we are aware of. Our test DC of the right CST ($DC = 0.77$) is lower than that reported in [8] ($DC = 0.83$). The main differences between two works are: they takes high resolution (7T) based input and semi-manual annotated reference, stacks four 2D models and is tested on only 5 subjects; while ours is applicable for a low-resolution dataset (1.5T), uses one 3D model and tested on a train-independent cohort of 1036 subjects. We suspect that the differences in the quality of the reference standard and the data are the main causes of this performance difference.

A limitation of our method is that we take a single tract ROI. This is mainly because of the large whole input size of $210 \times 211 \times 123 \times 6$ and the limitation of 3D convolution, which used for preserving the continuity of the tract. Another limitation is our low quality reference standard. Validation is difficult since the semi-manual annotation can not be obtained for such a large dataset.

For future work, our method will be applied in a dementia population. We will tackle the computation limitation of taking whole brain volume as input.

We conclude that our direct WM tract segmentation method has very good reproducibility and comparable performance to the reference standard. This is the first deep learning based method of WM tract segmentation developed on such a large-scale dataset. Our method can lead toward a faster, more lightweight way of diffusion measures analysis, thereby, reducing the time-consuming of segmentation, the complexity of pipeline setting and the required storage space.

References

1. OSullivan, M., et al.: Evidence for cortical disconnection as a mechanism of age-related cognitive decline. Neurology **57**(4), 632–638 (2001)
2. de Groot, M., et al.: Tract-specific white matter degeneration in aging: the Rotterdam study. Alzheimer's Dement **11**(3), 321–330 (2015)
3. Lawes, I.N.C., et al.: Atlas-based segmentation of white matter tracts of the human brain using diffusion tensor tractography and comparison with classical dissection. Neuroimage **39**(1), 62–79 (2008)
4. O'Donnell, L.J., Westin, C.F.: Automatic tractography segmentation using a high-dimensional white matter atlas. IEEE Trans. Med. Imaging **26**(11), 1562–1575 (2007)
5. Yendiki, A., Reuter, M., Wilkens, P., Rosas, H.D., Fischl, B.: Joint reconstruction of white-matter pathways from longitudinal diffusion MRI data with anatomical priors. Neuroimage **127**, 277–286 (2016)
6. Ronneberger, O., Fischer, P., Brox, T.: U-net: convolutional networks for biomedical image segmentation. In: Navab, N., Hornegger, J., Wells, W.M., Frangi, A.F. (eds.) MICCAI 2015. LNCS, vol. 9351, pp. 234–241. Springer, Cham (2015). https://doi.org/10.1007/978-3-319-24574-4_28

7. Milletari, F., et al.: V-net: Fully convolutional neural networks for volumetric medical image segmentation. In: 3D Vision (3DV), pp. 565–571. IEEE (2016)
8. Wasserthal, J., et al.: Direct white matter bundle segmentation using stacked u-nets. arXiv preprint arXiv:1703.02036 (2017)
9. Hofman, A., et al.: The Rotterdam study: 2016 objectives and design update. Eur. J. Epidemiol. **30**(8), 661–708 (2015)
10. Klein, S., Staring, M., Murphy, K., Viergever, M.A., Pluim, J.P.: Elastix: a toolbox for intensity-based medical image registration. IEEE Trans. Med. Imaging **29**(1), 196–205 (2010)
11. Leemans, A., et al.: Exploredti: a graphical toolbox for processing, analyzing, and visualizing diffusion MR data. Int. Soc. Mag. Reson. Med. **209**, 35–37 (2009)
12. Jenkinson, M., et al.: Improved optimization for the robust and accurate linear registration and motion correction of brain images. Neuroimage **17**(2), 825–841 (2002)
13. Dozat, T.: Incorporating nesterov momentum into adam (2016)
14. Choi, S.S., Cha, S.H., Tappert, C.C.: A survey of binary similarity and distance measures. J. Syst. Cybern. Inf. **8**(1), 43–48 (2010)
15. Kingma, D.P., Ba, J.: Adam: a method for stochastic optimization. arXiv preprint arXiv:1412.6980 (2014)
16. Landis, J.R., Koch, G.G.: The measurement of observer agreement for categorical data. Biometrics pp. 159–174 (1977)

Competition *vs.* Concatenation in Skip Connections of Fully Convolutional Networks

Santiago Estrada[1,2(✉)], Sailesh Conjeti[1,2], Muneer Ahmad[1,2], Nassir Navab[2], and Martin Reuter[1,3]

[1] German Center for Neurodegenerative Diseases (DZNE), Bonn, Germany
[2] Computer Aided Medical Procedures, Technische Universität München, München, Germany
santiago.estrada@tum.de
[3] Department of Radiology, Harvard Medical School, Boston, MA, USA

Abstract. Increased information sharing through short and long-range *skip* connections between layers in fully convolutional networks have demonstrated significant improvement in performance for semantic segmentation. In this paper, we propose Competitive Dense Fully Convolutional Networks (CDFNet) by introducing competitive maxout activations in place of naïve feature concatenation for inducing competition amongst layers. Within CDFNet, we propose two architectural contributions, namely competitive dense block (CDB) and competitive unpooling block (CUB) to induce competition at local and global scales for short and long-range skip connections respectively. This extension is demonstrated to boost learning of specialized sub-networks targeted at segmenting specific anatomies, which in turn eases the training of complex tasks. We present the proof-of-concept on the challenging task of whole body segmentation in the publicly available VISCERAL benchmark and demonstrate improved performance over multiple learning and registration based state-of-the-art methods.

1 Introduction

Fully convolutional neural networks (F-CNNs) are being increasingly adopted for pixel/voxel-wise semantic segmentation of images in an end-to-end fashion. F-CNNs are typically constructed with a dumb-bell like architecture comprising of the encoder and decoder blocks in sequence [1]. One of the main architectural advances has been the introduction of connectivity amongst and within these blocks, which has in turn improved parameter optimization and gradient flow. Computational graph elements associated with such a connectivity can be broadly categorized into long-range and short-range connections. Long-range connections were first introduced by Ronnerberger *et al.* [2] as skip connections between the encoder and decoder blocks and were demonstrated to improve information recovery and gradient flow. Short-range connections between convolutional layers were introduced in the seminal work on residual networks by

© Springer Nature Switzerland AG 2018
Y. Shi et al. (Eds.): MLMI 2018, LNCS 11046, pp. 214–222, 2018.
https://doi.org/10.1007/978-3-030-00919-9_25

He *et al.* [3]. This idea was taken further within the work of densely-connected neural networks [4], wherein multiple convolutional layers were stacked in sequence along with connections that iteratively concatenate the feature maps with outputs of the previous layers. Introducing these short-range dense connections alleviate vanishing gradients, encourage feature reusability and strengthen information propagation across the network [4].

One commonality between design of the computational graph within the aforementioned architectures is the use of concatenation layers to aggregate information through these connections. Such a design increases the size of the output feature map along the feature channels, which in turn results in the need to learn filters with a higher number of parameters. Goodfellow *et al.* introduced the idea of competitive learning through maxout activations [5], which was adapted by Liao and Carneiro [6] for competitive pooling of multi-scale filter outputs. Both [6] and [5] proved that the use of a maxout competitive unit boosts performance by creating a large number of dedicated sub-networks within a network that learns to target specific sub-tasks within the training task and reduces the number of parameters required. In this paper, we explore how such competitive units fare within a FCNN architecture targeted at biomedical image seg-

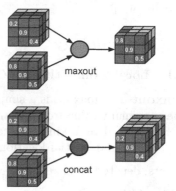

Fig. 1. Maxout activation: The maxout operation computes the maximum at each spatial location across feature maps. This is a more selective fusion operation than concatenation and results in a lower dimensional feature space.

mentation. We propose the Competitive Dense Fully Convolutional Network (CDFNet) by using competitive layers instead of concatenation by suitably adopting the DenseNet architecture proposed by Roy *et al.* in [7]. Particularly, we demonstrate that competitive units promote the formation of dedicated local sub-networks in each of the densely connected blocks within the encoder and the decoder paths. This in turn encourages sub-modularity through a network-in-network design that can learn more efficiently. Towards this, we propose two novel architectural elements targeted at introducing competition within the short- and long-range connections, as follows:

1. **Local Competition**: By introducing maxout activations within the short-range skip connections of each of the densely connected convolutional layers (at the same resolution), we encourage local competition during learning of filters and the multiple convolution layers in each block prevents filter co-adaptation.
2. **Global Competition**: We introduce a maxout activation between a long-range skip connection from the encoder and the features up-sampled from the prior lower-resolution decoder block. This promotes competition between finer feature maps with smaller receptive fields (skip connections) and coarser

feature maps from the decoder path that spans much wider receptive fields encompassing higher contextual information.

The proof-of-concept for CDFNet is shown on the challenging task of whole-body segmentation in contrast-enhanced abdominal Magnetic Resonance Imaging (abMRI) scans as a part of the publicly available VISCERAL segmentation benchmark [8].

2 Methodology

2.1 Local Competition - *Competitive Dense Block*

Maxout The maxout is a simple feed-forward activation function that chooses the maximum value from its inputs [5]. Within a CNN, a maxout feature map is constructed by taking the maximum across multiple input feature maps ($\mathbf{X}$) for a particular spatial location (say (i, j, k)), illustrated in Fig. 1. Assuming L inputs, denoted as $\mathbf{X} = \{\mathbf{x}^l\}_{l=1}^L$, with each $\mathbf{x}^l = \left[x_{ijk}^l\right]_{i,j,k=1}^{H,W,C}$, where H is height, W is width and C are number of channels for a particular feature map($\mathbf{x}^l$). The maxout($\mathbf{X}$) output is given by:

$$\text{maxout}(\mathbf{X}) = [y_{ijk}]_{i,j,k=1}^{H,W,C} \text{ where } y_{ijk} = \max\left\{x_{ijk}^1, \cdots, x_{ijk}^L\right\} \qquad (1)$$

Comparing to ReLU activation that allows for division of the input space into two regions through competition with constant value of 0, the maxout activation can divide into as many regions as L, with each region activated by a dedicated input. Such an activation is demonstrated to better estimate exponentially complex functions, as each individual region acts as a specialized sub-module focusing on dedicated tasks and allowing for data-driven self-organization within the network during training [9].

Competitive Dense Block (CDB) The dense convolutional block proposed in [4] introduces feed-forward connections from each layer to every other layer. The dense block *concatenates* feature-maps of all previous layers as input to the current layer and the output of the current layer is used as input to all subsequent layers within the block (dense connections). We replace the feature map *concatenations* with maxout activations to promote local competition amongst the layers. This is mathematically formulated in Eqs. 2–4 and illustrated in Fig. 2.

$$\mathbf{X}_l = H_3^l(\mathbf{y}_2) \quad \mathbf{X}_l = \tilde{H}_3^l(\mathbf{y}_2) \qquad (2)$$

$$\mathbf{y}_2 = [H_2^l(\mathbf{y}_1), \mathbf{y}_1, \mathbf{X}_{l-1}] \quad \mathbf{y}_2 = \text{maxout}(\tilde{H}_2^l(\mathbf{y}_1), \mathbf{y}_1) \qquad (3)$$

$$\underbrace{\mathbf{y}_1 = [H_1^l(\mathbf{X}_{l-1}), \mathbf{X}_{l-1}]}_{\text{Densely Connected Block}} \quad \underbrace{\mathbf{y}_1 = \text{maxout}(\tilde{H}_1^l(\mathbf{X}_{l-1}), \mathbf{X}_{l-1})}_{\text{Competitive Dense Block}} \qquad (4)$$

Here, $[\cdot]$ represents the concatenation operator and $\tilde{H}_j^l$ is a composite function of three consecutive operations: convolution, followed by ReLU and Batch

Normalization (BN). Such a sequence of operations ensures both improved convergence while simultaneously pre-conditioning inputs to the maxout activation by ensuring an even distribution of the input points [10] and an increase in the exploratory span of the created sub-networks [6]. It must be noted that as the convolutional layers span increasing receptive fields as we traverse through the block a soft constraint is imposed to implicitly prevent filter co-adaptation.

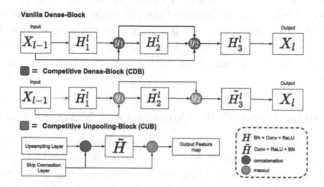

Fig. 2. Competitive Architectural Elements within CDFNet: first row) Vanilla Dense Block; second row) Competitive Dense Block and third row) Competitive Unpooling Block. The red and blue squares correspond to the blocks on Fig. 3

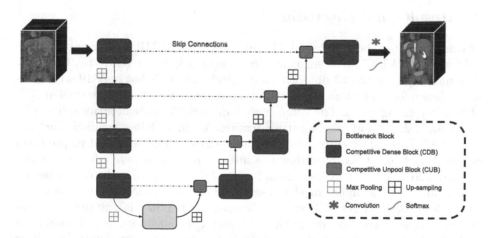

Fig. 3. Network Architecture: Competitive Dense Fully Convolutional Network (CDFNet), with 4 CDB on each of the encoder and decoder path and 4 CUB between them. CDB and CUB induce local and global competition within the network.

2.2   Global Competition - *Competitive Un-pooling Block* (CUB)

As mentioned in [2,11], the long-range skip connections between encoding and decoding paths is usually performed through the *concatenation* layer. To induce competition within this layer, a naïve solution would be to perform a maxout operation directly between the feature maps of the upsampling path and the skip connection as in the CDB design. However, we empirically observed that such architecture was unstable and resulted in loss of information. To counter this, we propose to first learn a joint feature-map (through a 1×1 convolutional layer $\tilde{H}$), which in turn competes with the features from the skip connection. Such a design (Fig. 2) improved feature selectivity between fine-grained with local span and coarser high-context information with much wider span coming from the up-sampling path.

2.3   Competitive Dense Fully Convolutional Network- CDFNet

We adopt the densely connected network for semantic segmentation architecture proposed in [7] and suitably introduce the CDB and CUB in place of the vanilla dense block and the unpooling layers respectively as illustrated in Fig. 3. In brief, the proposed CDFNet comprises of a sequence of four CDBs, constituting the encoder path (downsampling block) with four CDBs constituting the decoder path joined via a bottleneck layer. The skip connections from each of the encoder blocks feed into the CUB; that subsequently forwards features into the corresponding decoder block of the same resolution.

3   Results and Discussion

Dataset: We use the abdominal T1 contrast-enhanced MR scans from the publicly available VISCERAL segmentation benchmark [8] for validating CDFNet. The dataset presented 13 different anatomical structures but only 10 structures were chosen for evaluation (the left out organs were annotated in less than 30% of gold corpus volumes). The volumes were divided into patient-space splits of 15 scans for training and 5 held out for testing. Auxiliary labels available through the VISCERAL silver corpus from 70 anatomical scans were used to pre-train our models. It must be noted that the silver corpus labels were inherently noisy as they were generated by consensus fusion of the results of multiple competing algorithms [8]. The choice of this dataset for proof-of-concept is motivated by multiple factors (1) the task is very challenging due to potential soft organ motion (hence potential artefacts during acquisition), (2) spans a myriad of anatomies and (3) the high degree of class imbalance increases the complexity (*e.g.* liver to gallbladder has a ratio of 225:1). Moreover, the labels within the gold corpus are non-exhaustive due to potentially missing annotations in some scans.
Baselines and Comparative Methods: We compare our CDFNet with state-of-the art fully convolutional networks for semantic segmentation such as densely connected network (DenseNet) [11], U-Net [2] and SD-Net [12]. All the aforementioned networks were implemented maintaining consistency in the architecture

Table 1. Mean and standard deviation of the Dice scores for the different models and best algorithms from the VISCERAL Benchmark [8] on all, non-occluded and occluded organs.

Models	All	Non-occluded	Occluded
M-AR via MRF [8][5]	0.559 ± 0.301	0.777 ± 0.120	0.286 ± 0.208
M-AR w/DOSS [8][6]	–	0.809 ± 0.054	0.494 ± 0.238
UNet [2]	0.693 ± 0.200	0.828 ± 0.068	0.491 ± 0.146
SD-Net [12]	0.718 ± 0.179	0.835 ± 0.070	0.543 ± 0.138
DenseNet [11]	0.731 ± 0.184	$\mathbf{0.851 \pm 0.062}$	0.550 ± 0.153
CDFNet	$\mathbf{0.742 \pm 0.166}$	0.848 ± 0.060	$\mathbf{0.583 \pm 0.143}$

Table 2. Mean and standard deviation of the Dice scores for the different CDFNet baselines.

Networks	Local Competition	Global Competition	All	Non-occluded	Occluded
BL 0	✗	✗	0.731 ± 0.184	0.851 ± 0.062	0.550 ± 0.153
BL 1	✓	✗	0.729 ± 0.178	0.843 ± 0.056	0.559 ± 0.152
BL 2	✗	✓	0.739 ± 0.170	$\mathbf{0.852 \pm 0.061}$	0.570 ± 0.129
CDFNet	✓	✓	$\mathbf{0.742 \pm 0.166}$	0.848 ± 0.060	$\mathbf{0.583 \pm 0.143}$

i.e. four stages of encoders and corresponding decoders feeding into the classification layer. In addition to these, methods based on multi-atlas registration (M-AR) and label propagation from the original VISCERAL challenge (namely, M-AR via MRF and M-AR w/DOSS) [8] were also included for comparison.

We also test the importance of local and global competition by defining three ablative baselines: BL0: vanilla densely connected network proposed in [7] (*sans* any competitive blocks), BL1: network inducing local competition through CDB albeit with vanilla unpooling through concatenation and skip layers, and BL2: network inducing global competition through CUB with vanilla dense blocks. All the aforementioned architectures were trained with a composite loss function of median frequency balanced logistic loss and Dice loss [12], together with affine data augmentation. All networks were implemented on Keras [13] and trained until convergence using an NVIDIA Titan Xp GPU with 12 GB RAM with the following parameters: batch-size of 4, momentum set to 0.9, weight decay constant to 10^{-6}, with an initial learning rate of 0.01 and decreased by one order every 20 epochs.

Results: To better understand the behavior of the methods towards highly varying anatomies, we categorized the target organs into non-occluded and occluded organs (organs that are most susceptible to organ motion and not clearly visible due to poor lateral resolution). Table 1 presents the mean Dice scores of all organs, non-occluded organs and occluded organs as evaluated on the held-out test data. The results of our ablative testing against local and global competition is tabulated in Table 2. From Table 1 we observe that the proposed CDFNet demonstrates the best overall Dice score in comparison to all the other comparative methods and particularly performed well in segmenting occluded organs, with a statistically significant margin ($p < 0.001$) in comparison to the closest comparative method (DenseNet), without increase in the number of parameters.

It must also be noted that all the FCNN based methods significantly outperformed M-AR based methods which is consistent with observations made in [12]. From Table 2, we infer that introducing competition simultaneously at both local and global scales improves overall performance most notably for occluded organs. Particularly, BL2 with global competition through competitive unpooling improves significantly over BL0 demonstrating that features learned through the decoders do not co-adapt with features from the skip connections.

Figure 4 presents the structure-wise Dice scores comparing CDFNet to other FCNN architectures with additional information on the degree of class imbalance and percentage of gold corpus volumes that have the particular label. Particularly comparing CDFNet to DenseNet, we observe that smaller and occluded organs such as gallbladder, aorta and pancreas are better recovered as competition improves network's selectivity towards fine-grained structures. We also illustrate this behavior in an unseen test scan in Fig. 5(a-d), where the networks show stark contrast in the segmentation of smaller structures, while large organs such as the liver are segmented with comparative performance. We must note that the VISCERAL Gold Corpus benchmark is not exhaustive as demonstrated in Fig. 5(h) where the left and right kidneys were not annotated despite being visible in this scan. CDFNet successfully recovers these structures as shown in Fig. 5(g).

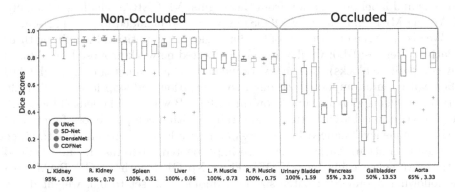

Fig. 4. Structure-wise Dice scores boxplot comparing CDFNet *vs.* other FCNN architectures, Additionally the percentage of gold corpus volumes that have the particular label and degree of class imbalance are given. Left and right are indicated as L. and R. and the P. stands for Psoas Muscle.

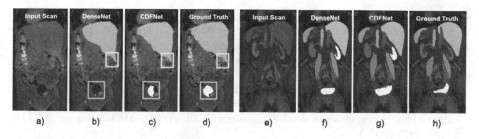

Fig. 5. Comparison of the Ground Truth *vs.* predictions. The red and yellow squares on (a-d) represent the organs where the proposed method CDFNet (c) improves the segmentation over DenseNet (b). The red arrows on left and right Kidney (e-h) show that the networks are generalizing even when they are not manually annotated on the ground truth.

4   Conclusion

In this paper, we introduced a novel network architecture, termed Competitive Dense Fully Convolutional Network (CDFNet) that introduced competition amongst filters to improve feature selectivity within a network. CDFNet introduced competition at a local scale by substituting concatenation layers with maxout activations that prevent filter co-adaptation and reduces the overall network complexity. It also induces competition at a global scale through competitive unpooling. We evaluated our proof-of-concept on the challenging task of whole-body segmentation and clearly demonstrated that small and highly occluded structures are recovered significantly better with CDFNet over other deep learning variants that employ concatenation layers.

References

1. Badrinarayanan, V., Kendall, A., Cipolla, R.: Segnet: a deep convolutional encoder-decoder architecture for image segmentation. IEEE Trans. Pattern Anal. Mach. Intell. **39**(12), 2481–2495 (2017)
2. Ronneberger, O., Fischer, P., Brox, T.: U-net: convolutional networks for biomedical image segmentation. In: Navab, N., Hornegger, J., Wells, W.M., Frangi, A.F. (eds.) MICCAI 2015. LNCS, vol. 9351, pp. 234–241. Springer, Cham (2015). https://doi.org/10.1007/978-3-319-24574-4_28
3. He, K., Zhang, X., Ren, S., Sun, J.: Deep residual learning for image recognition. In: Proceedings of the IEEE conference on computer vision and pattern recognition, pp. 770–778 (2016)
4. Huang, G., Liu, Z., Weinberger, K.Q., van der Maaten, L.: Densely connected convolutional networks. In: Proceedings of the IEEE conference on computer vision and pattern recognition, vol. 1, p. 3 (2017)
5. Goodfellow, I.J., Warde-Farley, D., Mirza, M., Courville, A., Bengio, Y.: Maxout networks. In: Proceedings of the 30th International Conference on International Conference on Machine Learning-Volume 28, pp. III-1319. JMLR. org (2013)

6. Liao, Z., Carneiro, G.: A deep convolutional neural network module that promotes competition of multiple-size filters. Pattern Recognit. **71**, 94–105 (2017)
7. Roy, A.G., Conjeti, S., Navab, N., Wachinger, C.: Quicknat: Segmenting MRI neuroanatomy in 20 s. arXiv preprint arXiv:1801.04161 (2018)
8. Jimenez-del Toro, O., Müller, H., Krenn, M., Gruenberg, K., Taha, A.A., Winterstein, M., Eggel, I., Foncubierta-Rodríguez, A., Goksel, O., Jakab, A.: Cloud-based evaluation of anatomical structure segmentation and landmark detection algorithms: visceral anatomy benchmarks. IEEE Trans. Med. Imaging **35**(11), 2459–2475 (2016)
9. Srivastava, R.K., Masci, J., Gomez, F., Schmidhuber, J.: Understanding locally competitive networks. arXiv preprint arXiv:1410.1165 (2014)
10. Liao, Z., Carneiro, G.: On the importance of normalisation layers in deep learning with piecewise linear activation units. In: 2016 IEEE Winter Conference on Applications of Computer Vision (WACV), pp. 1–8. IEEE (2016)
11. Jégou, S., Drozdzal, M., Vazquez, D., Romero, A., Bengio, Y.: The one hundred layers tiramisu: fully convolutional densenets for semantic segmentation. In: 2017 IEEE Conference on Computer Vision and Pattern Recognition Workshops (CVPRW), pp. 1175–1183. IEEE (2017)
12. Roy, A.G., Conjeti, S., Sheet, D., Katouzian, A., Navab, N., Wachinger, C.: Error Corrective Boosting for Learning Fully Convolutional Networks with Limited Data. In: Descoteaux, M., Maier-Hein, L., Franz, A., Jannin, P., Collins, D.L., Duchesne, S. (eds.) MICCAI 2017. LNCS, vol. 10435, pp. 231–239. Springer, Cham (2017). https://doi.org/10.1007/978-3-319-66179-7_27
13. Chollet, F., et al.: Keras. https://keras.io (2015)

Ensemble of Multi-sized FCNs to Improve White Matter Lesion Segmentation

Zhewei Wang[1], Charles D. Smith[2], and Jundong Liu[1(✉)]

[1] School of Electrical Engineering and Computer Science,
Ohio University, Athens, OH, USA
liuj1@ohio.edu
[2] Department of Neurology, University of Kentucky,
Lexington, KY, USA

Abstract. In this paper, we develop a two-stage neural network solution for the challenging task of white-matter lesion segmentation. To cope with the vast variability in lesion sizes, we sample brain MR scans with patches at three different dimensions and feed them into separate fully convolutional neural networks (FCNs). In the second stage, we process large and small lesion separately, and use ensemble-nets to combine the segmentation results generated from the FCNs. A novel activation function is adopted in the ensemble-nets to improve the segmentation accuracy measured by Dice Similarity Coefficient. Experiments on MICCAI 2017 White Matter Hyperintensities (WMH) Segmentation Challenge data demonstrate that our two-stage-multi-sized FCN approach, as well as the new activation function, are effective in capturing white-matter lesions in MR images.

1 Introduction

Multiple Sclerosis (MS) may result in lesions within patients' white matter tissues, which can be observed through Magnetic Resonance Imaging (MRI). Identifying and measuring the spatial and temporal disseminations of lesions are key components of diagnostic criteria for MS. Traditional approaches to segment MS lesions include the utilization of supervised classification [1] or unsupervised clustering [8,12,14] to separate lesions from the normal brain tissues, where the former are commonly modeled as either an additional class or the outliers to the latter.

In recent years, deep learning models, especially convolutional neural networks (CNN), have emerged as a new and more powerful paradigm in handling various artificial intelligence tasks, including image segmentation. Being able to process information from various spatial scales, the fully convolutional networks (FCN) [9] and its variants [10,11] have gained great popularity in recent years. U-Net [11] is arguably the most well-known FCN model in medical image analysis. It utilizes a deep CNN to encode discriminative features of the training images and relies on a deconvolution decoder to integrate the features together in producing the segmentation results.

Y. Shi et al. (Eds.): MLMI 2018, LNCS 11046, pp. 223–232, 2018.
https://doi.org/10.1007/978-3-030-00919-9_26

While U-net and its extensions [2–4, 10] are proven effective to segment fixed sized objects (e.g., organs or cells), they may not fare well for MS lesions, especially when the network is designed to optimize *Dice Similarity Coefficient* (DSC). MS lesions have a huge variability in size – large lesions can easily contain thousands of voxels, while many tiny ones are as small as only 1–2 voxels. As DSC is computed based on all foreground voxels, large lesions are more important and tend to be treated with favor, while small lesions could be overlooked without much penalty. Moreover, as DSC is not differentiable and therefore cannot be directly used for gradient descent, many neural network models [5, 6, 10, 13] take a probabilistic version of DSC, as an approximation to the discrete DSC, in their objective functions. Such approximation, however, deserves careful scrutiny, as the theoretical gaps between discrete optimizations and continuous optimization are generally difficult to overcome.

In this paper, we look into these two issues and propose a remedy based on a two-stage multi-sized FCNs architecture. To cope with the lesion variability issue, we process large and small lesions separately, and use ensemble nets to combine the segmentation results from different sized FCNs. The contributions of individual FCNs to the overall segmentation are automatically determined. To bridge the gap between discrete and continuous DSCs, we tackle the issue from the activation function perspective, and propose a new activation function to facilitate the network training and improve the segmentation accuracy.

2 Dice as Evaluation Metric and Objective Function: Issues

Let S be the segmentation result produced by a solution and R be the ground truth, both of which are binary maps defined on the entire image domain. DSC relies on the similarity of S and R to measure the segmentation accuracy:

$$DSC = \frac{2|S \cap R|}{|S| + |R|} \tag{1}$$

Segmentation Biases. As equal weights are assigned to all foreground voxels in S and R, seeking higher DSC would strive to capture large lesions, but tend to overlook small lesions, resulting in false-negative (type II) errors. When the input size of an FCN is set to the entire image or a large sub-volume, such effect can be easily observed. This situation can be regarded as a special type of data imbalance. When the inputs are set to small sub-volumes, global information would be limited within each input, and false positive (type I) error are prone to be generated. In addition, for the small patches that are mostly immersed within a large lesion, they may contain more lesion voxels than non-lesional ones. This leads to a different type of input imbalance, which could also result in erroneous segmentations. When DSC is used as a segmentation evaluation metric, all these biases are inherent to the system. To reduce them, processing the images with sub-volumes of different sizes can potentially provide a remedy.

Discrete vs. Continuous Dice. Defined on binary maps, DSC in Eq. 1 is not differentiable, therefore cannot be directly used as the objective function for FCNs. In practice, a probabilistic or continuous version DSC, called Dice loss [10], has been used as an approximation to lead the updates of segmentation. In Dice loss, segmentation S is relaxed to a probability map of real numbers between 0 and 1, and the loss is computed as:

$$\text{Dice loss} = -\frac{2\sum_i s_i r_i}{\sum_i s_i + \sum_i r_i} \tag{2}$$

where $s_i \in [0,1]$ is the label prediction at voxel i, and $r_i \in \{0,1\}$ is the corresponding binary ground truth.

There exists, however, a theoretical gap between the discrete optimization of DSC and the continuous optimization of Dice loss. An illustration example is given as follows.

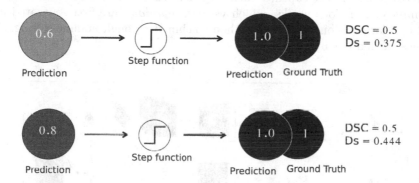

Fig. 1. An example to illustrate the gap between DSC and Dice loss (Ds). Refer to text for more details.

Consider two overlapping disks, one is the ground truth segmentation with intensity value of 1, and the other is the prediction with probabilities in the range of $[0,1]$. Assume the overlapping area between the ground truth and the prediction is half of the disk. To calculate DSC, the prediction map needs to be converted to binary through a Step function that uses 0.5 as the threshold. In Fig. 1, two prediction maps are shown, with the across-the-board probabilities of 0.6 and 0.8, respectively. The upper case (prediction = 0.6) has a Dice loss of 0.375, and that for the lower case (prediction = 0.8) is 0.444. The discrete DSCs for them, however, are both 0.5.

This example illustrates that decreases in the Dice loss do not necessarily lead to decreases (or even changes at all) in the values of DSC. This gap can pose serious difficulty in the network training procedure. Our approach to bridge the gap is through an activation function point of view, and the design will be presented in next section.

3 Remedy: Two-Stage-Multi-sized FCNs and a New Activation Function

As we mentioned in the previous section, when a single DSC-based FCN is utilized to segment lesions that have a vast variability in size, different types of segmentation biases may be generated. A combined remedy would be: (1) processing the images with sub-volumes of different sizes; and (2) treating large lesions and small lesions separately. While FCNs can handle images with arbitrary sizes, predetermined input size does affect the design of the network, especially the number of the layers. FCNs with small-sized input (we term them small-FCNs) and large-FCNs are more accurate for their respective sized lesions. With this in mind, the design of the fusion step should grant small-FCNs with more power to determine small lesions, while let large-FCNs be more authoritative about large lesions. This thought leads to the architecture of our two-stage-multi-sized FCNs model. In the first stage, we set up three FCN networks, for different sized neighborhoods, to best capture both large and small lesions. In stage two, the preliminary 3D lesions masks, which we term *opinions*, are first separated into small and large lesion groups, and then combined through nonlinear weighting schemes carried out by ensemble-nets.

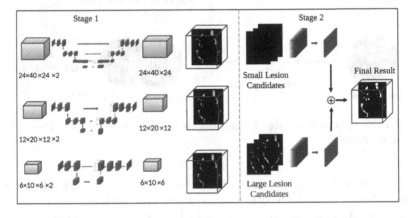

Fig. 2. The overall structure of our model for lesion segmentation.

Stage 1: Three Different Sized FCNs. In stage 1, we extract MR patches of three different sizes, and feed them into the corresponding FCNs. As each voxel may be covered by multiple patches, the prediction patches of each FCN are then sent back to the original image space to generate an overall probability map through averaging.

In order to fit our application and data, we made modifications to the 3D U-net [4] as follows. We keep the original design that two convolution layers are followed by one pooling/upsampling layer. The sizes of the convolution filters are set to $3 \times 3 \times 3$ except for the bottom layer of the U shape, in which the filter sizes are set to $1 \times 1 \times 1$. Every convolution layer is padded to maintain the same spatial dimension. The number of layers is reduced from 3D U-net as our input dimensions are smaller. The modified 3D U-net-like FCNs are shown in Fig. 2 Stage 1.

Stage 2: Ensemble of Preliminary Opinions. Three *opinions* are generated in Stage 1 for each MR image. Stage 2 is to merge them to produce an overall lesion segmentation. As we described in a previous section, each FCN in the first stage is more trustworthy in processing one specific type of lesions, i.e., small-FCNs generate more reliable segmentations for small lesions, while large-FCNs performs better on large lesions. To take the advantage of this fact, we separate the estimated lesions within each prediction map into small and large lesion groups and send them into two different ensemble nets for fusion. In this work, an empirical threshold of 1000-voxel has been used to decide the category (small or large) for any given lesion (a 3D connected component).

Ensemble Net. The functionality of the two ensemble nets can both be expressed as

$$\min_{w_1, w_2, w_3} D(\mathbf{y}, f(w_1\mathbf{x_1} + w_2\mathbf{x_2} + w_3\mathbf{x_3})) \tag{3}$$

where $\mathbf{x_1}$, $\mathbf{x_2}$, $\mathbf{x_3}$ are the contributing *opinions* from the three FCNs; $\mathbf{y}$ is the corresponding ground truth. $D(\cdot, \cdot)$ measures the distance between the combined opinion and the ground-truth. With different approaches for the combination, $f(\mathbf{x})$ can be formulated as either a linear or non-linear function that maps $\mathbf{x}$ to the probability space. As we explained before, the combining weights w_1, w_2 and w_3 should be individualized for small and large lesion groups, respectively. Learning such weights can also be conducted through neural networks. In both small and large lesion groups, if we concatenate the three *opinions* as three channels, and treat w_1, w_2 and w_3 as a filter of size $(1, 1, 1, 3)$, we can build an ensemble net of one convolution layer to learn the optimal weights in Eq. 3. The $f(\mathbf{x})$ function in Eq. 3 works as the activation function for this ensemble net.

We use Dice loss as the objective function of our ensemble-nets, to produce probability maps that match the ground-truth binary segmentations. As we explained in Sect. 2, a theoretical gap exists between the DSC and Dice loss. An observation is that activation functions that are closer to the Step function would be able to produce better approximations for the DSC, at least from the numerical point-of-view. In this regard, an "ideal" activation function should be differentiable and relatively steep around 0.5. Meanwhile, a reasonable capture or support range should be allowed to avoid vanishing gradients.

In FCN solutions for binary segmentation, the Sigmoid function is a commonly used activation function. In our ensemble nets, however, the inputs to the function $f(\mathbf{x})$ have a particular range of $[0, 1]$, and a steeper function, if tailored to the inputs, would be preferred over the Sigmoid in producing more accurate DSC approximations. With these two considerations, we propose a new activation function for our ensemble nets:

$$H(x) = \begin{cases} 1 & \text{if } x > 1 \\ 0 & \text{if } x < 0 \\ x + \frac{1}{2\pi}\sin(2\pi x - \pi) & \text{if } 0 \leq x \leq 1 \end{cases} \tag{4}$$

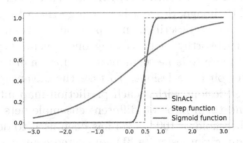

Fig. 3. Comparison of Step, SinAct and Sigmoid functions.

We term $H(x)$ SinAct function. Figure 3 shows a comparison of the Step, SinAct and Sigmoid functions. Compared with Sigmoid, the SinAct is steeper between 0 and 1. As we usually use 0.5 as the threshold to convert probability maps into binary results, being steep around 0.5 is a desired property. Another merit of SinAct function is that it evaluates to 0 when the input is equal or smaller than 0, and produces 1 when the input is equal to 1 and beyond. By contrast, the Sigmoid can approach infinitely close to 0 and 1, but would never reach the exact values.

4   Experiments

Data. The MR data used in this paper were obtained from the White Matter Hyperintensities (WMH) Segmentation Challenge at MICCAI 2017 (http://wmh.isi.uu.nl/). The training set of this challenge contains images of 60 subjects acquired at three sites [7]. For each subject, a pair of aligned T1-weighted and Fluid-attenuated inversion recovery (FLAIR) images are available. Several pre-processing steps are conducted on all image pairs. First, skulls are removed from both T1 and FLAIR images using FSL/BET tool. Second, the intensities of all images are individually normalized to the range of $[0, 1]$. 3D patches (sub-volumes) are extracted from the intensity-normalized brains using sliding windows. The patch sizes are set to $6 \times 10 \times 6$, $12 \times 20 \times 12$ and $24 \times 40 \times 24$ respectively, and the strides are half of the corresponding patch sizes. T1 and FLAIR patches from the same areas are concatenated as two channels and fed into the FCNs in Stage 1.

Implementation Details. With the sliding windows of the aforementioned patch sizes, we found the extracted patches containing no lesion at all ("empty patches") greatly outnumbered those with lesions inside. This would create a serious data imbalance in the training if we would use all the patches. To tackle this issue, we kept all the lesion patches, but only randomly picked an equal number of empty patches.

The three FCNs in Stage 1 are developed under Keras. ReLu is used as the activation function for all layers except the last one, where softmax is utilized to produce the final prediction. Dice loss is used as the network objective function and ADAM is adopted as the optimization method. The learning rate is set to $5e-6$, and it reduces 50% every 10 epochs. In total, each FCN is trained for 30 epochs. In Stage 2, lesions are separated into two groups, small and large lesions, and FCN ensembles are carried out within the individual groups. Volume size of 1000 voxels has been used as a hard threshold to determine the category for each 3D connected component. For the training subjects, the separation is based on their corresponding ground-truth, which means the component on the probability maps is assigned as a large lesion candidate if the corresponding groud truth component is larger than 1000 voxels. In the testing stage, a threshold of 0.5 is applied on the prediction probability map to produce a binary component first, then the map is assigned as either small or large based on the same threshold. To train our ensemble net, all three parameters in Eq. 3 are initialized to $1/3$. Each ensemble net is trained for 10 epochs.

Our experiment is carried out based on the training set of the WMH Segmentation Challenge through Monte Carlo cross-validation. 54 of the 60 subjects are randomly selected for training and the rest 6 subjects are used for testing. The whole experiments are repeated 5 times. The results are presented in next section.

4.1   Experimental Results

Evaluations of the individual components and overall network are carried out based on five performance metrics: *DSC*, *Hausdorff distance* (HD, 95th percentile), *Average volume difference* (AVD, in percentage), *Sensitivity for individual lesions* (Detection, in percentage) and *F-1 score for individual lesions*. The evaluation code was provided by the Challenge organizers, available under the Challenge website.

The final segmentation results are shown in Table 1. FCNs with fixed input sizes are the baseline models, and we take ensemble-nets through *majority vote* and Sigmoid as the competing ensemble solutions. Our SinAct-based ensemble net outperforms all other models in every evaluation metric except detection. In detection, FCNs with the smallest patch size of $6 \times 10 \times 6$ achieve the highest score, but they perform the worst in all other metrics, in part because of high false positive (type I) errors. Compared with *vote* and Sigmoid, our SinAct-based ensemble-net solution achieves higher accuracy (measured by DSC) and consistency (measured by HD and AVD) at the same time.

Table 1. Segmentation results on all lesions.

FCN	Ensemble	Results				
		Dice	HD	AVD	Detection	F1
$6 \times 10 \times 6$		77.74	17.82	21.72	**81.83**	57.41
$12 \times 20 \times 12$		79.78	4.65	19.28	72.43	69.91
$24 \times 40 \times 24$		80.39	3.95	18.43	73.55	71.03
3 FCNs	Vote	81.03	3.95	18.43	73.55	71.03
3 FCNs	Sigmoid	80.96	4.61	19.90	80.24	68.13
3 FCNs	SinAct	**81.26**	**2.58**	**17.54**	73.70	**71.65**

Table 2. Model performance on small and large lesions separately.

FCN	Lesion Size	Ensemble	Results				
			Dice	HD	AVD	Detection	F1
$6 \times 10 \times 6$	Small		59.30	18.06	47.87	**80.79**	55.85
$12 \times 20 \times 12$	Small		60.90	10.24	29.55	70.36	67.39
$24 \times 40 \times 24$	Small		61.20	9.35	29.67	64.22	66.04
3 FCNs	Small	Vote	63.64	9.63	28.69	71.93	69.52
3 FCNs	Small	Sigmoid	65.07	11.51	34.42	78.98	64.74
3 FCNs	Small	SinAct	**65.80**	**8.00**	**26.52**	72.47	**70.34**
$6 \times 10 \times 6$	Large		85.59	7.08	15.33	**98.89**	**90.02**
$12 \times 20 \times 12$	Large		84.92	6.40	14.10	77.87	66.54
$24 \times 40 \times 24$	Large		85.13	6.81	12.99	69.39	64.22
3 FCNs	Large	Vote	85.32	8.23	14.05	76.31	68.19
3 FCNs	Large	Sigmoid	**86.87**	**5.81**	12.58	88.59	84.66
3 FCNs	Large	SinAct	86.69	5.87	**12.33**	86.84	76.84

Table 2 provides evaluations of the models on small and large lesions separately. For both small and large lesion groups, almost all ensemble nets outperform the fixed-sized FCNs in DSC, which to certain extent validates our design of combining multi-sized FCNs. As our SinAct function provides more accurate DSC approximations at voxels with uncertain labels, it improves the membership decision most significantly at the boundary voxels. Among the three ensemble-nets, our SinAct net performs the best, in all metrics, for small lesions. For large lesions, SinAct is still better than *vote*, but achieves comparable performance with the Sigmoid. This disparity can be explained by the fact that boundary voxels account for high percentage for small lesions, but not so for large lesions. All in all, FCNs and the new activation function are shown to be effective in improving MS lesions segmentations from MRIs.

5 Conclusions

In this paper, we propose a two-stage-multi-sized FCNs strategy to enhance the segmentation of MS white matter lesions in MR images. The design is based on the rational that different sized lesions are best captured with appropriate sized FCNs. Ensemble-nets are constructed to combine the results from the FCNs, where SinAct, a new activation function, is adopted to improve the segmentation accuracy measured by DSC. Experiments show the effectiveness of both design approaches. Exploring more activation functions is the directions of our future efforts. We are also interested in applying the proposed strategy to other neuroimage analysis problems.

References

1. Anbeek, P., et al.: Automatic segmentation of different-sized white matter lesions by voxel probability estimation. Med. Image Anal. 8(3), 205–215 (2004)
2. Chen, Y., Shi, B., Wang, Z., Sun, T., Smith, C.D., Liu, J.: Accurate and Consistent Hippocampus Segmentation Through Convolutional LSTM and View Ensemble. In: Wang, Q., Shi, Y., Suk, H.-I., Suzuki, K. (eds.) MLMI 2017. LNCS, vol. 10541, pp. 88–96. Springer, Cham (2017). https://doi.org/10.1007/978-3-319-67389-9_11
3. Chen, Y., Shi, B., Wang, Z., Zhang, P., Smith, C.D., Liu, J.: Hippocampus segmentation through multi-view ensemble ConvNets. In: 14th IEEE, ISBI 2017, pp. 192–196 (2017)
4. Çiçek, Ö., et al.: 3D U-Net: learning dense volumetric segmentation from sparse annotation. In: MICCAI, pp. 424–432. Springer, Berlin (2016)
5. Drozdzal, M., et al.: The importance of skip connections in biomedical image segmentation. In: Deep Learning and Data Labeling for Medical Applications, pp. 179–187. Springer, Chem (2016)
6. Ekanayake, J., et al.: Generalised wasserstein dice score for imbalanced multi-class segmentation using holistic convolutional networks. In: Third International Workshop, BrainLes, MICCAI (2017)
7. Li, H., et al.: Fully convolutional network ensembles for white matter hyperintensities segmentation in MR images. arXiv preprint arXiv:1802.05203 (2018)
8. Liu, J., Smith, C.D., Chebrolu, H.: Automatic multiple sclerosis detection based on integrated square estimation. In: IEEE, CVPR Workshops, 20–25 June, 2009, pp. 31–38 (2009)
9. Long, J., et al.: Fully convolutional networks for semantic segmentation. In: Proceedings of CVPR, pp. 3431–3440 (2015)
10. Milletari, F., et al.: V-net: fully convolutional neural networks for volumetric medical image segmentation. In: 3D Vision (3DV). pp. 565–571. IEEE (2016)
11. Ronneberger, O., Fischer, P., Brox, T.: U-net: convolutional networks for biomedical image segmentation. In: MICCAI, pp. 234–241. Springer, Berlin (2015)
12. Souplet, J.C., et al.: An automatic segmentation of T2-FLAIR multiple sclerosis lesions. In: The MIDAS Journal-MS Lesion Segmentation (MICCAI 2008 Workshop). Citeseer (2008)

13. Sudre, C.H., et al.: Generalised dice overlap as a deep learning loss function for highly unbalanced segmentations. In: Deep Learning in Medical Image Analysis and Multimodal Learning for Clinical Decision Support, pp. 240–248. Springer, Berlin (2017)
14. Warfield, S., Tomas-Fernandez, X.: Lesion segmentation. In: Toga, A.W. (ed.) Brain Mapping, pp. 323–332. Academic Press, Waltham (2015)

Automatic Accurate Infant Cerebellar Tissue Segmentation with Densely Connected Convolutional Network

Jiawei Chen, Han Zhang, Dong Nie, Li Wang, Gang Li, Weili Lin, and Dinggang Shen[✉]

Department of Radiology and BRIC, University of North Carolina at Chapel Hill, Chapel Hill, USA
dgshen@med.unc.edu

Abstract. The human cerebellum has been recognized as a key brain structure for motor control and cognitive function regulation. Investigation of brain functional development in the early life has recently been focusing on both cerebral and cerebellar development. Accurate segmentation of the infant cerebellum into different tissues is among the most important steps for quantitative development studies. However, this is extremely challenging due to the weak tissue contrast, extremely folded structures, and severe partial volume effect. To date, there are very few works touching infant cerebellum segmentation. We tackle this challenge by proposing a densely connected convolutional network to learn robust feature representations of different cerebellar tissues towards automatic and accurate segmentation. Specifically, we develop a novel deep neural network architecture by directly connecting all the layers to ensure maximum information flow even among distant layers in the network. This is distinct from all previous studies. Importantly, the outputs from all previous layers are passed to all subsequent layers as contextual features that can guide the segmentation. Our method achieved superior performance than other state-of-the-art methods when applied to Baby Connectome Project (BCP) data consisting of both 6- and 12-month-old infant brain images.

1 Introduction

The first year of the human life represents the most dynamic phase of postnatal brain development, with rapid brain size growth and cognitive function development. Most of previous early development studies have focused on the cerebral cortex [1], with few on the development of cerebellum. In fact, the human cerebellum has been recognized as playing equal important roles in both motor control and various cognitive function regulations as the cerebral cortex, many of which are key to daily living [2]. Accurate segmentation of the cerebellum into white matter (WM), gray matter (GM), and cerebrospinal fluid (CSF) tissues is one of the most pivotal steps for quantitative analysis of early brain development, yet challenging for infant brain images. Manual segmentation of cerebellar tissues from 3D magnetic resonance (MR) images is extremely difficult and laborious, and often prone to biases or errors. It has been shown

© Springer Nature Switzerland AG 2018
Y. Shi et al. (Eds.): MLMI 2018, LNCS 11046, pp. 233–240, 2018.
https://doi.org/10.1007/978-3-030-00919-9_27

that, even manually segmented by experts, the results could still be less reproducible with unneglectable inter- and/or intra-operator variability. A more realistic and highly desired solution is computer-aided automatic cerebellum segmentation based on MR images; however, it is still challenging to date. Cerebellar cortex has far more complex structures with highly folded geometric patterns compared to the cerebral cortex, e.g., small cerebellar foliations (<0.5 mm) and comparable dense neurons. Moreover, due to ongoing maturation and largely immature myelination, the cerebellum has weak, even "isointense" contrast in MR images at 6–12 months of age. Furthermore, the small size of the cerebellum makes the partial volume effect more severe than that in the cerebral cortex; this becomes even worse for the already small-sized infant brain. Taking a 12-month-old cerebellum for example (Fig. 1, left), accurate WM, GM and CSF delineation in the blurred and isointense cerebellar cortex is among the most difficult medical image analysis problems [3]. To date, there are few studies on such topic.

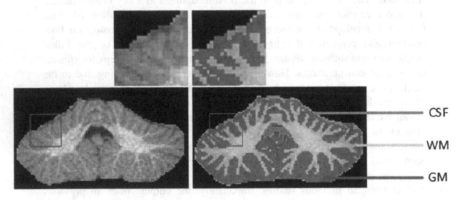

Fig. 1. Infant cerebellar MR image with low tissue contrast, scanned at 12 months of age.

Recently, deep convolutional neural networks (CNNs) [4] have achieved great successes in medical image segmentation [5, 6]. A U-shaped convolutional network [7], shorted for U-Net, was proposed for biomedical image segmentation, with a merit of preserving the resolution of the original images. The main spirit of the U-Net is that several expansive paths are built following a fully convolutional network, where respective deconvolution layers are employed to allow skipping the connections between low- and high-level features. Milletari *et al.* proposed a 3D fully convolutional network (FCN) [6] for volumetric image segmentation, but it suffers from a gradient vanishing problem that could undermine the model accuracy. To solve this issue, Chen *et al.* proposed a deep voxel-wise residual network [8], where more representative features are generated by integrating multimodal and multi-level contextual information to better guide tissue segmentation. Varying in topological structure, all these networks have similar short paths that connect only the previous and the later layers, making the input patches impossible to be fully convolved. To tackle this problem, a densely connected CNN (DenseNet) was proposed, where all layers are inter-connected directly and each layer receives extra inputs from all preceding layers and transits the feature representations to all subsequent layers [9]. The DenseNet has been extended for volumetric cardiac image segmentation in [10]. Inspired by the U-Net [7] and DenseNet [9], we propose a 3D, densely connected, U-shaped CNN to learn robust features for infant cerebellum segmentation. Specifically, in the contracting path, dense blocks are connected by the transition layers with a pooling operator to extract the context features. Our proposed network extends the densely connected convolution networks with an expansive path, along which deconvolution layers are placed to enforce a precise localization with the help from the context feature maps. The experimental results on the public Baby Connectome Project (BCP) dataset show a significant improvement by our proposed method in infant cerebellum segmentation compared to other state-of-the-art methods.

2 Method

2.1 Dataset and Preprocessing

We demonstrate the feasibility and superiority of our method with the MR images from 10 infants at the age of 12 months and 10 infants at the age of 6 months, selected from the BCP dataset. BCP was recently initiated for promoting the understanding of early brain development with state-of-the-art imaging sequences and protocols. The data were acquired by two 3T Siemens Prisma MRI scanners with the same settings at two different sites, Center for Magnetic Resonance Research (CMRR) at University of Minnesota and Biomedical Research Imaging Center (BRIC) at University of North Carolina at Chapel Hill. T1-weighted MR images were acquired with TR = 2400 ms, TE = 2.24 ms, flip angle = $8°$, and voxel resolution = $0.8 \times 0.8 \times 0.8$ mm^3.

Skull stripping and intensity inhomogeneity correction were performed to preprocess all the images. Ground-truth tissue segmentation results are important for model training and validation; however, manual labeling from the scratch is unrealistic. Therefore, we employed a widely adopted segmentation toolbox, LINKS [11], to obtain reasonable initial segmentation results, which were then manually edited to correct possible segmentation and geometric errors.

2.2 Network Architecture Design

Figure 2 shows the flowchart of the proposed method. The network consists of 6 dense blocks, each of which can be defined as a nonlinear mapping function:

$$x_l = H_l([x_0, x_1, \ldots, x_{l-1}]) \tag{1}$$

where $[x_0, x_1, \ldots, x_{l-1}]$ means the operation that directly connects the feature maps of all preceding layers (0, 1, ..., $l - 1$) and transits their own feature maps to all subsequent layers. It aims to improve the information flow between each pair of layers. The mapping function $H_l(.)$ is the composition of three subsequent operations: batch normalization (BN), rectified linear unit (ReLU, a nonlinear activation operator), and $3 \times 3 \times 3$ convolution. A feature map x_l can thus be obtained via the composite function $H_l([x_0, x_1, \ldots, x_{l-1}])$.

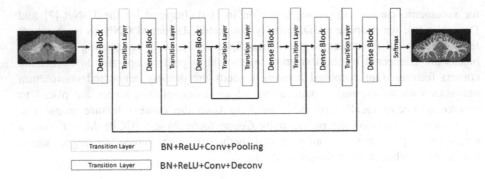

| Transition Layer | BN+ReLU+Conv+Pooling |
| Transition Layer | BN+ReLU+Conv+Deconv |

Fig. 2. Illustration of the proposed densely connected convolutional network.

These dense blocks are connected via transition layers into a U-shaped network with a contracting path and an expansive path. Along the contracting path, each transition layer between two dense blocks contains a batch normalization operator, a ReLU and an average pooling operator. The average pooling with a $2 \times 2 \times 2$ volumetric kernel and a stride of 2 aims to reduce the resolution of the input feature map while increasing its receptive field. In contrast to max-pooling, for average pooling operator, the switches that map the outputs of a pooling layer to the corresponding inputs are no longer required in back-propagation, which can reduce memory consumption in the training stage.

On the other hand, in the expansive path, the average-pooling operator in a transition layer is replaced by a deconvolution operator to restore the resolution of the input feature maps. In addition, the deconvolution operator also allows one to assemble the context information from a lower resolution feature map to a higher resolution one. Furthermore, to ensure accurate segmentation along the image boundary, the deconvolutional feature map is combined along the expansive path with its mirrored image in the contracting path as the inputs of subsequent convolution layer. At the final layer, the convolution with a $1 \times 1 \times 1$ kernel is employed to produce four feature maps (i.e., WM, GM, CSF and background) and they are then converted into probability maps by the following voxel-wise soft-max:

$$p_k(\boldsymbol{x}) = \exp(f_k(\boldsymbol{x})) / \sum_{i=1}^{C} \exp(f_i(\boldsymbol{x})) \tag{2}$$

where $\boldsymbol{x}$ is the position of a voxel, C is the total number of different tissues, and $f_k(\boldsymbol{x})$ is the intensity of the k-th feature map at voxel $\boldsymbol{x}$.

2.3   Network Training

The T1-weighted cerebellar MR intensity images of the training subjects (see Sect. 3 for cross validation parameters) and the corresponding cerebellar tissue segmentation ground truth are employed to train the network. The image of each subject is divided into patches with a size of $32 \times 32 \times 32$. Along the contracting path, the number of kernels is doubled at each transition layer, starting from 64 to 256. Along the expansive path, such a number is halved at each transition layer. In addition, the convolution layer is performed on the zero-padding maps to make the size of outputs identical to that of the inputs. Finally, these kernel parameters are optimized via a stochastic gradient descent algorithm implemented by Caffe [12], where the initial learning rate is 0.05 and is automatically decreased by 10% after each epoch.

3 Experimental Results

In the experiment, the training data is only derived from the subjects at the age of 12 months, where eight subjects are used for training, one subject for validation, and the remaining one for testing. For each subject, 2,000 patches are randomly selected; thus, for eight training subjects, we have a total of 16,000 patches for training, while, for one validation subject, we have 2,000 patches to monitor the overfitting issue. Then, the learning rate will decrease by 10% every 6,000 iterations. The performance is evaluated using Dice Ratio (DR), measuring the proportion of overlap voxels between the automatic segmentation map I_S and the ground truth map I_G:

$$DR = \frac{2|I_S \cap I_G|}{|I_S| + |I_G|} \tag{3}$$

3.1 Performance on 12-Month-Old Subjects

To validate our proposed method, we compare it with two state-of-the-art methods: LINKS [11] and U-Net [7] in the task of cerebellum segmentation for 12-month-old infants.

We first make qualitative comparisons with the results from LINKS and U-Net. A typical set of results is shown in Fig. 3. For the results from U-Net, there are several topological errors in the WM structure, while our proposed method obtains clearer and more reasonable WM structure. By comparing the 3D surface renderings of the GM-WM interface among all the methods, we can see more "handles" (indicating segmentation errors) in the GM-WM interface structures generated by U-Net. To emphasize the differences among these methods, we zoom in a typical region at the cerebellar lobule VI. It can be observed that the competing methods led to quite confusing boundary between WM and GM in this region, while our proposed method obtained a clearer and more reasonable WM structure.

For quantitative comparisons, we employ leave-one-out validation in the comparison experiment and evaluate the performance by the means and standard deviations (std) of the DRs among all the three methods. Our method achieved significantly higher DR for all three tissue types than other two methods (Table 1).

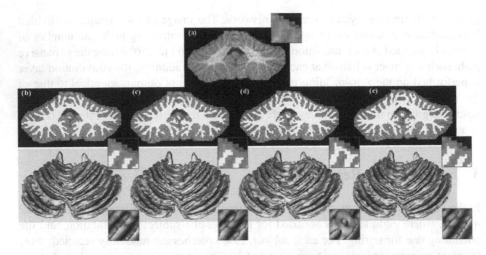

Fig. 3. Tissue segmentation results based on a randomly selected 12-month-old infant. The first row shows a T1-weighted MR image. The second row shows the segmentation results from manual labeling (ground truth), LINKS [11], U-Net [7], and our method. The third row shows the surface rendering results of the GM-WM interface derived from respective methods.

Table 1. Performance on 10 12-month-old subjects with leave-one-out cross-validation.

	WM	GM	CSF
LINKS	0.856±0.040	0.880±0.007	0.843±0.052
U-Net	0.862±0.023	0.886±0.005	0.846±0.034
Proposed	**0.908±0.020**	**0.894±0.003**	**0.856±0.014**

3.2 Performance on 6-Month-Old Infants

To test the generalization ability of our method, the model trained on ten 12-month-old subjects are directly applied to ten 6-month-old subjects. Of note, cerebellum segmentation on this age group is more challenging. For example, the T1-weighted MR image in Fig. 4(a) reaches the peak of isotropic intensity, for which even manual segmentation can be quite challenging. While other competing methods were significantly affected (see much worse result in Fig. 4(b, c)), our proposed method could still reliably and consistently generate decent tissue segmentation results, with much improved GM-WM surface reconstruction results. Such results indicate that densely connected convolutional network is capable to learn robust feature representations and provide comprehensive contextual guidance information for tissue classification.

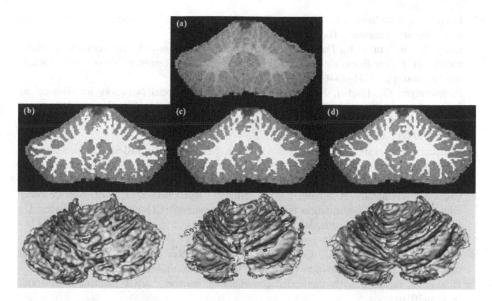

Fig. 4. Tissue segmentation results on a randomly selected 6-month-old infant. The first row shows a T1-weighted MR image. The second row shows the segmentation results by LINKS [11], U-Net [7], and our method. The last row shows the surface renderings results from the three methods.

4 Conclusions

In this paper, we developed a U-shaped densely connected convolutional network for infant cerebellar tissue segmentation. We directly connected all the layers with each other to ensure maximum information flow among even distant layers in the network, which provides comprehensive contextual guidance information for tissue classification in this challenging task. Compared to U-Net, our proposed network consists of dense blocks, thus avoiding gradient vanishing problem. Experimental results show that our method outperforms other state-of-the-art methods, even in the extremely challenging case of 6-month-old infant cerebellar tissue segmentation.

Acknowledgements. This work was supported by the National Institutes of Health (MH109773, MH100217, MH070890, EB006733, EB008374, EB009634, AG041721, AG042599, MH088520, MH108914, and MH107815). This work also utilizes approaches developed by an NIH grant (1U01MH110274) and the efforts of the UNC/UMN Baby Connectome Project Consortium.

References

1. Li, G., Lin, W., Gilmore, J.H., Shen, D.: Spatial patterns, longitudinal development, and hemispheric asymmetries of cortical thickness in infants from birth to 2 years of age. J. Neurosci. **35**(24), 9150–9162 (2015)
2. Wolf, U., Rapoport, M.J., Schweizer, T.A.: Evaluating the affective component of the cerebellar cognitive affective syndrome. J. Neuropsychiatry Clin. Neurosci. **21**(3), 245–253 (2009)

3. Poretti, A., Boltshauser, E., Huisman, T.A.: Pre-and postnatal neuroimaging of congenital cerebellar abnormalities. The Cerebellum **15**(1), 5–9 (2016)
4. Long, J., Shelhamer, E., Darrell, T.: Fully convolutional networks for semantic segmentation. In: Proceedings of the IEEE Conference on Computer Vision and Pattern Recognition, pp. 3431–3440 (2015)
5. Ronneberger, O., Fischer, P., Brox, T.: U-Net: Convolutional Networks for Biomedical Image Segmentation. In: Navab, N., Hornegger, J., Wells, W.M., Frangi, A.F. (eds.) MICCAI 2015. LNCS, vol. 9351, pp. 234–241. Springer, Cham (2015). https://doi.org/10. 1007/978-3-319-24574-4_28
6. Milletari, F., Navab, N., Ahmadi, S.A.: V-net: Fully convolutional neural networks for volumetric medical image segmentation. In: 2016 Fourth International Conference on 3D Vision (3DV), pp. 565–571. IEEE (2016)
7. Çiçek, Ö., Abdulkadir, A., Lienkamp, S.S., Brox, T., Ronneberger, O.: 3D U-Net: Learning Dense Volumetric Segmentation from Sparse Annotation. In: Ourselin, S., Joskowicz, L., Sabuncu, M.R., Unal, Gozde, Wells, W. (eds.) MICCAI 2016. LNCS, vol. 9901, pp. 424–432. Springer, Cham (2016). https://doi.org/10.1007/978-3-319-46723-8_49
8. Chen, H., Dou, Q., Yu, L., Qin, J., Heng, P.A.: VoxResNet: Deep voxelwise residual networks for brain segmentation from 3D MR images. NeuroImage (2017)
9. Huang, G., et al.: Densely connected convolutional networks. arXiv preprint arXiv:1608. 06993 (2016)
10. Yu, L., Cheng, J.-Z., Dou, Q., Yang, X., Chen, H., Qin, J., Heng, P.-A.: Automatic 3D Cardiovascular MR Segmentation with Densely-Connected Volumetric ConvNets. In: Descoteaux, M., Maier-Hein, L., Franz, A., Jannin, P., Collins, D.L., Duchesne, S. (eds.) MICCAI 2017. LNCS, vol. 10434, pp. 287–295. Springer, Cham (2017). https://doi.org/10. 1007/978-3-319-66185-8_33
11. Wang, L., Gao, Y., Shi, F., Li, G., Gilmore, J.H., Lin, W., Shen, D.: LINKS: learning-based multi-source Integration frameworK for segmentation of infant brain images. Neuroimage **108**, 160–172 (2015)
12. Jia, Y., et al.: Caffe: Convolutional architecture for fast feature embedding. In: Proceedings of the 22nd ACM International Conference on Multimedia, pp. 675–678 (2014)

Nuclei Detection Using Mixture Density Networks

Navid Alemi Koohababni[1,4(✉)], Mostafa Jahanifar[2],
Ali Gooya[3], and Nasir Rajpoot[1,4]

[1] Department of Computer Science, University of Warwick, Coventry, UK
n.alemi-Koohbanani@warwick.ac.uk
[2] Department of Biomedical Engineering, Tarbiat Modares University, Tehran, Iran
[3] Department of Electronic and Electrical Engineering, University of Sheffield,
Sheffield, UK
[4] Alan Turing Institute, London, UK

Abstract. Nuclei detection is an important task in the histology domain as it is a main step toward further analysis such as cell counting, cell segmentation, study of cell connections, etc. This is a challenging task due to complex texture of histology image, variation in shape, and touching cells. To tackle these hurdles, many approaches have been proposed in the literature where deep learning methods stand on top in terms of performance. Hence, in this paper, we propose a novel framework for nuclei detection based on Mixture Density Networks (MDNs). These networks are suitable to map a single input to several possible outputs and we utilize this property to detect multiple seeds in a single image patch. A new modified form of a cost function is proposed for training and handling patches with missing nuclei. The probability maps of the nuclei in the individual patches are next combined to generate the final image-wide result. The experimental results show the state-of-the-art performance on complex colorectal adenocarcinoma dataset.

Keywords: Mixture density network · Histology · Nuclei detection

1 Introduction

Precise localizing the nucleus in histology images is a main step for successive medical image analysis such as cell segmentation, counting and morphological analysis [1]. Unfortunately, robust cell detection is a challenging task due to nucleus clutters, large variation in shape and texture, nuclear pleomorphism, touching cells and poor image quality [2]. Since manual detection of nucleus for further diagnostic assessment imposes a high workload on pathologists, computer assisted methods have attracted a lot of interest in recent years [3]. To this end, many automatic cell detection algorithms are proposed in literature. Parvin et al. [4] introduced the iterative voting methods which use oriented kernels to localize cell centers, where the voting direction and areas were updated in each iteration.

© Springer Nature Switzerland AG 2018
Y. Shi et al. (Eds.): MLMI 2018, LNCS 11046, pp. 241–248, 2018.
https://doi.org/10.1007/978-3-030-00919-9_28

Qi et al. [5] utilize a single path voting mechanism that is followed by clustering step. Similarly, Hafiane et al. [6] detect the nuclei by clustering the segmented centers using an iterative voting algorithm. Multiscale Laplacian-of-Gaussian (LOG) [7] and construction of concave vertex graph [8] can also be found in the literature. A popular approach to handle touching cells is based on the watershed algorithm [1,9]. However, due to the large variations in microscopy modality, nucleus morphology, and the inhomogeneous background, it remains to be a challenging topic for these non-learning methods. Data-driven methods utilizing hand-crafted features have also been extensively applied for cell detection due to their promising performance. Interested readers are referred to [10] for more details about methods which rely on hand crafted features and classic supervised methods.

Deep learning has shown an outstanding performance in computer vision analysis of both natural and biomedical images. Deep learning methods extract the appropriate features from an image without the need for laborious feature engineering and parameter tunning. Ciresan et al. [11] applied a deep neural network (DNN) as a pixel classifier to differentiate between mitotic and non-mitotic nuclei in breast cancer histopathology images. Xie et al. [12] proposed a structured regression convolution neural network (CNN) for nuclei detection wherein the gaussian distribution is fitted on the nucleus center to construct the probability map which is considered as an image mask, then a weighted mean squared loss is minimized via pixel-wise back-propagation. Xu et al. [13] proposed a stacked sparse autoencoder strategy to learn high level features from patches of breast histopathology images and then classify these patches as nuclear or non-nuclear. Sirinukunwattana et al. [14] proposed a locality sensitive deep learning approach for nuclei detection in the H&E stained colorectal adenocarcinoma histology images. In this approach, a spatially constrained CNN is first employed to generate a probability map for a given input image using local information. Then the centroids of nucleus are detected by identifying local maximum intensities.

In this paper, we propose a simple yet effective method based on Mixture Density Networks (MDN) introduced by Bishop [15] for solving inverse problems, where we have multiple targets for an individual input. MDN learns the distribution of nucleus within an image hypothesizing that each nuclei has a Gaussian distribution with a maximum value on its center. Here we formalize the concept of MDN for cell detection problem. Due to MDN's flexibility to localize nucleus, we show that it has a better performance when compared with the other cell detection algorithms on a challenging colon cancer dataset.

Our contributions in this paper are the followings: (i) We define the problem of nuclei detection as mapping a single input image patch into the probability density function (pdf) of the nuclei center, from which the observed locations have been sampled. The pdf is modeled as a Gaussian Mixture Model (GMM) and its parameters are learned via a back-propagation. In addition, a Bernoulli distribution is trained whose parameter predicts if the local patch contains any nucleus and thus the fit of the GMM is liable. (ii) We show the network can detect the nuclei even when trained with a sparse annotated samples, whereas using other methods result in a poor performance. (iii) we demonstrate the capability of algorithm to learn the distribution of nuclei center from the training data without the need to define fixed variance size for all nucleus as some methods do [12,14].

The rest of this paper is organized as follows: A brief review of MDN and its generalization to our problem is presented in Sect. 2. The experimental results and comparison to the state of-the-art are described and discussed in Sect. 3, and finally, some concluding remarks are drawn in Sect. 4.

2 Mixture Density Networks

For a general task of supervised learning our goal is to model a conditional distribution $p(t|x)$ (for image patch x and nucleus center t), which is considered Gaussian for many problems and a least square energy function is often obtained using maximum likelihood. These assumptions can lead to a poor performance in many application having plausible non-Gaussian distributions. One of such applications is one to many mapping where one input corresponds to several outputs. The assumption of having a Gaussian posterior distribution forces the model to predict only one output discarding other target values at best. Moreover, The network prediction is the average of all target values which is incorrect [15]. To address this problem, we can consider a general framework for modeling the conditional posterior probability distribution by modeling it as a mixture density represented as a linear combination of kernel functions:

$$p(t|x) = \sum_{k=1}^{K} \alpha_k(x)\phi_k(t|x) \tag{1}$$

where K is the number of components in the mixture and α_is are mixing coefficients. We assume that kernel functions $\phi(t|x)$ are isotropic Gaussian:

$$\phi_k(t|x) = \frac{1}{(2\pi)^{c/2}\sigma_k^c(x)} \exp\left\{-\frac{\|t - \mu_k(x)\|^2}{2\sigma_k^2(x)}\right\} \tag{2}$$

where $\mu_k(x)$ and $\sigma_k^2(x)$ are the mean and the variance of the kth Gaussian, respectively, and c is the dimension of target variable.

Here, the parameters of the mixture model are considered to be functions of input image patch x. This can be achieved by using a conventional neural network as a function that takes x as input. These layers are then combined with other fully connected layers to from the Mixture Density Network (MDN), (see Fig. 1). Building the MDN increases the number of parameters from c output to $(c+2) \times K$. There are some restrictions on these parameters that can be found in detail in [15].

To define the error function, the standard negative logarithm of the maximum likelihood is used. Therefore the original loss function for the network is [15]:

$$E(W) = -\sum_{n=1}^{N} \ln p(t_n|x_n) = -\sum_{n=1}^{N} \ln\left(\sum_{k=1}^{K} \alpha_k(x_n)\phi(t_n|x_n)\right) \tag{3}$$

where summation over n applies to all dataset. In the next section, we modify this cost function so that it becomes more suitable to handle image patches with multiple and/or missing nuclei.

2.1   Extending MDN for Nuclei Detection

For nuclei detection, deep learning approaches are either provided with small patches each containing one nuclei [13,14] or designed as pixel wise structured logistic regression [12,16]. Here, we formulate the cell detection as the problem of mapping one to many outputs, as each input vector (image) can have multiple variables defined as the locations (coordinates) of the nuclei.

To adjust the MDN for nuclei detection, we modify the Eq. (3) to take one input (image patch) and all of its corresponding target coordinates of the nuclei during training. This equation can only be used when all input patches contain nuclei (when we have at least one target variable for each image), whereas there are many patches with no nucleus. To address this problem, we add a Bernoulli variable to our loss function to ignore mixture parameters:

$$
E(W) = -\sum_{i=1}^{I} \sum_{n=1}^{N_i} \ln \left\{ \sum_{k=1}^{K} \alpha_k(x_i, w) N(t_{ni}|\mu_k(x_i, w), \sigma_k^2(x_i, w) \right\}
$$
$$
- \ln \begin{cases} e(x_i) & \text{if } x_i \text{ has any nucleus} \\ 1 - e(x_i) & \text{Otherwise} \end{cases} \tag{4}
$$

where I is the number of the training images, N_i is the number of nucleus within each image and t_{ni} is the coordinate of nth point within the image patch i. e_i is a Bernoulli variable that specifies the probability of the patch containing any nucleus and the variance covering the dilation.

Pointset for each nuclei: During the training of the network, we use a dilated point set located within 6 pixels from the nucleus center. This augments the training data and increases the training efficiency. We sample 10 points from a Gaussian distribution with the mean on nucleus centroid.

Network Architecture: In this paper, a CNN model was selected because of its capability to deal directly with raw images, without the need of preprocessing and an explicit features extraction process. The network is trained to capture the important aspects of the input data. By optimizing the dense representation of the input data in the feature maps, the performance of the fully connected part (MDN) is improved.

For having a rich feature and better convergence, Resnet [17] with 18 layers is utilized. In this architecture 'relu' activation function are replaced with 'elu'. We did not use very deep Resnet architecture as its training requires huge amount of data. Two fully connected layers are added after average-pooling to construct the whole architecture of MDN (See Fig. 1).

To provide an appropriate input size to the network, the original images were cropped to patches of size 50×50. The network architecture consists of 2 fully

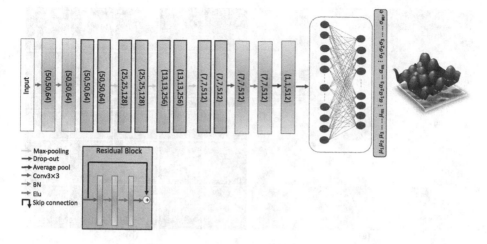

Fig. 1. The schematic architecture of the proposed method.

connected layers (256 and $((c + 2) \times K) + 1$), respectively). We set the number of mixtures to 100, therefore the MDN should predict 401 values (for each mixture 400 values and 1 value for the Bernoulli distribution). After acquiring network predictions, the patches with no nucleus having the low value of e are ignored (threshold for e is set to 0.5). We choose the most significant Gaussians by applying a threshold of 0.001 on the mixture coefficients (α_i). Afterward, the probability maps are generated using α_i,s, σ_i,s and μ_i,s. Finally to extract the centroids of the nuclei within the remaining patches, local maxima are sought.

3   Experimental Results

Dataset: For our experiments, we use the Colorectal cancer (CRC) dataset provided by [14]. It involves 100 H&E images of colorectal adenocarcinomas of size 500×500 which are cropped from CRC whole slide images. The total number of 29756 nuclei were annotated for detection purpose. All the images are obtained at 20X magnification. This dataset is randomly divided into two halves for training and testing. The cell detection on this dataset is challenging due to touching cells, blurred (or weak) cell boundaries and inhomogeneous background noise.

Results and Discussion: Figure 2 shows the probability maps and the centroid locations along with the ground truth circles overlaid on the original images. As shown, the network could learn the locations of complex nuclei such as epithelial as well as congested area where lymphocyte nuclei lie. The broader view of the two challenging images and their corresponding probability maps are depicted in Fig. 3. For visual assessment, the annotated centroids (yellow circles) and predicted locations (red dots) are also shown in Fig. 3.

For the quantitative evaluation we use the same two-fold cross validation explained in [14]. Precision, Recall and F1 score are used for validating the

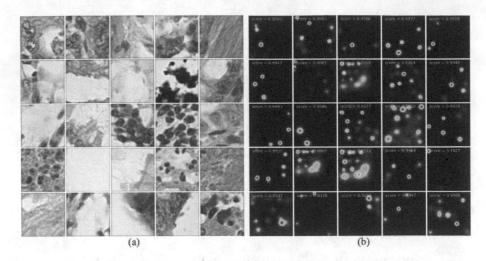

(a)   (b)

Fig. 2. The image patches with their corresponding generated probability maps. (a) The ground truth nuclei locations is overlaid on the images. (b)The corresponding probability map generated using our proposed MDN. The score on top of each image is showing the probability of that patch containing any nucleus.

detection performance. Each detected nucleus within the radius of 6 pixels from the annotated center is considered as true positive. The final results are shown in Table 1. The algorithm has low false negatives which leads to higher recall compared to other methods. In other word, high recall highlights its performance in detecting relatively more cells compared to its counterparts. Overall the F1 score is high, which shows a good detection performance in the proposed MDN based framework.

Due to its probabilistic output, one advantage of the proposed method is its ability to handle images with weak and sparse annotations. We demonstrate this through the following procedure. Firstly we equally divide the dataset into training and validation sets and then remove 30% of the available annotations from the training set and compare the results with SR-CNN. The quantitative results in Table 2, obtained using this sparsely annotated data, show that the proposed method can achieve a better performance.

Table 1. Comparison of precision, recall and F1 scores with other approaches.

Method	Precision	Recall	F1 score
Proposed	0.788	0.882	0.832
SC-CNN [14]	0.781	0.823	0.802
SR-CNN [12]	0.790	0.834	0.811
SSAE [13]	0.617	0.644	0.630

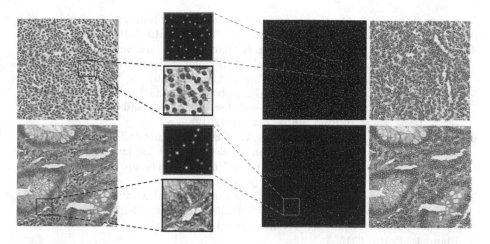

Fig. 3. The original images on the left most column and their corresponding MDN outputs. For better visualization of congested lymphocyte nuclei (first row) and complex tumor epithelial, regions of interest are enlarged in the green boxes. The right most column shows the ground truth specified in yellow circles with detected nuclei as red dot.

Table 2. Comparison of precision, recall and F1 scores using weakly annotated data.

Method	Precision	Recall	F1 score
Proposed	0.67	0.75	0.71
SR-CNN [12]	0.59	0.63	0.60

4   Conclusion

In this study, we used a probabilistic approach for detecting nucleus. MDN has been used in literature for one to many regression tasks. Here, we proposed a framework for employing MDN for nuclei detection. Firstly the features learned using a CNN taking images as input. Then, the MDN learns the distribution of nucleus within the image patch using a mixture of Gaussian. Our method is capable of utilizing weak annotated data while preserving a good performance. Finally, we showed that the proposed method can detect nucleus in colorectal histology images with a higher F1 score when compared to other approaches.

References

1. Grau, V., Mewes, A., Alcaniz, M., Kikinis, R., Warfield, S.K.: Improved watershed transform for medical image segmentation using prior information. IEEE Trans. Med. Imaging **23**(4), 447–458 (2004)
2. Quelhas, P., Marcuzzo, M., Mendonça, A.M., Campilho, A.: Cell nuclei and cytoplasm joint segmentation using the sliding band filter. IEEE Trans. Med. Imaging **29**(8), 1463–1473 (2010)

3. Schmitt, O., Hasse, M.: Radial symmetries based decomposition of cell clusters in binary and gray level images. Pattern Recognit. **41**(6), 1905–1923 (2008)

4. Parvin, B., Yang, Q., Han, J., Chang, H., Rydberg, B., Barcellos-Hoff, M.H.: Iterative voting for inference of structural saliency and characterization of subcellular events. IEEE Trans. Image Process. **16**(3), 615–623 (2007)

5. Qi, X., Xing, F., Foran, D.J., Yang, L.: Robust segmentation of overlapping cells in histopathology specimens using parallel seed detection and repulsive level set. IEEE Trans. Biomed. Eng. **59**(3), 754–765 (2012)

6. Hafiane, A., Bunyak, F., Palaniappan, K.: Fuzzy clustering and active contours for histopathology image segmentation and nuclei detection. In: International Conference on Advanced Concepts for Intelligent Vision Systems, pp. 903–914. Springer, Berlin (2008)

7. Akakin, H.C., et al.: Automated detection of cells from immunohistochemically-stained tissues: application to Ki-67 nuclei staining. In: Medical Imaging 2012: Computer-Aided Diagnosis. Volume 8315, International Society for Optics and Photonics (2012) 831503

8. Yang, L., Tuzel, O., Meer, P., Foran, D.J.: Automatic image analysis of histopathology specimens using concave vertex graph. In: International Conference on Medical Image Computing and Computer-Assisted Intervention,pp. 833–841. Springer, Berlin (2008)

9. Jung, C., Kim, C.: Segmenting clustered nuclei using H-minima transform-based marker extraction and contour parameterization. IEEE Trans. Biomed. Eng. **57**(10), 2600–2604 (2010)

10. Thomas, R.M., John, J.: A review on cell detection and segmentation in microscopic images. In: 2017 International Conference on Circuit, Power and Computing Technologies (ICCPCT), pp. 1–5. IEEE (2017)

11. Cireşan, D.C., Giusti, A., Gambardella, L.M., Schmidhuber, J.: Mitosis detection in breast cancer histology images with deep neural networks. In: International Conference on Medical Image Computing and Computer-Assisted Intervention, pp. 411–418. Springer, Berlin (2013)

12. Xie, Y., Xing, F., Shi, X., Kong, X., Su, H., Yang, L.: Efficient and robust cell detection: a structured regression approach. Med. Image Anal. **44**, 245–254 (2018)

13. Xu, J., Xiang, L., Liu, Q., Gilmore, H., Wu, J., Tang, J., Madabhushi, A.: Stacked sparse autoencoder (SSAE) for nuclei detection on breast cancer histopathology images. IEEE Trans. Med. Imaging **35**(1), 119–130 (2016)

14. Sirinukunwattana, K., Raza, S.E.A., Tsang, Y.W., Snead, D.R., Cree, I.A., Rajpoot, N.M.: Locality sensitive deep learning for detection and classification of nuclei in routine colon cancer histology images. IEEE Trans. Med. Imaging **35**(5), 1196–1206 (2016)

15. Bishop, C.M.: Mixture density networks. Technical report. Citeseer (1994)

16. Xie, W., Noble, J.A., Zisserman, A.: Microscopy cell counting and detection with fully convolutional regression networks. Comput. Methods Biomech. Biomed. Eng.: Imaging Vis. **6**(3), 283–292 (2018)

17. He, K., Zhang, X., Ren, S., Sun, J.: Deep residual learning for image recognition. In: Proceedings of the IEEE Conference on Computer Vision and Pattern Recognition, pp. 770–778 (2016)

Attention-Guided Curriculum Learning for Weakly Supervised Classification and Localization of Thoracic Diseases on Chest Radiographs

Yuxing Tang[1(✉)], Xiaosong Wang[1(✉)], Adam P. Harrison[1], Le Lu[1], Jing Xiao[2], and Ronald M. Summers[1]

[1] National Institutes of Health, Clinical Center, Bethesda, MD, USA
`yuxing.tang@nih.gov, rms@nih.gov`
[2] Ping An Technology Co., Ltd., Shenzhen, China

Abstract. In this work, we exploit the task of joint classification and weakly supervised localization of thoracic diseases from chest radiographs, with only image-level disease labels coupled with disease severity-level (DSL) information of a subset. A convolutional neural network (CNN) based attention-guided curriculum learning (AGCL) framework is presented, which leverages the severity-level attributes mined from radiology reports. Images in order of difficulty (grouped by different severity-levels) are fed to CNN to boost the learning gradually. In addition, highly confident samples (measured by classification probabilities) and their corresponding class-conditional heatmaps (generated by the CNN) are extracted and further fed into the AGCL framework to guide the learning of more distinctive convolutional features in the next iteration. A two-path network architecture is designed to regress the heatmaps from selected seed samples in addition to the original classification task. The joint learning scheme can improve the classification and localization performance along with more seed samples for the next iteration. We demonstrate the effectiveness of this iterative refinement framework via extensive experimental evaluations on the publicly available ChestXray14 dataset. AGCL achieves over 5.7% (averaged over 14 diseases) increase in classification AUC and 7%/11% increases in Recall/Precision for the localization task compared to the state of the art.

1 Introduction

The chest X-ray (radiograph) is a fast and painless screening test that is commonly performed to diagnose various thoracic abnormalities, such as pneumonias, pneumothoraces and lung nodules. It is one of the most cost-effective imaging examinations and imparts minimal radiation exposure to the patient while displaying a wide range of visual diagnostic information. Identifying and distinguishing the various chest abnormalities in chest X-rays is a challenging task even

---

Y. Tang and X. Wang—Equal contribution.

This is a U.S. government work and not under copyright protection in the U.S.; foreign copyright protection may apply 2018
Y. Shi et al. (Eds.): MLMI 2018, LNCS 11046, pp. 249–258, 2018.
https://doi.org/10.1007/978-3-030-00919-9_29

to the human observer. Therefore, its interpretation has been performed mostly by board-certified radiologists or other physicians. There are huge demands on developing computer-aided detection (CADe) methods to assist radiologists and other physicians in reading and comprehending chest X-ray images.

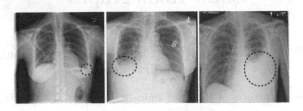

Fig. 1. Left: *small* left pleural effusion. **Middle**: *moderate* right effusion. **Right**: *large* left pleural effusion.

Currently, deep learning methods, especially convolutional neural networks (CNN) [4,9], have become ubiquitous. They have achieved compelling performance across a number of tasks in the medical imaging domain [10,13]. Most of these applications typically involve only one particular type of disease or lesion, such as automated classification of pulmonary tuberculosis [5], pneumonia detection [7], and lung nodule segmentation [3]. Wang *et al.* [11] recently introduced a hospital-scale chest X-ray (ChestX-ray14) dataset containing 112,120 frontal-view X-ray images, with 14 thoracic disease labels text-mined from associated radiology reports using natural language processing (NLP) techniques. Furthermore, a weakly-supervised CNN based multi-label thoracic disease classification and localization framework was proposed in [11] using only image-level labels. Li *et al.* [6] presented a unified network that simultaneously improves classification and localization with the help of extra bounding boxes indicating disease location.

In addition to the disease labels that represent the presence or absence of certain disease, we also want to utilize the attributes of those diseases contained in the radiology reports. Disease severity level (DSL) is one of the most critical attributes, since different severity levels are correlated with highly different visual appearances in chest X-rays (see examples in Fig. 1). Radiologists tend to state such disease severity levels (*i.e.*, *[minimal, tiny, small, mild]*, *[middle-size, moderate]*, *[remarkable, large, severe]*, etc.) when describing the findings in chest X-rays. This type of disease attribute information can be exploited to enhance and enrich the accuracy of NLP-mined disease labels, which consequently may facilitate to build more accurate and robust disease classification and localization framework than [11]. More recently, Wang *et al.* [12] proposed the TieNet (Text-Image Embedding Network), which was an end-to-end CNN-RNN architecture for learning to embed visual images and text reports for image classification and report generation. However, the disease attributes were not explicitly modeled in the TieNet framework.

In this paper, we propose an attention-guided curriculum learning (AGCL) framework for the task of joint thoracic disease classification and weakly supervised localization, where only image-level disease labels and severity level information of a subset are available. Note, we do not use bounding boxes for training. In AGCL, we use the disease severity level to group the data samples as a means to build the curriculum for *curriculum learning* [1]. For each disease category, we begin by learning from severe samples, progressively adding moderate and mild samples as the CNN matures and converges gradually by seeing samples from "easy" to "hard". The intuition behind curriculum learning is to mimic the common human process of gradual learning, starting from the easiest or obvious samples to harder or more ambiguous ones, which is notably the case for medical students learning to read radiographs. Furthermore, we use the CNN generated disease heatmaps (*visual attention*) of "confident" *seed* images to guide the CNN in an iterative training process. The initial seeds are composed of: (1) images of severe and moderate disease level, and (2) images with high classification probability scores from the current CNN classifier. A two-path multi-task learning network architecture is designed to regress the heatmaps from selected seed samples in addition to the original classification task. In each iteration, the joint learning scheme can harvest more seeds of high quality as the network fine-tuning process iterates, resulting in increased guidance and more discriminative CNN for better classification and localization.

We test our proposed method on the public ChestXray14 dataset to evaluate the multi-label disease classification and localization performance. Comprehensive experimental results demonstrate the effectiveness of our framework in acquiring high-quality seeds, and the visual attention generated from seed images are evidently beneficial in guiding the learning procedure to improve both the classification and localization accuracy.

2   Method

2.1   A CNN Based Classification and Localization Framework

The proposed AGCL approach starts by initializing a CNN pre-trained from ImageNet and then fine-tuning it on the ChestX-ray14 dataset on all C ($C = 14$) disease categories. This is similar to [11] except that the transition layer is discarded. This serves as the baseline of our method for multi-label classification and localization. The flowchart of the baseline framework is shown in Fig. 2(a).

2.2   Disease Severity-Level Based Curriculum Learning

Generally, the knowledge to be acquired by students is meticulously designed in a curriculum, so that "easier" concepts are introduced first, and more in-depth knowledge is systematically acquired by mastering concepts with increasing difficulty. The "easy-to-hard" principle of curriculum learning [1] has been helpful for both image classification and weakly supervised object detection [8] in computer vision. The curriculum that controls what training data should be fed to the model is usually built based on prior information, such as object size (the larger, the easier) or other more sophisticated human supervision.

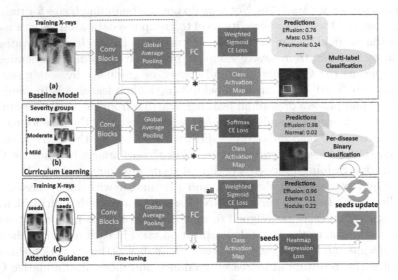

Fig. 2. Overall architecture of attention-guided curriculum learning (AGCL).

We mine the disease severity level (DSL) attributes from radiology reports using a similar NLP techniques introduced in [11]. Severity descriptions that correlated to the disease keyword are extracted using the dependency graph built on each sentence in the report. DSL attributes are then collected whenever available from the whole training set and are grouped into three clusters, namely *mild*, *moderate* and *severe*. We treat the severity attributes as prior knowledge to build the curriculum. The prediction layers of the baseline model are replaced with a randomly initialized 2-way fully connected (FC) layer and a softmax cross-entropy loss, and we fine-tune the baseline model to a binary classification network for each disease category. The training samples are presented to the network in order of decreasing severity levels (increasing difficulties) of a certain disease, that is from severe samples to moderate to mild gradually as the CNN becomes more adept at later iterations during training. The negative samples come from *normal* cases (without any diseases mentioned in the radiology report) in the dataset and the number of negative samples for each category is balanced with the number of positive samples of that category. Note that we fine-tune from the weights learned from the baseline model in Sect. 2.1 because (1) the images annotated with all severity levels account for only about 25% of the training samples, which is not sufficient for training a deep CNN with millions of parameters, and (2) the baseline model is expected to have captured an overall concept distribution of the target dataset, which could be a useful starting point for curriculum learning.

The disease-specific class activation map [14] (CAM, or heatmap) H^c of a chest X-ray image for a positive disease class c is:

$$H^c(x, y) = \sum_{d=1}^{D} \mathbf{w}_c(d) * f(x, y, d),$$ (1)

where $\mathbf{w}_c(d)$ is the weights of the FC layer corresponding to the positive disease category $c \in \mathbb{C} = \{1, ..., C\}$ in each binary classification network, and $f(x, y, d)$ is the activation of the d-th $(d \in \{1, ..., D\})$ neuron of the last convolutional layer at a spatial coordinate (x, y), where D is number of feature maps.

The heatmaps can be further employed as visual attention guidance for the CNN in the succeeding iterative refinement steps described in Sect. 2.3. The reason to split the network into individual binary models per disease instead of fine-tuning as a whole is that the severity levels tend to be inconsistent among different diseases in a multi-label situation. Moreover, the binary models are empirically found to be more discriminative and spatially accurate on generating disease-specific heatmaps.

2.3 Attention Guided Iterative Refinement

In this section, we explore and harvest highly "confident" seed images. We assume their computed disease-specific heatmaps could highlight the regions that potentially contribute more to the final disease recognition than the non-seed images. The highlighted regions represent the Region of Interest (ROI), or in other words, *visual attention* of disease patterns. In addition to the curriculum learning for each disease category shown in Fig. 2(b), we introduce a heatmap regression path (shown in Fig. 2(c)) to enforce the attention-guided learning of better convolutional features, which in turn generate more meaningful heatmaps. By using such an iterative refinement loop, we demonstrated that both the classification and localization results could be simultaneously and significantly improved over the baseline.

Harvesting Seeds: Ideally, image samples with *severe* and *moderate* disease severity levels could potentially be selected as seeds (denoted as $\mathbb{S}_1$) since their visual appearances are relatively easier to recognize than *mild* ones. Additional selection criterion requires that an image is labeled with a certain disease c and is correctly classified by the corresponding binary classifier introduced in Sect. 2.2 with a probability score larger than a threshold t (seeds collected as $\mathbb{S}_2$). We believe that the disease-specific heatmaps (seed attention maps) generated by Eq. (1) from those *seeds* image samples ($\mathbb{S} = \mathbb{S}_1 \cup \mathbb{S}_2$) shall exhibit higher precision in localizing disease patterns than other samples.

Attention Guidance from Seeds: We create a branch in the original classification network to guide the learning of better convolutional features using the seed attention maps. This branch shares all the convolutional blocks with the baseline model in Sect. 2.1 and includes an additional heatmap regression path. The regression loss is modeled as the sum of the channel-wise smooth $L1$ losses over feature channels between the heatmap generated by the current network $(\hat{H}^c)$ and the seed attention map of the last iteration (H^c).

$$Loss_{reg}(I) = \sum_{d=1}^{D} \sum_{x,y} smooth_{L_1}(\hat{H}^c(x,y) - H^c(x,y)), \forall I \in \mathbb{S} \qquad (2)$$

in which

$$smooth_{L_1}(z) = \begin{cases} 0.5z^2, & \text{if } |z| < 1 \\ |z| - 0.5, & \text{otherwise.} \end{cases} \qquad (3)$$

The final objective function to be optimized is a weighted sum of the sigmoid cross-entropy loss for multi-label classification ($Loss_{cls}$) and the heatmap regression loss ($Loss_{reg}$) for localization:

$$Loss_{final}(I) = Loss_{cls}(I) + \lambda \sum_{c=1}^{C} \mathbf{1}_c Loss_{reg}(I), \qquad (4)$$

where $\mathbf{1}_c = 1$ if an image I is a seed for disease category $c \in C$, otherwise $\mathbf{1}_c = 0$. λ is used to balance the classification and regression loss so that they have roughly equal contributions. We empirically set λ to 0.005.

Harvesting Additional Seeds: Once the network is retrained with the attention guidance, the curriculum learning procedures will be conducted again to harvest new confident seeds. All non-seed positive training images in each disease category will be inputted to their corresponding binary classifiers, among which highly scored images are harvested as additional seeds. Together with the initial seeds, their heatmaps are further fed to refinement framework as additional visual attention to guide the CNN to focus on disease-specific attended regions in the chest X-rays. Consequently, more and more confident seeds could be harvested while the accuracy of classification and localization improves gradually.

3   Experiments

We extensively evaluate the proposed AGCL approach on the ChestX-ray14 dataset [11], which contains 112,120 frontal-view chest X-ray images of 30,805 unique patients, with 14 thoracic disease labels, extracted from associated radiology reports using NLP techniques. A small subset of 880 images within the dataset are annotated by board-certified radiologists, resulting in 984 bounding box locations containing 8 types of disease. We further extracted severity attributes along with the disease keywords. For classification, we use the same patient-level data splits provided in the dataset, which uses roughly 70% of the images for training, 10% for validation and 20% for testing. The disease localization is evaluated on all the 984 bounding boxes (not used for training).

We resize the original 3-channel 1024 × 1024 images to 512 × 512 pixels due to the trade-off between higher resolution and affordable computational load. ResNet-50 [2] is employed as the backbone of the proposed CNN architectures[1]. For the baseline method and all the AGCL steps, we optimize the network using SGD with momentum and stop training after the validation loss reaches a plateau. The learning rate is set to be 0.001 and divided by 10 every 10 epochs. The AGCL is implemented using the Caffe framework.

Table 1. Per-category multi-label classification AUC comparison on the test set of ChestX-ray14. BSL: baseline model. PT: Pleural Thickening. AVG: Average AUC.

Disease	Atelectasis	Cardiomegaly	Effusion	Infiltration	Mass	Nodule	Pneumonia
[11]	.7003	.8100	.7585	.6614	.6933	.6687	.6580
[12]	.7320	.8440	.7930	.6660	.7250	.6850	.7200
BSL	.7268	.8545	.7899	.6788	.7527	.7143	.6934
AGL	.7353	.8656	.8113	.6823	.7722	.7178	.7100
AGCL-1	.7500	.8644	.8028	.6748	.7590	.7064	.7130
AGCL-2	**.7557**	**.8865**	**.8191**	**.6892**	**.8136**	**.7545**	**.7292**

Disease	Pneumothorax	Consolidation	Edema	Emphysema	Fibrosis	PT	Hernia	AVG
[11]	.7993	.7032	.8052	.8330	.7859	.6835	.8717	.7451
[12]	.8470	.7010	.8290	.8650	.7960	.7350	.8760	.7724
BSL	.8260	.7052	.8148	.8698	.7892	.7260	.8500	.7708
AGL	.8423	.7042	.8366	.8874	**.8180**	.7499	.8543	.7777
AGCL-1	.8413	.7209	.8321	.8771	.7922	.7472	**.9012**	.7844
AGCL-2	**.8499**	**.7283**	**.8475**	**.9075**	.8179	**.7647**	.8747	**.8027**

Disease Classification: We quantitatively evaluate the disease classification performance using the AUC (area under the ROC curve) score for each category. We ablate the curriculum learning step in the AGCL framework to assess its effect. It is denoted by AGL (attention-guided learning), where seeds are only initialized with high scored images from the baseline model. The per-disease AUC comparisons of the benchmark [11], our baseline method, AGL, and AGCL with one refinement step (AGCL-1) and two refinement steps (AGCL-2) are shown in Table 1. A higher AUC score implies a better classifier.

Compared with the benchmark results [11], our baseline model achieves higher AUC scores for all the categories except *Hernia*, which contains a very limited number (< 200) of samples. AGL consistently achieves better performance than the baseline model, demonstrating the effectiveness of attention-guided learning in our framework. Furthermore, the proposed AGCL improves upon AGL by introducing more confident heatmaps from seed images using curriculum learning. The iterative refinement process using AGCL is proven to be effective given the fact that AGCL-2 achieves better classification results than

---

[1] Up-to-date results using the DenseNet-121: https://arxiv.org/abs/1807.07532.

AGCL-1. We experimentally find that AGCL-3 has similar results as AGCL-2, which we believe the iterative refinement process has reached the convergence.

Table 2. Comparison of disease localization results using $T(IoBB) = 0.25$. GT: number of ground-truth bounding boxes. BSL: baseline model.

Disease	GT	Detected Box			True Positive			Recall			Precision		
		BSL	AGL	AGCL	BSL	AGL	AGCL	BSL	AGL	AGCL	BSL	AGL	AGCL
Atelectasis	180	734	687	**620**	138	162	**190**	0.46	0.58	**0.66**	0.19	0.24	**0.31**
Cardiomegaly	146	394	342	**390**	369	320	**366**	0.99	0.99	**1.00**	0.94	0.94	**0.94**
Effusion	153	743	544	**546**	205	218	**228**	0.55	0.64	**0.72**	0.28	0.40	**0.42**
Infiltration	123	595	616	**501**	221	232	**242**	0.76	0.80	**0.87**	0.42	0.38	**0.48**
Mass	85	291	262	**278**	106	116	**148**	0.65	0.69	**0.79**	0.36	0.44	**0.53**
Nodule	79	296	293	**295**	16	28	**28**	0.19	0.32	**0.32**	0.05	0.10	**0.09**
Pneumonia	120	558	535	**526**	175	189	**210**	0.76	0.80	**0.82**	0.31	0.35	**0.40**
Pneumothorax	98	394	359	**347**	79	80	**106**	0.45	0.46	**0.49**	0.20	0.22	**0.31**
Total	984	3935	3617	**3498**	1309	1345	**1518**	0.66	0.68	**0.73**	0.33	0.37	**0.44**

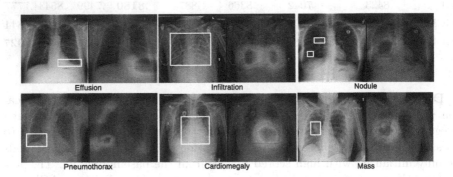

Fig. 3. Selected examples of disease localization results (heatmaps overlaid on X-ray images; red color indicates stronger responses) on the ChestXray14 test set using our proposed AGCL framework. The ground-truth bounding boxes are shown in green, and the disease labels are given under each pair of images.

Weakly Supervised Disease Localization: We generate bounding boxes from the disease-specific heatmap for each image with corresponding disease, following the benchmark method applied in [11,14], and evaluate their qualities against ground-truth (GT) bounding boxes annotated by radiologists. A box is considered as a true positive (TP) if its Intersection of the GT Over the detected Bounding Box area ratio (IoBB [11], similar to Area of Precision or Purity) is larger than a threshold $T(IoBB)$. Table 2 shows the comparison of the baseline model, AGL and AGCL-2 (denoted as AGCL in the table).

Overall, AGCL achieves the best localization results by generating the least number of bounding boxes (3498) but with the most number of true positives (1518), namely the highest precision (0.44). It recalls 73% of the ground-truth boxes by proposing an average of 3.5 boxes per image. AGCL employs more seed images than AGL by incorporating disease severity level (DSL) based curriculum learning, which improves upon AGL as shown in Table 2. The relative performance improvements of AGCL are more significant for *Effusion*, *Mass* and *Infiltration*, where more *moderate* and *severe* samples are labeled than other disease types. *Nodule* is often labeled as *small* therefore curriculum learning barely helps. However, visual attention based iterative learning (AGL) outperformed the baseline model even for very difficult diseases such as *Nodule* and *Pneumothorax*. We show some qualitative localization heatmap examples in Fig. 3.

4 Conclusion

In this paper, we exploit to utilize the NLP-mined disease severity level information from radiology reports to facilitate the curriculum learning for more accurate thoracic disease classification and localization. In addition, an iterative attention-guided refinement framework is developed to further improve the classification and weakly-supervised localization performance. Extensive experimental evaluations on the ChestXray14 database validate the effectiveness on significant performance improvement derived from both the overall framework and each of its components individually. Future work includes formulating structured reports, extracting richer information from the reports such as coarse location of lesions and using follow up studies, and mining common disease patterns, to help develop more precise predictive models.

Acknowledgments. This research was supported by the Intramural Research Program of the National Institutes of Health Clinical Center and by the Ping An Technology Co., Ltd. through a Cooperative Research and Development Agreement. The authors thank NVIDIA for GPU donation.

References

1. Bengio, Y., Louradour, J., et al.: Curriculum learning. In: ICML (2009)
2. He, K., et al.: Deep residual learning for image recognition. In: IEEE CVPR (2016)
3. Jin, D., Xu, Z., et al.: CT-realistic lung nodule simulation from 3D conditional generative adversarial networks for robust lung segmentation. In: MICCAI (2018)
4. Krizhevsky, A., Sutskever, I., Hinton, G.E.: Imagenet classification with deep convolutional neural networks. In: NIPS (2012)
5. Lakhani, P., Sundaram, B.: Deep learning at chest radiography: automated classification of pulmonary tuberculosis by using convolutional neural networks. Radiology **284**(2), 574–582 (2017)

6. Li, Z., Wang, C., Han, M., Xue, Y., Wei, W., Li, L.J., Fei-Fei, L.: Thoracic disease identification and localization with limited supervision. In: IEEE CVPR (2018)
7. Rajpurkar, P., Irvin, J., Zhu, K., Yang, B., et al.: CheXNet: radiologist-level pneumonia detection on chest X-rays with deep learning. arXiv:1711.05225 (2017)
8. Shi, M., Ferrari, V.: Weakly supervised object localization using size estimates. In: ECCV (2016)
9. Tang, Y., Wang, J., Gao, B., et al.: Large scale semi-supervised object detection using visual and semantic knowledge transfer. In: IEEE CVPR (2016)
10. Tang, Y., et al.: Semi-automatic RECIST labeling on CT scans with cascaded convolutional neural networks. In: MICCAI (2018)
11. Wang, X., Peng, Y., Lu, L., Lu, Z., Bagheri, M., Summers, R.M.: ChestX-ray8: hospital-scale chest X-ray database and benchmarks on weakly-supervised classification and localization of common thorax diseases. In: IEEE CVPR (2017)
12. Wang, X., Peng, Y., et al.: TieNet: text-image embedding network for common thorax disease classification and reporting in chest X-rays. In: IEEE CVPR (2018)
13. Yan, K., et al.: Deeplesion: automated mining of large-scale lesion annotations and universal lesion detection with deep learning. J. Med. Imaging 5(3), 036501 (2018)
14. Zhou, B., Khosla, A., Lapedriza, A., Oliva, A., Torralba, A.: Learning deep features for discriminative localization. In: IEEE CVPR (2016)

Graph of Hippocampal Subfields Grading for Alzheimer's Disease Prediction

Kilian Hett[1,2(✉)], Vinh-Thong Ta[1,2,3], José V. Manjón[4], and Pierrick Coupé[1,2]

[1] Univ. Bordeaux, LaBRI, UMR 5800, PICTURA, 33400 Talence, France
[2] CNRS, LaBRI, UMR 5800, PICTURA, 33400 Talence, France
kilian.hett@labri.fr
[3] Bordeaux INP, LaBRI, UMR 5800, PICTURA, 33600 Pessac, France
[4] Universitat Politècnia de València, ITACA, 46022 Valencia, Spain

Abstract. Numerous methods have been proposed to capture early hippocampus alterations caused by Alzheimer's disease. Among them, patch-based grading approach showed its capability to capture subtle structural alterations. This framework applied on hippocampus obtains state-of-the-art results for AD detection but is limited for its prediction compared to the same approaches based on whole-brain analysis. We assume that this limitation could come from the fact that hippocampus is a complex structure divided into different subfields. Indeed, it has been shown that AD does not equally impact hippocampal subfields. In this work, we propose a graph-based representation of the hippocampal subfields alterations based on patch-based grading feature. The strength of this approach comes from better modeling of the inter-related alterations through the different hippocampal subfields. Thus, we show that our novel method obtains similar results than state-of-the-art approaches based on whole-brain analysis with improving by 4 percent points of accuracy patch-based grading methods based on hippocampus.

Keywords: Hippocampal subfields · Patch-based grading
Graph-based method · Alzheimer's disease classification
Mild Cognitive Impairment

1 Introduction

Alzheimer's disease (AD) is the most prevalent dementia for the older adults. This disease leads to an irreversible form of neurodegenerative process causing mental dysfunctions. Neuroimaging studies performed on AD patients has

Data used in preparation of this article were obtained from the Alzheimer's Disease Neuroimaging Initiative (ADNI) database (adni.loni.usc.edu). As such, the investigators within the ADNI contributed to the design and implementation of ADNI and/or provided data but did not participate in analysis or writing of this report. A complete listing of ADNI investigators can be found at: http://adni.loni.usc.edu/wp-content/uploads/how_to_apply/ADNI_Acknowledgement_List.pdf.
K. Hett et al.: the Alzheimer's Disease Neuroimaging Initiative

© Springer Nature Switzerland AG 2018
Y. Shi et al. (Eds.): MLMI 2018, LNCS 11046, pp. 259–266, 2018.
https://doi.org/10.1007/978-3-030-00919-9_30

revealed that AD causes structural brain changes. These changes are character-ized by an accelerated neural and synapse losses, which are advanced when the diagnosis is established. A presymptomatic phase of AD is named mild cognitive impairment (MCI). Patients having MCI suffer from amnesia and light mental issues that do not impact their daily life. Moreover, MCI patients can return to a cognitive normal status or progress to dementia. Predicting this conversion is a challenging task but can make easier the design of clinical trials and accelerate the development of new therapies.

It has long been known that in-vivo imaging with magnetic resonance imaging (MRI) can detect structural alterations such as atrophy of grey matter volume. Thus, several methods were proposed. On the one hand, voxel-based morphom-etry (VBM) methods were designed to detect the most discriminant regions at a voxel scale [18]. On the other hand, region-based methods were proposed to ana-lyze specific brain structures. These analysis are usually conducted with volume, shape or thickness measurements [18]. It is interesting to note that both of VBM and region-based approaches have demonstrated that the medial temporal lobe especially the hippocampus is the area having the earliest alterations. However, although the hippocampus volume is one of the criterion that can be used to confirm the diagnosis of AD in clinical routines, it does not provide acceptable performance for the prediction of AD conversion. Recently, more advanced meth-ods were proposed to detect subtler structural modifications of the hippocampus [11]. Among them, patch-based grading (PBG) framework was proposed to bet-ter capture subtle brain alterations caused by AD [2]. The main idea of PBG methods is to detect modifications in a cubic fixed-size area named patch. PBG methods applied to the hippocampus have demonstrated state-of-the-art perfor-mances for AD detection and prediction compared to others methods based on the hippocampus [2,5,14].

However, the hippocampus is not a heterogeneous structure. Indeed, the hip-pocampus is composed of different subfields having distinct characteristics. A common definition of hippocampal subfields [17] divided them into the subicu-lum, the cornu ammonia (CA), and the dentate gyrus (DG). The CA represents the most prominent area. It is usually divided into four regions: CA1, CA2, CA3, and CA4. The CA1 is also composed of several layers, such as the stratum pyra-midale (SP), stratum radiatum (SR), stratum molecular (SM), and stratum lacunosum (SL). Moreover, postmortem and animal-based studies showed that hippocampal subfields are not impacted equally. Those studies showed that CA1 and subiculum are the most impacted at the last stages of AD [6,15]. Conse-quently, we assume that a straightforward whole hippocampus analysis could limit the prediction performances. An analysis of the hippocampus at a finner scale such as hippocampal subfields may improve prediction.

To confirm this assumption, we propose a novel method to better capture AD signature within hippocampal subfields. Our method integrates patch-based grading features into a new graph-based model that provides efficient representa-tion of the inter-related alterations through the hippocampus. We demonstrate that our novel approach improves patch-based grading method applied into the

Table 1. Description of the dataset used in this work. Data are provided by ADNI.

Characteristic/Group	CN	sMCI	pMCI	AD
Number of subjects	213	90	126	130
Ages (years)	75.7 ± 5.0	74.9 ± 7.5	73.7 ± 7.0	74.1 ± 7.7
Sex (M/F)	108/105	58/32	68/58	64/66
MMSE	29.1 ± 1.0	27.6 ± 1.7	26.5 ± 1.6	23.5 ± 1.9

hippocampus by 4% points of accuracy and obtains state-of-the-art results compared to last advanced methods based on whole brain analysis for AD prediction.

2   Materials and Methods

Dataset. Data used in this work were obtained from Alzheimer's Disease Neuroimaging Initiative (ADNI) dataset[1]. ADNI is a North American campaign launched in 2003 with aims to provide MRI, positron emission tomography scans, clinical neurological measures and other biomarkers. The data used in this study are all the baseline T1-weighted (T1-w) MRI of the ADNI1 phase. This dataset includes AD patients, MCI and cognitive normal (CN) subjects. The group of MCI is composed of subjects who have abnormal memory dysfunctions and embed two groups; the first one is composed with patients having stable MCI (sMCI) and the second one with patients having progressive MCI (pMCI) who converted in the following 36 months after the baseline. The information of the dataset used in our work is summarized in Table 1.

Preprocessing. First, each image was preprocessed with a method based on an advanced pipeline providing: (a) a denoising step with an adaptive non-local mean filter [8], (b) an affine registration in the MNI space [1], (c) a correction of the image inhomogeneities [16] and (d) an intensity normalization. Second, segmentation of hippocampal subfields was performed with HIPS. This method is based on a combination of non-linear registration and patch-based label fusion [10]. This method uses a training library based on a dataset composed of high resolution T1w images manually labeled according to the protocol proposed by [17]. Consequently, to perform the segmentation, the ADNI images are up-sampled with a local adaptive super resolution method to fit in the training image resolution [3]. The method provides automatic segmentation of hippocampal subfields gathered into 5 regions: Subiculum, CA1SP, CA1SR-L-M, CA2-3 and CA4/DG. Finally, visual quality control was conducted to remove all wrong segmentations from the dataset. Moreover, to prevent any bias in the dataset, the quality control was performed without the pathological status of each subject.

Computation of patch-based grading biomarkers. To capture anatomical similarities of alterations caused by AD, we use the patch-based grading

---

[1] http://adni.loni.ucla.edu.

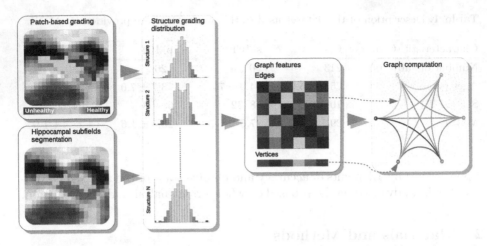

Fig. 1. Illustration of the graph construction. From left to right, for each hippocampal region an estimation of the density probability of PBG values is computed. Next, histograms are used to built our graph of hippocampal subfields grading. Graph edges represent the distances between structure grading distribution while vertices represents the mean grading value for a given hippocampal regions (*i.e.*, hippocampus, subiculum, CA1-SP, etc.)

framework [2]. PBG framework provides at each voxel a score between -1 and 1 related to the alteration severity. The patch-based grading value g at x_i is defined as:

$$g_{x_i} = \frac{\sum_{t_j \in K_i} w(P_{x_i}, P_{t_j}) p_t}{\sum_{t_j \in K_i} w(P_{x_i}, P_{t_j})}, \tag{1}$$

where P_{x_i} and P_{t_j} represent the cubic patches surrounding the voxel i of the test subject image x and the voxel j of the template image t, respectively. The template t comes from a training library composed of CN subjects and AD patients. p_t is the pathological status set to -1 for patches extracted from AD patients and to 1 for those extracted from CN subjects. K_i is a set of the most similar P_{t_j} patches to P_{x_i} found in the training library. The anatomical similarity between the test subject x and the training library is estimated by a weight function $w(P_{x_i}, P_{t_j}) = \exp(-||P_{x_i} - P_{t_j}||_2^2/(h^2 + \epsilon))$, where $h^2 = \min_{t_j} ||P_{x_i} - P_{t_j}||_2^2$ and $\epsilon \to 0$.

Graph construction. First, the grading process is carried out over the whole hippocampus. Afterwards, the corresponding hippocampal subfield segmentations is used to fuse grading values and to built our graph (see Fig. 1). An undirected graph is defined as $G = (V, E, \Gamma, \omega)$, where $V = \{v_1, ..., v_N\}$ is the set of vertices for the N considered hippocampal regions (*i.e.*, the whole hippocampus and each on its hippocampal subfields) and $E = V \times V$ is the set of edges. Thus, in our model the vertices represents the mean of the grading values for a given hippocampus region while the edges are based on grading distribution distances between two hippocampal regions.

The probability distributions of PBG values are estimated with a histogram H_v for each hippocampus region v. The number of bins is set following the Sturge's rule. For each vertex we assign a function $\Gamma : V \to \mathbb{R}$ defined as $\Gamma(v) = \mu_{H_v}$, where μ_{H_v} is the mean of H_v. For each edge we assign a weight given by the function $\omega : E \to \mathbb{R}$ defined as $\omega(v_i, v_j) = \exp(-d(H_{v_i}, H_{v_j})^2/\sigma^2)$ where d is the Wasserstein distance with L_1 norm that showed best performance during our experiments.

In this work, we used the Elastic Net regression (EN) method that provides a sparse representation of the most discriminative edges and vertices, and thus enables to reduce the feature dimensionality by capturing the key regions and the key relationships between the different hippocampus regions (see Fig. 1). Finally, after z-score normalization, a concatenation of the two feature vectors is given as input of EN feature selection method.

Details of implementation. The most similar patches were extracted with a patch-match method [4]. We used the parameters proposed in [5] for the sizes of the patches and K_i. This results in a hippocampus grading computation in about 1 second. Next, the age effect is corrected using linear regression estimated on CN population. The EN method is computed with the SLEP package [7]. The classifications were obtained with the random forest method (RF) [2]. All features were normalized using z-score before selection and classification methods. In our experiments, we performed sMCI versus pMCI classification. The EN features selection and the classifier were trained with CN and AD. Indeed, as shown in [14], using CN and AD to train the feature selection method and the classifier enables to better discriminate sMCI and pMCI subjects. Furthermore, it also enables to limit bias and over-fitting problem without cross-validation step. However, 100 runs were performed to decrease the inner variability of RF. Mean area under curve (AUC), accuracy (ACC), balanced accuracy (BACC), sensibility (SEN), and specificity (SPE) are provided as results in Tables 2 and 3.

3   Results and Discussions

First, a comparison of the prediction performances was conducted with PBG applied into the whole hippocampus as proposed in [2], the hippocampal subfields with EN selection, and our proposed method (see Table 2). The average of PBG values into each region (*i.e.*, whole hippocampus and hippocampal subfields) were used. For hippocampal subfields features, the most relevant subfields selected are the subiculum, and the two definitions of CA1 (*i.e.*, CA1-SP and CA1-SRLM, see Fig. 2). It is very interesting that hippocampal subfields selected by EN method are in line with previous studies which have shown CA1 and subiculum are the subfields having the most significant atrophy in late stages of AD[6,15]. PBG based on the whole hippocampus structure obtains 76.8% of AUC, 70.3% of ACC and is more specific than sensitive. The averages of PBG

---

[2] http://code.google.com/p/randomforest-matlab.

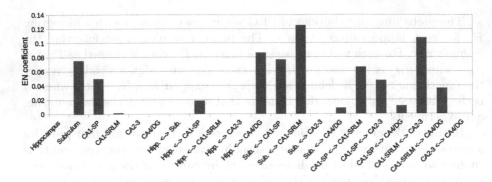

Fig. 2. Graphic representing the coefficients estimated by EN method from the vector of features computed by our graph-based method after z-score normalization. The first six labels represent hippocampal regions and the others represents relationships of these regions. It is interesting to note that selected structures are in line with previous hippocampal subfields investigations.

Table 2. Comparison of different hippocampal PBG approaches is presented. First, PBG applied within the whole hippocampus is provided as the baseline. Second, the best hippocampal subfield features selected by EN method. Finally, results provided by our graph-based of hippocampal subfields grading. This comparison shows that our proposed method improves AUC, ACC, BACC, and SEN compared to other approaches. All results are given in percentage.

Methods	AUC	ACC	BACC	SEN	SPE
Hippocampus	76.8±0.2	70.3±0.0	70.6±0.0	69.0±0.0	72.2±0.0
Hipp. subfields EN	77.1±0.2	71.1±0.4	71.4±0.4	69.5±0.6	**73.2±0.5**
Proposed method	**78.2±0.2**	**74.7±0.4**	**74.3±0.5**	**77.1±0.5**	71.4 ± 0.9

values within subiculum, CA1-SP, and CA1-SRLM obtain 77.1% of AUC, 71.1% of ACC and improve specificity compare to the hippocampus. Thus, the concatenation of mean grading values based on each hippocampal subfields selected with a EN method slightly increases the prediction performances of AD. However, our proposed graph-based method improves by 1.4 percent points with AUC and 4.4 percent points of ACC compared to the hippocampus. Our graph-based method also improves by 1.1 percent points with AUC and 3.6 percent points with ACC compared to the use of the most discriminant hippocampal subfields. Moreover, in both cases, our proposed method increases the sensibility of AD conversion.

Second, a comparison of our novel graph-based method based on hippocampal subfields and state-of-the-art methods based on the hippocampus, using similar ADNI1 dataset, is provided in the upper part of Table 3. In this comparison, we included the original PBG method [2], a method based on multiple instance learning [13], and an advanced PBG method based on a sparse representation [14]. The results demonstrate that our novel graph-based method obtains better results than all compared methods applied to the hippocampus. Indeed, to the

Table 3. Comparison with state-of-the-art methods based on the hippocampus region and approaches based on a whole brain analysis using similar ADNI1 dataset and the same definition of sMCI/pMCI. These results show that our proposed method obtains best results compared to methods applied within the hippocampus. Moreover, compared to approaches based on a whole brain analysis, our method obtains competitive results. All results are given in percentage.

Methods	Registration	AUC	ACC	SEN	SPE
Hippocampus					
Original grading [2]	Affine	–	71.0	70.0	71.0
Multiple instance grading [13]	Affine	–	70.4	66.5	<u>73.1</u>
Sparse-based grading [14]	Non linear	–	69.0	–	–
Proposed method	Affine	**78.2**	<u>74.7</u>	<u>77.1</u>	71.4
Whole brain					
Voxel-based [9]	Non linear	76.6	74.7	**88.8**	51.6
Sparse-based grading [14]	Non linear	–	**75.0**	–	–
Deep ensemble learning [12]	Non linear	75.4	74.8	70.9	**78.8**

best of our knowledge, state-of-the-art methods applied on hippocampus have obtained 71% of ACC for sMCI versus pMCI classification while our graph-based of hippocampal subfields grading obtains 74.7% of ACC.

Finally, in the lower part of Table 3 a comparison with state-of-the-art methods applied on the whole brain is provided. Our method is compared with a VBM approach [9], the advanced PBG method based on a sparse representation [14] and a recent deep ensemble learning method [12]. This comparison shows that our novel graph of hippocampal subfields grading obtains comparable ACC and AUC than the last advanced approaches.

4   Conclusions

In this work, we proposed a new approach to better capture AD signature into the hippocampus. Our method is based on a graph-based representation of inter-related hippocampal subfields alterations. Alterations were captured with a patch-based grading framework while the relationships of alterations between the different subfields are based on histogram distances. We demonstrate that our method improves patch-based grading method based on hippocampus by 4 percent points for sMCI versus pMCI classification. Moreover, our novel approach obtains competitive results compared to state-of-the-art methods based on a whole brain analysis.

Acknowledgement. This study has been carried out with financial support from the French State, managed by the French National Research Agency (ANR) within the project DeepVolbrain and in the frame of the investments for the future program IdEx Bordeaux (HL-MRI ANR-10-IDEX-03-02), Cluster of excellence CPU, TRAIL

(BigDataBrain ANR-10-LABX- 57) and the Spanish DPI2017-87743-R grant from the Ministerio de Economia, Industria y Competitividad of Spain.

References

1. Avants, et al.: A reproducible evaluation of ANTs similarity metric performance in brain image registration. NeuroImage **54**(3), 2033–2044 (2011)
2. Coupé, P., et al.: Scoring by nonlocal image patch estimator for early detection of Alzheimer's disease. NeuroImage: Clin. **1**(1), 141–152 (2012)
3. Coupé, et al.: Collaborative patch-based super-resolution for diffusion-weighted images. NeuroImage **83**, 245–261 (2013)
4. Giraud, et al.: An optimized patchmatch for multi-scale and multi-feature label fusion. NeuroImage **124**, 770–782 (2016)
5. Hett, K., et al.: Adaptive fusion of texture-based grading: application to Alzheimer's disease detection. In: International Workshop on Patch-based Techniques in Medical Imaging, pp. 82–89. Springer, Berlin (2017)
6. Kerchner, et al.: Hippocampal CA1 apical neuropil atrophy and memory performance in Alzheimer's disease. NeuroImage **63**(1), 194–202 (2012)
7. Liu, et al.: Slep: sparse learning with efficient projections. Ariz. State Univ. **6**(491), 7 (2009)
8. Manjón, et al.: Adaptive non-local means denoising of MR images with spatially varying noise levels. J. Magn. Reson. Imaging **31**(1), 192–203 (2010)
9. Moradi, et al.: Machine learning framework for early MRI-based Alzheimer's conversion prediction in MCI subjects. NeuroImage **104**, 398–412 (2015)
10. Romero, et al.: Hips: a new hippocampus subfield segmentation method. NeuroImage **163**, 286–295 (2017)
11. Sørensen, L., et al.: Differential diagnosis of mild cognitive impairment and Alzheimer's disease using structural MRI cortical thickness, hippocampal shape, hippocampal texture, and volumetry. NeuroImage: Clin. **13**, 470–482 (2017)
12. Suk, et al.: Deep ensemble learning of sparse regression models for brain disease diagnosis. Med. Image Anal. **37**, 101–113 (2017)
13. Tong, et al.: Multiple instance learning for classification of dementia in brain MRI. Med. Image Anal. **18**(5), 808–818 (2014)
14. Tong, et al.: A novel grading biomarker for the prediction of conversion from mild cognitive impairment to Alzheimer's disease. IEEE Trans. Biomed. Eng. **64**(1), 155–165 (2017)
15. rujillo-Estrada, et al.: Early neuronal loss and axonal/presynaptic damage is associated with accelerated amyloid-β accumulation in aβpp/ps1 Alzheimer's disease mice subiculum. J. Alzheimer's Dis. **42**(2), 521–541 (2014)
16. Tustison, et al.: N4 ITK: improved N3 bias correction. IEEE Trans. Med. Imaging **29**(6), 1310–1320 (2010)
17. Winterburn, et al.: A novel in vivo atlas of human hippocampal subfields using high-resolution 3 T magnetic resonance imaging. NeuroImage **74**, 254–265 (2013)
18. Wolz, et al.: Multi-method analysis of MRI images in early diagnostics of Alzheimer's disease. PloS One **6**(10), e25446 (2011)

Deep Multiscale Convolutional Feature Learning for Weakly Supervised Localization of Chest Pathologies in X-ray Images

Suman Sedai[✉], Dwarikanath Mahapatra, Zongyuan Ge, Rajib Chakravorty, and Rahil Garnavi

IBM Research - Australia, Melbourne, VIC, Australia
ssedai@au1.ibm.com

Abstract. Localization of chest pathologies in chest X-ray images is a challenging task because of their varying sizes and appearances. We propose a novel weakly supervised method to localize chest pathologies using class aware deep multiscale feature learning. Our method leverages intermediate feature maps from CNN layers at different stages of a deep network during the training of a classification model using image level annotations of pathologies. During the training phase, a set of *layer relevance weights* are learned for each pathology class and the CNN is optimized to perform pathology classification by convex combination of feature maps from both shallow and deep layers using the learned weights. During the test phase, to localize the predicted pathology, the multiscale attention map is obtained by convex combination of class activation maps from each stage using the *layer relevance weights* learned during the training phase. We have validated our method using 112000 X-ray images and compared with the state-of-the-art localization methods. We experimentally demonstrate that the proposed weakly supervised method can improve the localization performance of small pathologies such as nodule and mass while giving comparable performance for bigger pathologies e.g., Cardiomegaly.

Keywords: Weakly supervised learning · X-ray pathology classification

1 Introduction

Chest X-ray is very economical and the most commonly used imaging modality for screening and diagnosis of many lung diseases. There is an exponential growth in the number of X-ray images taken in hospitals that must be reviewed by radiologists. Manual examination of scans is time consuming and subjective. Therefore, automated systems that can assess chest X-ray images will greatly

© Springer Nature Switzerland AG 2018
Y. Shi et al. (Eds.): MLMI 2018, LNCS 11046, pp. 267–275, 2018.
https://doi.org/10.1007/978-3-030-00919-9_31

assist radiologists and health care centers in managing patients and critical operations. Moreover, automated localization and annotation of pathologies and disease areas within the scan and providing those visualization to radiologist would allow clinicians to better understand the system's assessment and evaluate its reliability.

Existing object localization methods are based on patch classification [6], region-based convolution networks [2,3], fully convolutional neural networks [9–11]. These approaches are *fully supervised* approach i.e., they require location-level annotation of object being detected during training phase. Acquiring such annotations is a tedious process and is expensive to perform over large datasets. *Weakly supervised* methods on the other hand, can predict the location of object of interest with only image level annotation in training time. Therefore, it bypasses the need for the bounding box location annotation of pathologies. In this paper, we propose a novel weakly supervised method based on Convolutional neural network (CNN) by leveraging the intermediate feature maps of CNN to localize the chest pathologies in X-ray images.

Early works on weakly supervised methods use *multiple instance learning* and *bag of words* for chest pathology localization in X-ray images [1] and cancer cell detection in histopathology images [13]. Recent work have shown that CNN trained using image level annotation alone can be used to localize the object of interest [7,14]. The global pooling of convolution layers in CNN retains spatial information about the discriminative regions in the image which can be used to compute the class activation map (CAM) [14]. CAM gives the relative importance of the layer activation at different 2D spatial locations, can be used as saliency map to localize the object. In medical imaging domain, CAM based methods have been developed for tuberculosis detection in X-ray images [5]. In another work, soft attention map obtained from CAM have been combined with LSTM network to detect lung nodule in chest X-ray images [8]. Recently, [12] used weakly supervised method and CAM to localize the chest pathologies. These approaches, however, only use activation maps from the deepest convolution layers where the resolution of feature maps have been reduced to minimum amongst all the layers, which means localization ability of the network is dependent on the spatial resolution of the last convolution layer [14].

However, using feature maps from only highest convolution layers may adversely affect the localization of small pathologies. Successful localization of small pathologies, such as nodule, may increase the accuracy in incidental findings during routine check-ups and, therefore, the efficacy of chest x-ray based investigation. Therefore, we propose a weakly supervised localization method based on CNN using multiscale learning of feature maps at both shallower and deeper layers. The proposed method also learns the layer-wise relevance weights which determines the relative importance of each layer to classify a given pathology. The learned layer-wise relevance information is then used to combine the feature maps from individual layers. Thus, allowing pathologies to obtain multiscale attention map from different layers according to their relevance in classification process. The main advantage of the proposed method is its ability to localize

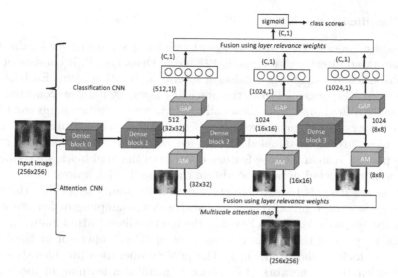

Fig. 1. Proposed chest X-ray pathology localization framework: the classification CNN (C-CNN) combines the intermediate feature maps using learned *layer relevance weights*. The attention CNN (A-CNN) computes the *multiscale attention map* using the feature maps and the learned *layer relevance weights*.

chest pathologies of different sizes, and particularly those with small sizes which are often more challenging, using weak labels (image level annotation) only.

2   Methodology

Our proposed method learns pathology localization from image-level supervision where training images are known to contain the instance of pathology class but their locations in the image are unknown. As shown in Fig. 1, the designed network uses the base network of DenseNet blocks. The network switches between 2 modes during training and test phases; (1) Classification CNN (C-CNN) and (2) Attention CNN (A-CNN), respectively. We first train the C-CNN by enforcing both shallower and deeper convolutional layers to contribute to the overall classification of pathologies. We introduce a class specific *layer relevance weights* to combines the feature maps from these layers and the classification is performed by only the *convex combination* of the responses from the feature maps. In prediction phase, A-CNN combines the convolutional feature maps from individual layers using the learned *layer relevance weights* to obtain the *multiscale attention map*. The proposed *multiscale attention map* is robust against pathology size as it encapsulates the feature maps from both coarse and fine layers.

2.1 Classification-CNN

We present a general framework for multiscale feature learning for localization. The network architecture we chose is 121 layers Densenet [4]. It consists of four dense blocks where each block consists of several convolution layers. Each layer in the *dense block* is connected to all the preceding layers by iterative concatenation of previous *feature maps*. This allows all layers to access *feature maps* from their preceding layers which encourages heavy feature reuse. The feature maps at end of each block are down-sampled and passed to the next block and the global average pooling response of the feature maps from the final block are connected to a densely connected network to obtain the classification scores.

The issue with this base architecture is that its ability to localize the small pathologies is compromised due to successive down-sampling of feature maps. We modify this architecture to leverage the intermediate feature maps. In order to do so, we plug in the *global average pooling* (GAP) operator at the end of each dense block as shown in Fig 1. The pooling operation provides structural regularization to the network [14], hence it facilitates learning of meaningful feature maps.

Let F_b be the feature maps from block b. The dimension of F_b is dependent on the number of convolution layers on the block. As shown in Fig. 1, $F_1 \in \mathbb{R}^{512 \times 32 \times 32}$, $F_2 \in \mathbb{R}^{1024 \times 16 \times 16}$ and $F_3 \in \mathbb{R}^{1024 \times 8 \times 8}$. We apply *global average pooling* operation to F_1, F_2 and F_3 to obtain the pooled feature maps of dimension $\mathbb{R}^{512 \times 1 \times 1}$, $\mathbb{R}^{1024 \times 1 \times 1}$ and $\mathbb{R}^{1024 \times 1 \times 1}$. These pooled feature maps are flattened and passed through separate fully connected layer to obtain the block-specific C dimensional *logits* vectors i.e., $L_b = [l_b^1, \cdots, l_b^C], b = 1, \cdots, B$. The *logit* response from all the layers have same dimension (equal to the number of category for classification) and now can be combined using class specific convex combination to obtain the probability score for the class p_c.

$$p_c = \sigma \left(\sum_{b=1}^{B} w_b^c \times l_b^c \right) \qquad (1)$$

where σ is *sigmoid* function; w_b^c is the *layer relevance weight* assigned to the bth block to predict the cth class and follows the *convex* weight constraint as described below.

2.2 Class Aware Training of Convolutional Features

We are given the training data set $\{I_n, \mathbf{y}_n\}_{n=1}^{N}$ where I_n is the input image and $\mathbf{y}_n$ is a label vector. For brevity, we drop the subscript n. The label vector is given by $\mathbf{y} = [y_1, \cdots, y_C]; y_i \in \{0, 1\}$ indicates the presence of the cth pathology class in the image and C is a number of pathology classes. Let W be the weights of the C-CNN including the *layer relevance weights* w_b^c. We initialize the layer relevance weights w_b^c to $1/B$ and the remaining network weights with Xavier initialization. We then optimize the network weights W by minimizing the class-balanced cross entropy loss with a *convex* weight constraint:

$$\underset{W}{\text{minimize}} \quad L(W) = \sum_{c=1}^{C} \left(-\beta_c \sum_{y_c=1} \log p_c - \sum_{y_c=0} (1 - \beta_c)\log (1 - p_c) \right)$$

$$\text{subject to} \quad w_b^c \geq 0 \text{ and } \sum_{b=1}^{B} w_b^c = 1 \; c = 1,\ldots,C.$$

where β_c is a balancing factor which denotes the percentage of '0' samples in the ground truth i.e, $\beta_c = \frac{|y_c=0|}{|y_c|}$. The balancing factor is used to mitigate the effect of large number of '0' samples. The *convex* weights constraint enables the probabilistic combination of *logits* from each block as shown by Eq. 1. As a result, the learned weights encodes the relevance of each block in classifying a given pathology. The proposed network is trained using mini-batch gradient descent and the Adam optimizer with momentum and a batch size of 32. The learning rate is set to 10^{-3} which is decreased by a factor of 0.1 whenever the *validation loss* reaches plateau.

2.3 Pathology Localization by Attention CNN (A-CNN)

C-CNN presented above enables individual blocks in the network to learn relevant feature maps with respect to each other. A-CNN uses the weights learned from C-CNN to compute the *multiscale attention map* of pathologies (Fig. 1). First, the attention map for each block are computed using the CAM technique. The *multiscale attention map* is then obtained using convex combination of attention map at each block. The CAM at each block can be computed using the weighted average of the feature maps of the block using the learned fully connected weights. Let $V_j^c(b)$ denote the sampled FC weights which connects j^{th} feature map from b^{th} block to the cth class. The attention map of the cth class at the bth dense-block can be computed as:

$$S_b^c = \sum_{j=1}^{N_f(b)} V_j^c(b)F_j^b \tag{2}$$

where $N_f(b)$ is the number of feature maps at the b-th block. The *multiscale attention map* for each class can now be obtained as a convex combination of intermediate attention maps:

$$S_c = \sum_{i=1}^{B} w_b^c R(S_b^c), c = 1,\ldots,C \tag{3}$$

where $R()$ is a function that takes an intermediate attention map S_b^c and resizes it to the same spatial resolution as the input image and w_b^c is the layer relevance weights of A-CNN. The resulting attention map S_c encapsulates the feature maps from all the blocks through class specific probabilistic combination of attention maps from individual block using the weights learned during training phase.

3   Experiments

We use the ChestX-ray14 dataset [12], which is the largest collection of public chest X-ray dataset by far. It consists of 112,120 frontal-view chest X-ray images of 30,805 unique patients. Each image is labeled with one or more types of 14 common thorax diseases. Also, for a subset of 983 images, bounding box annotations of 8 pathologies are provided for the evaluation of weakly supervised localization methods.

We randomly split the dataset into 70% for training, 10% for validation and 20% for test using patient id to ensure there is no patient overlap. We also make sure that the images with bounding box annotations falls only in the test set. The images are downscaled to the size of 256×256 before feeding to the network. The classification network is then trained using the method described in Sect. 2.2. During test phase, we compute the multiscale attention map of each pathology using the method described in Sect. 2.3. The attention map of the pathology gives approximate spatial location of the pathology in the input image. The attention map is converted to the bounding box by simple thresholding of the attention map and enclosing the resulting masks with the rectangles. We then evaluate the performance of the predicted bounding boxes against the ground truth bounding boxes.

Table 1. Localization accuracy and average false positive (AFP) of our A-CNN compared to the state of the art weakly supervised localization methods RN-CAM [12] and DN-CAM.

| | Localization accuracy/(AFP) | | | | | |
| | T(IOU)>0.3 | | | T(IOU) >0.5 | | |
Pathology	RN-CAM	DN-CAM	A-CNN	RN-CAM	DN-CAM	A-CNN
Atelectasis	0.24 (1.0)	0.17 (0.9)	**0.30** (0.8)	0.05 (1.0)	0.01 (1.1)	**0.1** (0.9)
Cardiomegaly	0.45 (0.7)	**0.86** (0.2)	0.84 (0.2)	0.17 (0.8)	**0.51** (0.4)	0.47 (0.5)
Effusion	**0.3** (0.9)	0.14 (0.9)	0.25 (0.8)	**0.11** (0.9)	0.01 (0.9)	0.03 (0.9)
Infiltration	0.27 (0.7)	0.21 (0.6)	**0.32** (0.7)	0.06 (0.7)	0.10 (0.7)	**0.12** (0.8)
Mass	0.15 (0.7)	0.17 (0.6)	**0.48** (0.5)	0.01 (0.7)	0.05 (0.8)	**0.2** (0.8)
Nodule	0.03 (0.6)	0.03 (0.6)	**0.27** (0.7)	0.01 (0.6)	0.01 (0.8)	**0.11** (0.7)
Pneumonia	0.16 (1.1)	0.20 (0.9)	**0.4** (0.8)	0.03 (1.1)	0.09 (0.9)	**0.10** (0.8)
Pneumothorax	0.13 (0.5)	0.11 (0.6)	**0.31** (0.8)	0.03 (0.5)	0.04 (0.6)	**0.08**(0.8

We compare our method with the baseline Resnet-CAM(RN-CAM) [12] and Densenet-CAM (DN-CAM). Both networks use only the feature maps from the deepest convolution layers to localize the pathologies. We use intersection over union (IOU) ratio between the predicted and ground truth bounding boxes as the detection criteria. We consider positive detection when IOU is greater than a given threshold value. IOU is commonly used measure in evaluation of object detection [3,12]. We evaluate our localization method (Λ-CNN) for two different thresholds of 0.3 and 0.5.

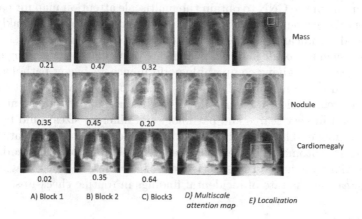

Fig. 2. Localization examples of few pathologies using the proposed *multiscale attention map*. The layer relevance weights are shown below the attention maps.

Table 1 compares the pathology detection accuracy and average false positive (AFP) of our proposed method compared with RN-CAM [12] and with the DN-CAM both without using intermediate feature maps i.e., they use feature maps from only the deepest layer for localization. The proposed method outperforms Resnet for all pathologies except for comparable performance for effusion. Our method also gives improved localization accuracy compared to Densenet for every pathology except cardiomegaly where the performance is comparable. Particularly, the proposed method gives notably improved accuracy for most challenging cases of small pathologies such as *mass* 0.48 and *nodule* 0.27 in comparison to both RN-CAM and DN-CAM. Figure 2 shows the examples of localization and *multiscale attention map* produced by our proposed method along with the attention map produced at individual dense block of the network and corresponding *layer relevance weight*. The proposed *multiscale attention map* is obtained by class specific probabilistic combination of feature maps from both coarser and deeper blocks, therefore can capture small and large pathologies using a single network. It can be observed that the *layer relevance weights* put emphasis on shallower blocks for smaller pathologies and larger weights on deeper blocks for larger pathology classes.

4   Conclusion

In this paper, we propose a novel weakly supervised method based on class aware multiscale convolutional feature learning to localize chest pathologies in X-ray images. The classification CNN learns to classify pathology responses from the intermediate feature maps along with the class specific layer relevance weights for coarser and deeper layers. In the test phase, the learned layer relevance weights are used to perform the probabilistic combination of the intermediate feature maps from the CNN to obtain the multiscale attention map for pathology localization. Experimental results demonstrate that the proposed weakly supervised method significantly improves the localization performance of small sized pathologies, such as *nodule* and *mass* which are particularly challenging to locate in X-ray scans, while giving comparable performance for bigger pathologies such as effusion and cardiomegaly. The proposed method has a very practical use in multitude of real-world problems where the availability of quality annotation for localization in very scarce and pathologies of different sizes could be present in the same image. These conditions frequently occur in medical data such as X-ray images. Automated systems, powered by the proposed method, have a great potential to enhance the effectiveness of a computer aided diagnosis system by increasing the rate of incidental findings in routine check-ups.

References

1. Avni, U., Greenspan, H., Goldberger, J.: X-ray categorization and spatial localization of chest pathologies. In: Fichtinger, G., Martel, A., Peters, T. (eds.) Proceedings of the MICCAI, pp. 199–206 (2011)
2. Ding, J., Li, A., Hu, Z., Wang, L.: Accurate pulmonary nodule detection in computed tomography images using deep convolutional neural networks. In: Descoteaux, M., Maier-Hein, L., Franz, A., Jannin, P., Collins, D.L., Duchesne, S. (eds.) Proceedings of the MICCAI, pp. 559–567 (2017)
3. Girshick, R.: Fast R-CNN. In: IEEE ICCV, pp. 1440–1448 (2015)
4. Huang, G., Liu, Z., v. d. Maaten, L., Weinberger, K.Q.: Densely connected convolutional networks. In: IEEE Conference on CVPR, pp. 2261–2269 (2017)
5. Hwang, S., Kim, H.E.: Self-transfer learning for weakly supervised lesion localization. In: Ourselin, S., Joskowicz, L., Sabuncu, M.R., Unal, G., Wells, W. (eds.) Proceedings of the MICCAI, pp. 239–246 (2016)
6. Liao, S., Gao, Y., Lian, J., Shen, D.: Sparse patch-based label propagation for accurate prostate localization in CT images. IEEE Trans. Med. Imaging **32**(2), 419–434 (2013)
7. Oquab, M., Bottou, L., Laptev, I., Sivic, J.: Is object localization for free? - weakly-supervised learning with convolutional neural networks. In: IEEE Conference on CVPR, pp. 685–694 (2015)
8. Pesce, E., Ypsilantis, P., Withey, S., Bakewell, R., Goh, V., Montana, G.: Learning to detect chest radiographs containing lung nodules using visual attention networks. CoRR, arXiv:1712.00996 (2017)
9. Ronneberger, O., Fischer, P., Brox, T.: U-net: convolutional networks for biomedical image segmentation. In: Navab, N., Hornegger, J., Wells, W.M., Frangi, A.F. (eds.) Proceedings of the MICCAI, pp. 234–241 (2015)
10. Sedai, S., Tennakoon, R., Roy, P., Cao, K., Garnavi, R.: Multi-stage segmentation of the fovea in retinal fundus images using fully convolutional neural networks. In: ISBI, pp. 1083–1086 (2017)
11. Sedai, S., Mahapatra, D., Hewavitharanage, S., Maetschke, S., Garnavi, R.: Semi-supervised segmentation of optic cup in retinal fundus images using variational autoencoder. In: MICCAI, pp. 75–82 (2017)

12. Wang, X., Peng, Y., Lu, L., Lu, Z., Bagheri, M., Summers, R.M.: Chestx-ray8: Hospital-scale chest x-ray database and benchmarks on weakly-supervised classification and localization of common thorax diseases. CoRR, arXiv:1705.02315 (2017)
13. Xu, Y., Zhu, J.Y., Chang, E.I.C., Lai, M., Tu, Z.: Weakly supervised histopathology cancer image segmentation and classification. Med. Image Anal. **18**(3), 591–604 (2014)
14. Zhou, B., Khosla, A., Lapedriza, A., Oliva, A., Torralba, A.: Learning deep features for discriminative localization. In: IEEE Conference on CVPR, pp. 2921–2929 (2016)

Combining Heterogeneously Labeled Datasets For Training Segmentation Networks

Jana Kemnitz[1,2,3(✉)], Christian F. Baumgartner[3], Wolfgang Wirth[1,2], Felix Eckstein[1,2], Sebastian K. Eder[1], and Ender Konukoglu[3]

[1] Paracelsus Medical University Salzburg, Salzburg, Austria
[2] Chondrometrics GmbH Ainring, Ainring, Germany
[3] Computer Vision Lab, ETH Zurich, Zurich, Switzerland
j.kemnitz@outlook.com

Abstract. Accurate segmentation of medical images is an important step towards analyzing and tracking disease related morphological alterations in the anatomy. Convolutional neural networks (CNNs) have recently emerged as a powerful tool for many segmentation tasks in medical imaging. The performance of CNNs strongly depends on the size of the training data and combining data from different sources is an effective strategy for obtaining larger training datasets. However, this is often challenged by heterogeneous labeling of the datasets. For instance, one of the dataset may be missing labels or a number of labels may have been combined into a super label. In this work we propose a cost function which allows integration of multiple datasets with heterogeneous label subsets into a joint training. We evaluated the performance of this strategy on thigh MR and a cardiac MR datasets in which we artificially merged labels for half of the data. We found the proposed cost function substantially outperforms a naive masking approach, obtaining results very close to using the full annotations.

1 Introduction

Accurate segmentation of complex and anatomical structures in medical images is the one of most critical parts in the image analysis pipeline. Segmentation results affect all the subsequent processes of image analysis such as object representation, feature measurement, the development of imaging biomarkers and ultimately the resulting diagnosis and treatment of diseases [1, 2].

The recent reemergence of convolutional neural networks (CNNs) allows automatic segmentation of anatomical structures with unprecedented accuracy [3, 4]. However, the performance of CNNs depends strongly on the size of the training data [3]. Since fully annotated datasets are still often relatively small, a possible strategy is to combine multiple datasets from different sources for training.

© Springer Nature Switzerland AG 2018
Y. Shi et al. (Eds.): MLMI 2018, LNCS 11046, pp. 276–284, 2018.
https://doi.org/10.1007/978-3-030-00919-9_32

Apart from possible domain shifts, a problem that may arise in practice is that different datasets may be following different labeling protocols and may thus contain different subsets of labels. For instance, detailed labels in one dataset may be combined into a "super label" in another dataset, or a label may be completely missing from the one of the datasets. Note that the latter case can be thought of as the missing label forming a super label with the background.

Combining heterogeneously labeled datasets has previously been investigated in the context of atlas-based segmentation employing majority voting, semilocally weighted voting, performance level estimation and multi-protocol label fusion [5]. However, to our knowledge incorporating such data for training segmentation networks still remains a open challenge [3].

A naive approach to address this problem would be to simply set training cost function (e.g. crossentropy loss) to zero at pixel locations where the desired label is not available. This means that in those locations the network would be free to predict any label. However, this is not taking full advantage of the available information. For instance, for training images for which one label is missing, we know that in those locations the network should only predict background or the missing label, but not any other labels. Similarly, if a training image combines two anatomic labels into one, in those regions only those two structures should be predicted, but not, for example, background.

In this paper, we propose a simple and effective cost function which allows integrating such information into the training process and thus takes advantage of the full extent of available training information. We evaluate the proposed cost function on two datasets: thigh MR images from the Osteoarthritis Initiative (OAI) [6] and publicly available cardiac MR data from the ACDC challenge [7]. For both datasets we simulate incomplete labels by merging a number of labels for parts of the datasets.

2   Methods

The goal of the proposed method is to learn the parameters of a segmentation network which can assign a label $y_i \in \mathcal{L}_a = \{\ell_0, \ldots, \ell_L\}$ for each pixel i of an image X. Generally, for training we may have multiple datasets which have been annotated with different subsets of those labels. To describe the proposed method, we focus on the simpler problem, where we assume that we have only two training datasets D_1, D_2 of which D_1 was annotated with all target labels, while D_2 contains one super label $\mathcal{L}_s = \{\ell_0, \ldots, \ell_S\}$ that corresponds to S of the labels in $\mathcal{L}_a$. That is D_2 contains the following labels $\{\{\ell_0, \ldots, \ell_S\}, \ell_{S+1}, \ldots, \ell_L\} = \{\mathcal{L}_s, \ell_{S+1} \ldots, \ell_L\}$. For notational simplicity we define a binary mask $m_i \in \{0, 1\}$ which is 0 at all pixels that have label $\mathcal{L}_s$ and 1 otherwise. In other words, $m_i = 1$ only where full information is available. This simplified problem, with two datasets and one super label, can be easily extended to more complex scenarios.

The commonly used cross entropy function for a single fully annotated image is given by

$$C^{xent} = \sum_i \sum_{\ell \in \mathcal{L}_a} p(y_i = \ell) \log q(y_i = \ell | X), \tag{1}$$

where p denotes the ground-truth probability distribution and q denotes the networks softmax output. In the following we consider a naive extension of this cost function disregarding pixels with incomplete information, and our proposed cost function which takes into account the possible predictions of super labels. An overview of the strategies is shown in Fig. 1.

2.1   Naive Masking

Apart from completely disregarding datasets with incomplete labeling, the simplest strategy is to mask out regions with incomplete information in the crossentropy loss function:

$$C^{naive} = \sum_i m_i \sum_{\ell \in \mathcal{L}_a} p(y_i = \ell) \log q(y_i = \ell | X), \tag{2}$$

using the mask m_i defined earlier. While still using images from both datasets D_1, D_2 for training, this formulation disregards the information contained in $\mathcal{L}_s$, that it corresponds to $\{\ell_0, \ldots, \ell_S\}$ and not to any other label. In practice, we found that this often leads to undesired structure labels or background leaking into those regions.

2.2   Super Label Aware Crossentropy Loss

In order to overcome this limitation, we propose adding an additional term to the crossentropy loss also taking into account the super labels as follows:

$$
\begin{aligned}
C_i^{slac} &= m_i \sum_{\ell \in \mathcal{L}_a} p(y_i = \ell) \log q(y_i = \ell) + (1 - m_i) \sum_{\ell \in \mathcal{L}_s} p(y_i = \ell) \log \sum_{\ell \in \mathcal{L}_s} q(y_i = \ell), \\
&= m_i \sum_{\ell \in \mathcal{L}_a} p(y_i = \ell) \log q(y_i = \ell) + (1 - m_i) \log \sum_{\ell \in \mathcal{L}_s} q(y_i = \ell),
\end{aligned}
\tag{3}
$$

where we omitted the sum over i and the conditioning on X for brevity. Here, the second term encourages the network to predict $q(y_i = \mathcal{L}_s) = \sum_{\ell \in \mathcal{L}_s} q(y_i = \ell)$, in regions where the training image is labeled with the super label. The simplification in the second equality is due the fact that by definition $\sum_{\ell \in \mathcal{L}_s} p(y_i = \ell) = 1$ where $m_i = 1$.

3   Experiments and Results

3.1   Data

We evaluated segmentation accuracy of the cost functions introduced above on two data sets.

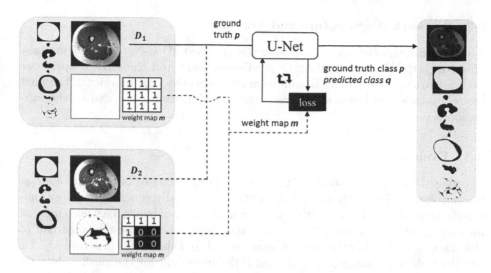

Fig. 1. Thigh MRI trainings paths of the U-Net for segmentation with a) training data D_1 annotated with all target labels, while training dataset D_2 contains the following labels $\{\{\ell_0,\ldots,\ell_S\},\ell_{S+1},\ldots,\ell_L\} = \{\mathcal{L}_s,\ell_{S+1}\ldots,\ell_L\}$; both with binary mask $m_i \in \{0,1\}$ which is 0 at all pixels that have label $\mathcal{L}_s$ and 1 otherwise.

Thigh MRI: The thigh MRI data consist of 139 patient scans of the osteoarthritis initiative (OAI) [6], a publicly available data base created for imaging biomarker validation in knee osteoarthritis. MRIs were acquired using a 3T system (slice thickness 5 mm; in-plane resolution 0.98 mm; no inter-slice gap) and segmentations were available for patient from previous studies [8,9]. The dataset was divided into training, test and validation set comprising 99, 20 and 20 subjects, respectively. All muscle MRI slices where cropped and centered towards the femoral bone of the right knee to simplify the segmentation problem with a resulting image size of 256 × 256 pixels.

Cardiac MRI: The cardiac MRI data from the ACDC challenge [7] consists 100 patient scans each including a short-axis cine-MRI acquired on 1.5T and 3T systems with resolutions ranging from 0.70 mm to 1.92 mm in-plane and 5–10 mm through-plane. Segmentation for the background, the myocardium (Myo), the left ventricle (LV) and the right ventricle (RV) were available for the end-diastolic (ED) and end-systolic (ES) phases of each patient. The dataset was divided into training, test and validation set comprising 60, 25 and 15 subjects, respectively. All images were resampled to a common resolution of 1.37 × 1.37 mm² and resampled centrally placed into images of constant size, padding with zeros where necessary.

3.2   Network Architecture and Training

All experiments were performed using the modified 2D U-Net architecture proposed in [11]. We used mini-batch gradient descent and the ADAM optimizer with a learning rate of 0.01 to minimize the respective cost functions. The final model was selected based on the respective loss functions evaluated on the validation set.

3.3   Evaluation

In order to evaluate the ability of the loss functions discussed in Sect. 2 to address the problem of differently labeled datasets, we artificially generated a fully annotated dataset D_1 and a dataset D_2 for which a number of labels have been merged into super labels. For both the cardiac and thigh datasets we relabeled half of the training and validation sets as summarized in Table 1. To generate D_2, for the thigh data we merged the AD and IMF labels, and for the cardiac data we created a "heart" super label containing all of the structures apart from background. The final performance was evaluated on the fully labeled test sets using the Dice score (DSC), average symmetric surface distance (ASSD) and Hausdorff distance (HD).

Table 1. Simulated data D_1 (completely labeled) and D_2 (containing a super label $\mathcal{L}_s$) for thigh and cardiac MR segmentation.

Thigh	D_1	D_2	Cardiac	D_1	D_2
Background	x	x	background	x	x
Femoral bone (FB)	x	x	left ventricular (LV)	x	$\mathcal{L}_s$
Quadriceps (QC)	x	x	right ventricular (RV)	x	$\mathcal{L}_s$
Flexors (FX)	x	x	myocardium (Myo)	x	$\mathcal{L}_s$
Sartorius (ST)	x	x			
subcutaneous fat (SCF)	x	x			
Adductors (AD)	x	$\mathcal{L}_s$			
Intermuscular fat (IMF)	x	$\mathcal{L}_s$			

In addition to the network training with the two cost functions $\mathcal{C}^{naive}$ and $\mathcal{C}^{slac}$ we also evaluated two baseline methods: (1) we trained only on the complete dataset D_1 with the normal crossentropy cost function $\mathcal{C}^{xent}$ to obtain a lower bound on the performance, and (2) we trained with $\mathcal{C}^{xent}$ on the entire unaltered training sets to obtain an upper bound.

Table 2. Thigh and cardiac MR segmentation accuracy measure in mean (std) for the evaluated cost functions $\mathcal{C}^{naive}$ and $\mathcal{C}^{slac}$ (best performance in bold font) and the lower bound (LB) and upper bound (UB) for all structures.

	Thigh					
	Femoral bone (FB)			**Quadriceps (QC)**		
	DSC	ASSD	HD	DSC	ASSD	HD
$\mathcal{C}^{xent}$ (LB)	0.971 (0.014)	0.60 (0.77)	7.00 (12.17)	0.952 (0.056)	1.32 (0.79)	14.40 (6.32)
$\mathcal{C}^{naive}$	**0.978 (0.008)**	0.45 (0.58)	5.40 (12.50)	0.977 (0.006)	0.81 (0.35)	10.60 (8.42)
$\mathcal{C}^{slac}$	0.974 (0.008)	**0.38 (0.09)**	**2.05 (1.70)**	**0.980 (0.010)**	**0.61 (0.23)**	**7.78 (3.79)**
$\mathcal{C}^{xent}$ (UB)	0.978 (0.006)	0.32 (0.09)	1.86 (1.15)	0.979 (0.008)	0.67 (0.31)	7.37 (5.16)
	Flexors (FX)			**Sartorius (ST)**		
	DSC	ASSD	HD	DSC	ASSD	HD
$\mathcal{C}^{xent}$ (LB)	0.905 (0.065)	2.30 (1.28)	16.56 (4.88)	0.809 (0.117)	4.22 (2.53)	36.44 (25.82)
$\mathcal{C}^{naive}$	**0.957 (0.019)**	1.05 (0.58)	11.20 (6.51)	0.903 (0.052)	1.76 (1.32)	15.90 (11.07)
$\mathcal{C}^{slac}$	**0.957 (0.021)**	**0.90 (0.35)**	**9.36 (4.16)**	**0.967 (0.010)**	**0.33 (0.09)**	**2.10 (1.52)**
$\mathcal{C}^{xent}$ (UB)	0.968 (0.013)	0.75 (0.33)	6.70 (3.71)	0.945 (0.055)	0.92 (1.08)	14.07 (24.17)
	Subcutaneous fat (SCF)			**Adductors (AD)**		
	DSC	ASSD	HD	DSC	ASSD	HD
$\mathcal{C}^{xent}$ (LB)	0.936 (0.132)	0.92 (1.37)	11.29 (15.28)	0.809 (0.117)	4.22 (2.53)	36.44 (25.82)
$\mathcal{C}^{naive}$	0.965 (0.035)	0.48 (0.19)	6.33 (12.38)	0.908 (0.039)	1.13 (0.51)	10.8 (8.66)
$\mathcal{C}^{slac}$	**0.974 (0.008)**	**0.41 (0.09)**	**6.11 (11.18)**	**0.967 (0.010)**	1.09 (0.45)	9.05 (4.48)
$\mathcal{C}^{xent}$ (UB)	0.975 (0.014)	0.38 (0.12)	5.19 (11.93)	0.945 (0.055)	0.92 (1.08)	14.07 (24.17)
	Intermuscular fat (IMF)			**Average**		
	DSC	ASSD	HD	DSC	ASSD	HD
$\mathcal{C}^{xent}$ (LB)	0.608 (0.093)	2.62 (1.09)	32.67 (10.24)	0.847 (0.100)	2.05 (1.42)	18.96 (11.81)
$\mathcal{C}^{naive}$	0.744 (0.076)	1.55 (0.34)	27.00 (7.31)	0.919 (0.077)	1.04 (0.46)	12.52 (6.70)
$\mathcal{C}^{slac}$	**0.823 (0.031)**	**0.92 (0.16)**	**18.00 (3.29)**	**0.940 (0.054)**	**0.66 (0.28)**	**7.78 (5.20)**
$\mathcal{C}^{xent}$ (UB)	0.821 (0.046)	1.03 (0.36)	21.96 (7.06)	0.943 (0.020)	0.71 (0.31)	9.29 (7.20)
	Cardiac					
	Left ventricle (ED)			**Left ventricle (ES)**		
	DSC	ASSD	HD	DSC	ASSD	HD
$\mathcal{C}^{xent}$ (LB)	0.960 (0.018)	0.37 (0.38)	5.85 (3.77)	0.914 (0.040)	0.81 (0.69)	8.30 (3.59)
$\mathcal{C}^{naive}$	0.951 (0.018)	0.64 (0.56)	8.01 (5.78)	0.919 (0.040)	1.00 (1.16)	10.11 (5.69)
$\mathcal{C}^{slac}$	**0.962 (0.018)**	**0.42 (0.54)**	**5.88 (3.64)**	**0.923 (0.052)**	**0.77 (0.84)**	**7.20 (3.16)**
$\mathcal{C}^{xent}$ (UB)	0.962 (0.017)	0.39 (0.48)	5.49 (2.95)	0.934 (0.034)	0.53 (0.40)	7.76 (3.34)
	Right ventricle (ED)			**Right ventricle (ES)**		
	DSC	ASSD	HD	DSC	ASSD	HD
$\mathcal{C}^{xent}$ (LB)	0.876 (0.171)	1.69 (3.37)	16.28 (14.57)	0.828 (0.140)	1.81 (2.26)	15.96 (7.84)
$\mathcal{C}^{naive}$	0.909 (0.039)	0.91 (0.54)	14.52 (6.78)	0.809 (0.089)	2.06 (0.91)	15.87 (5.51)
$\mathcal{C}^{slac}$	**0.922 (0.048)**	**0.83 (0.98)**	**13.57 (6.13)**	0.827 (0.116)	1.76 (1.33)	**15.15 (5.96)**
$\mathcal{C}^{xent}$ (UB)	0.927 (0.043)	0.82 (0.90)	13.74 (6.33)	0.834 (0.108)	1.74 (1.43)	15.93 (5.73)
	Myocardium (ED)			**Myocardium (ES)**		
	DSC	ASSD	HD	DSC	ASSD	HD
$\mathcal{C}^{xent}$ (LB)	0.873 (0.031)	0.47 (0.18)	8.17 (5.08)	0.882 (0.042)	0.75 (0.47)	11.80 (5.85)
$\mathcal{C}^{naive}$	0.852 (0.044)	0.66 (0.32)	11.27 (6.58)	0.863 (0.055)	0.86 (0.51)	11.78 (5.85)
$\mathcal{C}^{slac}$	**0.878 (0.030)**	**0.54 (0.29)**	**9.99 (8.46)**	**0.891 (0.035)**	**0.67 (0.42)**	**10.06 (5.68)**
$\mathcal{C}^{xent}$ (UB)	0.881 (0.026)	0.51 (0.21)	8.90 (6.36)	0.896 (0.039)	0.61 (0.32)	10.74 (6.39)

continued

Table 2. continued

	Thigh					
	Femoral bone (FB)			Quadriceps (QC)		
	DSC	ASSD	HD	DSC	ASSD	HD
	Average					
	DSC	ASSD	HD			
$\mathcal{C}^{xent}$ (LB)	0.889 (0.074)	0.89 (1.32)	11.06 (6.78)			
$\mathcal{C}^{naive}$	0.884 (0.048)	1.02 (1.67)	12.08 (6.03)			
$\mathcal{C}^{slac}$	**0.901 (0.050)**	**0.83 (0.73)**	**10.31 (5.51)**			
$\mathcal{C}^{xent}$ (UB)	0.906 (0.045)	0.77 (0.62)	10.43 (5.18)			

The results obtained with the investigated costs functions are summarized in Table 2. Example segmentations for both datasets are shown in Fig. 2. With the proposed cost function $\mathcal{C}^{slac}$ we achieved segmentation results very close to using the full annotations (upper bound) in both thigh and cardiac datasets.

3.4   Discussion and Conclusion

In this work we proposed a cost function to enable the integration of multiple datasets with heterogeneous label subsets into a joint training. We evaluated the performance of this strategy on thigh MR and a cardiac MR datasets in which we artificially merged labels for half of the data. We found the proposed cost function substantially outperforms a naive masking approach and achieved results very close to using the full annotations. This novel cost function improves the segmentation performance compared to a naive masking precisely in those single labeled regions merged into a super label by avoiding undesired label or background leaking (see Fig. 2, Table 2). As expected we found that the proposed cost function led to the biggest improvement over the naive masking approach in regions were labels were merged into super labels.

One specific motivation of this work was to investigate the potential of this novel loss term in the scope of the OAI database where several datasets with heterogeneous label subsets are available from previous studies [8,9,12]. This new loss term will allow us to merge all this heterogeneous label subsets into a joint training.

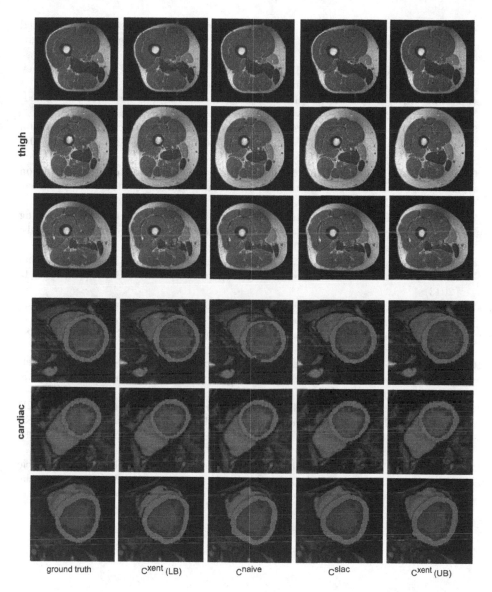

Fig. 2. Examples of thigh and cardiac ground truth and predicted segmentation using the evaluated cost functions $\mathcal{C}^{naive}$ and $\mathcal{C}^{slac}$ and the lower bound (LB) and upper bound (UB).

References

1. Shen, D., Wu, G., Suk, H.: Deep learning in medical image analysis. Annu. Rev. Biomed. Eng. **19**(1), 221–48 (2017)

2. Prescott, J.W.: Quantitative imaging biomarkers: the application of advanced image processing and analysis to clinical and preclinical decision making. J. Digit. Imaging **26**(1), 97–108 (2013)
3. Litjens, G., Kooi, T., Bejnordi, B.E., Setio, A.A.A., Ciompi, F., et al.: A survey on deep learning in medical image analysis. Med. Image Anal. **42**, 60–88 (2017)
4. Ronneberger, O., Fischer, P., Brox, T.: U-net: convolutional networks for biomedical image segmentation. In: MICCAI, pp. 234–41 (2015)
5. Iglesias, J.E., Sabuncu, M.R., Aganj, I., Bhatt, P., Casillas, C., et al.: An algorithm for optimal fusion of atlases with different labeling protocols. NeuroImage **106**, 451–63 (2014)
6. Peterfy, C.G., Schneider, E., Nevitt, M.: The osteoarthritis initiative: report on the design rationale for the magnetic resonance imaging protocol for the knee. Osteoarthr. Cartil. **16**(12), 1433–41 (2008)
7. Bernard, O., Lalande, A., Zotti, C., Cervenansky, F., Yang, X. et al.: Deep learning techniques for automatic MRI cardiac multi-structures segmentation and diagnosis: is the problem solved? IEEE Trans. Med. Imaging (2018)
8. Ruhdorfer, A., Dannhauer, T., Wirth, W., Hitzl, W., Kwoh, C.K.: Cross-sectional and longitudinal side differences in thigh muscles. Arthr. Care Res. **65**(7), 1034–42 (2013)
9. Ruhdorfer, A., Wirth, W., Dannhauer, T., Eckstein, F.: Longitudinal (4 year) change of thigh muscle and adipose tissue distribution in chronically painful vs painless knees - data from the osteoarthritis initiative. Osteo. Cartil. **23**(8) 1348–56 (2015)
10. Cicek, Ö., Abdulkadir, A., Lienkamp, S.S., Brox, T., Ronneberger, O.: 3D U-Net: learning dense volumetric segmentation from sparse annotation. In: MICCAI, pp. 424–32 (2016)
11. Baumgartner, C.F., Koch, L.M., Pollefeys, M., Konukoglu, E.: An exploration of 2D and 3D deep learning techniques for cardiac MR image segmentation. In: Proceedings of the Statistical Atlases and Computational Models of the Heart (STACOM), ACDC Challenge, MICCAI17 Workshop (2017)
12. Kemnitz, J., Wirth, W., Eckstein, F., Culvenor, A.G.: The Role of Thigh Muscle and Adipose Tissue in Knee Osteoarthritis Progression in Women: Data from the Osteoarthritis Initiative. Osteo. Cartil. (2018) Epub ahead of print

SoLiD: Segmentation of *Clostridioides Difficile* Cells in the Presence of Inhomogeneous Illumination Using a Deep Adversarial Network

Ali Memariani[✉] and Ioannis A. Kakadiaris

Computational Biomedicine Lab, Department of Computer Science,
University of Houston, Houston, TX, USA
{amemaria,ikakadia}@central.uh.edu

Abstract. Segmentation of cells in scanning electron microscopy images is a challenging problem due to the presence of inhomogeneous illumination. Classical pre-processing methods for illumination normalization destroy the texture and add noise to the image. In this paper, we present a deep cell segmentation method using adversarial training that is robust to inhomogeneous illumination. Specifically, we apply a model based on U-net as the segmenter and a deep ConvNet as the discriminator for the adversarial training called SoLiD: "Segmentation of *clostridioides difficile* cells in the presence of inhomogeneous iLlumInation using a Deep adversarial network". We also present an image augmentation algorithm to obtain the training images required for SoLid. The results indicate that SoLiD is robust to inhomogeneous illumination. The segmentation performance is compared to the U-net and the dice score is improved by 44%.

Keywords: Cell segmentation · Deep adversarial training · Data augmentation · U-net

1 Introduction

Clostridioides difficile infection (CDI) is the most common cause of death due to infectious gastroenteritis in the USA and a significant source of morbidity [2]. Extraction of cell-related information (e.g., length, location, deformation) in scanning electron microscopy (SEM) images is an important task in CDI research studies [4]. However, analysis of SEM images is challenging due to noise and inhomogeneous illumination. Classical illumination normalization techniques could reduce the effect of illumination as a pre-processing step. However, they destroy the texture and add noise to the image [6,11].

Deep learning algorithms have outperformed the state of the art in many biomedical image processing tasks [15]. Fully convolutional networks have been

© Springer Nature Switzerland AG 2018
Y. Shi et al. (Eds.): MLMI 2018, LNCS 11046, pp. 285–293, 2018.
https://doi.org/10.1007/978-3-030-00919-9_33

applied for image segmentation [9]. Specifically, U-net is widely used for biomedical image segmentation tasks [14]. However, to the best of our knowledge the challenges above have prevented the introduction of a deep network for automatic segmentation in SEM images with inhomogeneous illumination (Fig. 1).

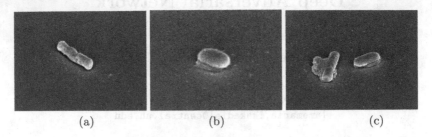

(a)   (b)   (c)

Fig. 1. Inhomogeneous illumination makes the segmentation of scanning electron microscopy images challenging. Examples of illumination challenges are depicted as follows: (a) shadows on the cell body, (b) shadows in the periphery, and (c) bright spots in the area around the cell.

Generative adversarial networks (GANs) were presented to synthesize images similar to the real world images [5]. Adversarial training can improve image segmentation by producing label maps that are similar to the manual ground truth [10]. Recently, adversarial networks have gained more attention in the segmentation of MRI images [1,7,8,13,16] where the datasets and the annotations are available. In this paper, we present SoLiD, "Segmentation of *clostridioides difficile* cells in the presence of inhomogeneous iLlumInation using a Deep adversarial network" with the following contributions: (i) an image augmentation algorithm to generate synthetic cell images for training deep ConvNets; (ii) a deep adversarial algorithm to train a cell segmentation network using the synthetic images. SoLiD advantages are as follows: (i) SoLiD is capable of synthesizing more than 20,000 training images while preserving the background texture and cell shapes. (ii) SoLiD is robust to inhomogeneous illumination which is a challenge in SEM images.

The rest of the paper is organized as follows: Sect. 2 describes SoLid algorithm. Section 3 presents the experimental results comparing the segmentation performance of SoLiD with the state-of-the-art provided by U-net. Finally, section 4 draws the conclusions. The algorithm is applied to a dataset of *Clostridioides difficile* images. The results indicate that using the adversarial training step significantly improves the performance of the segmentation without increasing its complexity.

2   Methods

SoLiD consists of two deep ConvNets, namely the segmenter and the discriminator. The segmenter predicts a label map for the pixels while the discriminator distinguishes between the predicted label maps and the ground truth.

Algorithm 1: Adversarial training of SoLiD

    Input   : Augmented training cells, Training labels
    Output: Trained segmenter network, Trained discriminator network

1 **begin**
2   **for** *number of pretraining iterations* **do**
3   Select a batch of labels G
4   Train the discriminator with the cross-entropy loss $L_C(D(G), 1)$
5   **end**
6   **for** *number of adversarial iterations* **do**
7   Select a batch of training images and their labels $\{I, G\}$
8   Feed forward the batch to the segmenter and predict the segmentation $S(I)$. Compute the segmentation cross-entropy loss $L_C(S(I), G)$
9   Feed the predicted labels to the discriminator and compute the adversarial loss $L_C(D(S(I)), 0)$
10   Given the labels G, compute the discriminator cross-entropy loss $L_C(D(G), 1)$
11   Compute L_D and backpropagate the discriminator (Eq. 2)
12   Compute L_S and backpropagate the segmenter (Eq. 1)
13   **end**
14 **end**

The input to the segmenter is a cell image. The segmenter includes a convolution path and a deconvolution path similar to U-net. The convolution path extracts a feature map for segmentation using convolution layers while the deconvolution path increases the resolution, creating a label map. The generated label map may differ significantly from the ground truth since the segmenter does not consider the smoothness of the labels, resulting in a non-continuous segmentation.

A second ConvNet (discriminator) is used to train the segmenter to produce label maps similar to the ground truth. The discriminator is a regular ConvNet classifier trained on the ground truth and predicted segmentations. During training, it learns to classify the input image into two classes: "artificially generated" or "ground truth", and backpropagates the gradients.

Segmenter Network: The segmenter network consists of six convolutional units: the first three units include a 3×3 convolution layer, a ReLU layer and a 2×2 max pooling layer with a stride of two downsampling the image (contracting units). The next three units (expanding units) include an upsampling of the features followed by a 2×2 deconvolution. Each contracting unit doubles the number of feature channels while each expanding unit halves the number of channels. The segmenter minimizes a loss function L_S:

$$L_S = W_C * L_C(S(I), G) + L_C(D(S(I)), 1) \tag{1}$$

where $L_C(S(I), G)$ is a cross-entropy term between the predicted labels S corresponding to the image I and the ground truth G. The second term

---

Algorithm 2: Data augmentation algorithm.

Input : Manually annotated acquired images
Output: Synthetic images

1 **begin**
2   Randomly select a background patch and feed it to the texture synthesis algorithm [3].
3   Synthesize a background image with the same resolution as the original image.
4   **for** *every synthesized background image* **do**
5   Select the number of cells to be placed into the image.
6   **for** *the selected number of cells and their labels, randomly* **do**
7   Select a cell in the acquired image set with inhomogeneous illumination.
8   Rotate the cell with a random angle θ.
9   Warp the cell with a 2D affine transform with a random geometric transformation matrix T.
10   Select a random location for the cell centroid and place the cell into the background image.
11   **end**
12   **end**
13 **end**

$L_C\big(D(S(I)),1\big)$ is the adversarial loss term, computed by the discriminator. The label map of image I generated by the segmenter is denoted by $S(I)$ and D is the discriminator network described in the next section. The adversarial loss forces the segmenter to produce label maps that would be considered as ground truth by the discriminator. To distinguish touching cells, the segmenter considers the boundaries of the cells (cell wall) as a separate class. Hence, the segmenter loss is one-hot encoded with three classes. The number of cell wall samples are considerably less compared to the other classes. To compensate for the bias in the training set, the segmenter cross-entropy loss is weighted (W_C). The minority class receives a higher classification weight.

The segmenter network may misclassify a large portion of cells due to inhomogeneous illumination. We present the adversarial training to evaluate such misclassifications and improve the segmenter (Algorithm 1). A discriminator ConvNet is applied to compute the likelihood of the predicted segmentation map being an actual label map.

Discriminator Network: The discriminator improves the generated labels by sending feedback to the generator if the segmentation labels are significantly different from the ground truth. It does not increase the complexity of the network since it is used only during training. It consists of five convolutional layers with valid padding, followed by ReLU activations and average pooling. Furthermore, two fully connected layers are placed at the end of the discriminator.

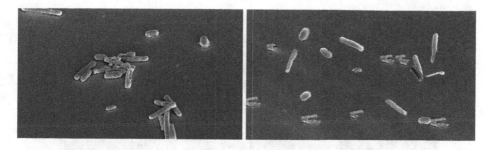

Fig. 2. Depiction of samples of the acquired (L) and the synthesized (R) images.

To avoid saturation, the last layer of the discriminator does not have a thresholding operator so it produces an unscaled output. Computing scores between 0 and 1 may cause the discriminator to generate values close to 0 for generated label maps, in which case the gradient would be too small to update the generator and eventually saturate the network [5].

The discriminator (D) computes the cross-entropy of the ground truth label maps (G) and 1, and the cross-entropy of the generated label maps $(S(I))$ and 0, minimizing the following loss function:

$$L_D = L_C(D(G), 1) + L_C(D(S(I)), 0). \tag{2}$$

During the training, the discriminator improves the segmenter network, penalizing the segmentation labels that do not look like manual labels. Therefore, the adversarial result has properties such as smoothness and robustness to inhomogeneous illumination.

Data Augmentation: Deep networks require large numbers of training data. Therefore, data augmentation becomes important in the analysis of microscopy images, since their acquisition is expensive and time-consuming [15]. We present a data augmentation algorithm capable of synthesizing large numbers of images with the same background texture and cell shapes in the images captured by SEM.

First, SEM-acquired images are manually annotated to three classes, namely cell body, cell wall, and background. The image quilting technique by Efros and Freeman is applied to synthesize similar background images [3]. Then, the cells are randomly warped and placed into the image. Warping the cells ensures that the training data are different from the testing data. Algorithm 2 depicts the steps of the augmentation algorithm.

3 Experimental Results

To develop and validate SoLiD, we applied UH-Cdiff1 a dataset of *C. difficile* cell images acquired via SEM imaging with pixel dimensions 411 × 711 and

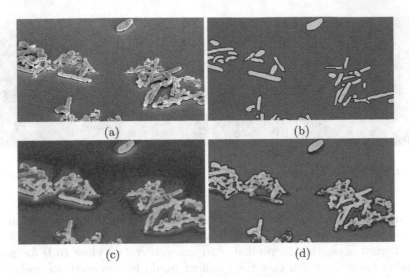

Fig. 3. The segmentation results from SoLiD are qualitatively compared to the result from U-net: (a) A sample cell image obtained by scanning electron microscopy; (b) the corresponding manual annotation; (c) the segmentation obtained by U-net (Note that U-net is not robust shadows around the cells and inhomogeneous illumination in the background, and the cell boundaries are missing.); (d) SoLiD is robust to the mentioned illumination challenges and successfully distinguishes the cells from the background. The figure is best viewed in color.

10,000x magnification [12]. A set of 22 images (308 cells) with inhomogeneous illumination, similar contrast, and cell density were selected for the experiments. Furthermore, many cells are clustered together and in many cases, the cells were partially deformed due to laboratory treatment, making the detection challenging (Fig. 2).

The cells were manually annotated using a simple GUI and the annotations were verified by a laboratory expert. Then, the background portions of the images were used to synthesize background images of size 411×711. The image augmentation algorithm was applied to generate cells with inhomogeneous illumination. Patches of size 128×128 were selected to form a training set with more than 17,000 samples. The segmentation method is implemented in TensorFlow 1.4.0 and the results are compared to U-net. Figure 3 depicts the qualitative comparison of the segmentation obtained by the two methods. The effect of inhomogeneous illumination can be observed as bright areas around the cells, bright spots on the cell body, and shadows in the background.

Pixel labels are assigned according to the maximum score values obtained by the segmenter network. One-vs-all is applied to obtain binary masks for the detected cells. Then, we computed the dice score for the cells to measure the performance of cell segmentation. The ROC curve and the area under the curve (AUC) are computed for the entire image to measure the classification performance over all three classes. The cells cover a smaller portion of the images in the dataset compared to the background. Furthermore, both methods correctly classified major pixels of the background. Therefore, AUC values tend to be higher than dice score values. Table 1 indicates that SoLiD is more robust to inhomogeneous illumination compared to U-net. Figure 4 depicts the corresponding ROC curves (in logarithmic scale) where SoLiD is positioned above U-net, indicating the better performance of SoLiD in segmenting SEM images.

Table 1. Comparative results between the segmentation performance of SoLiD and the state-of-the-art in semantic segmentation by U-net. The dice score represents the performance of the methods segmenting the cells correctly while AUC depicts the performance over the whole image.

Method	Cell dice score	AUC
U-net [14]	0.50	0.93
SoLiD	**0.72**	**0.99**

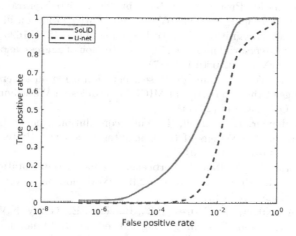

Fig. 4. The ROC curve indicates that SoLiD outperforms U-net [14] in distinguishing between the background, cell walls, and the cells. Note that the false positive rate is in logarithmic scale.

4   Conclusion

A deep adversarially trained cell segmentation method called SoLiD is presented which is capable of segmenting cells in SEM images with inhomogeneous illumination. SoLiD outperforms the state of the art in segmentation accuracy of cell images while maintaining the same complexity during the deployment. In this work, we did not focus on separating overlapping cells. This task will be addressed in the future.

Acknowledgments. This work was supported in part by the Hugh Roy and Lillie Cranz Cullen Endowment Fund.

References

1. Dai, W., et al..: SCAN: Structure correcting adversarial network for organ segmentation in chest X-rays. arXiv preprint arXiv:1703.08770 (2017)
2. DuPont, H.L., Garey, K., Caeiro, J.P., Jiang, Z.D.: New advances in Clostridium difficile infection: changing epidemiology, diagnosis, treatment and control. Curr. Opin. Infect. Dis. **21**(5), 500–507 (2008)
3. Efros, A.A., Freeman, W.T.: Image quilting for texture synthesis and transfer. In: Computer Graphics and Interactive Techniques, pp. 341–346. New York, NY, USA (2001)
4. Endres, B.T., et al.: A novel method for imaging the pharmacological effects of antibiotic treatment on Clostridium difficile. Anaerobe **40**, 10–14 (2016)
5. Goodfellow, I., et al.: Generative adversarial nets. In: Proceedings of the Advances in Neural Information Processing Systems, pp. 2672–2680. Montral, Canada (2014)
6. Han, H., Shan, S., Chen, X., Gao, W.: A comparative study on illumination preprocessing in face recognition. Pattern Recognit. **46**(6), 1691–1699 (2013)
7. Kohl, S., et al.: Adversarial networks for the detection of aggressive prostate cancer. arXiv preprint arXiv:1702.08014 (2017)
8. Li, Z., Wang, Y., Yu, J.: Brain tumor segmentation using an adversarial network. In: Proceedings of the International MICCAI Brainlesion Workshop, pp. 123–132. Quebec City, QC, Canada (2017)
9. Long, J., Shelhamer, E., Darrell, T.: Fully convolutional networks for semantic segmentation. In: Proceedings of the Computer Vision and Pattern Recognition, pp. 3431–3440. Boston, MA (2015)
10. Luc, P., Couprie, C., Chintala, S., Verbeek, J.: Semantic segmentation using adversarial networks. In: Proceedings of the NIPS Workshop on Adversarial Training, pp. 1–9. Barcelona, Spain (2016)
11. Memariani, A., Nikou, C., Endres, B.T., Bassères, E., Garey, K.W., Kakadiaris, I.A.: DeTEC: detection of touching elongated cells in SEM images. In: Proceedings of the Advances in Visual Computing, pp. 288–297 (2016)
12. Memariani, A., Nikou, C., Endres, B., Bassères, E., Garey, K., Kakadiaris, I.A.: DETCIC: detection of elongated touching cells with inhomogeneous illumination using a stack of conditional random fields. In: Proceedings of the International Joint Conference on Computer Vision, Imaging and Computer Graphics Theory and Applications, pp. 574–580 (2018)
13. Moeskops, P., Veta, M., Lafarge, M.W., Eppenhof, K.A., Pluim, J.P.: Adversarial training and dilated convolutions for brain MRI segmentation. In: Proceedings of the Deep Learning in Medical Image Analysis and Multimodal Learning for Clinical Decision Support, pp. 56–64. Quebec City, QC, Canada (2017)
14. Ronneberger, O., Fischer, P., Brox, T.: U-net: convolutional networks for biomedical image segmentation. In: Proceedings of the Medical Image Computing and Computer-Assisted Intervention, pp. 234–241. Munich, Germany (2015)

15. Shen, D., Wu, G., Suk, H.I.: Deep learning in medical image analysis. Annu. Rev. Biomed. Eng. **19**, 221–248 (2017)
16. Xue, Y., Xu, T., Zhang, H., Long, L.R., Huang, X.: SegAN: adversarial network with multi-scale l_1 loss for medical image segmentation. Neuroinformatics **16**, 383–392 (2018)

On the Adaptability of Unsupervised CNN-Based Deformable Image Registration to Unseen Image Domains

Enzo Ferrante[1]([✉]), Ozan Oktay[2], Ben Glocker[2], and Diego H. Milone[1]

[1] Research Institute for Signals, Systems and Computational Intelligence, Sinc(i), FICH-UNL/CONICET, Santa Fe, Argentina
eferrante@sinc.unl.edu.ar
[2] Biomedical Image Analysis Group, Imperial College London, London, UK

Abstract. Deformable image registration is a fundamental problem in medical image analysis. During the last years, several methods based on deep convolutional neural networks (CNN) proved to be highly accurate to perform this task. These models achieved state-of-the-art accuracy while drastically reducing the required computational time, but mainly focusing on images of specific organs and modalities. To date, no work has reported on how these models adapt across different domains. In this work, we ask the question: can we use CNN-based registration models to spatially align images coming from a domain different than the one/s used at training time? We explore the adaptability of CNN-based image registration to different organs/modalities. We employ a fully convolutional architecture trained following an unsupervised approach. We consider a simple transfer learning strategy to study the generalisation of such model to unseen target domains, and devise a one-shot learning scheme taking advantage of the unsupervised nature of the proposed method. Evaluation on two publicly available datasets of X-Ray lung images and cardiac cine magnetic resonance sequences is provided. Our experiments suggest that models learned in different domains can be transferred at the expense of a decrease in performance, and that one-shot learning in the context of unsupervised CNN-based registration is a valid alternative to achieve consistent registration performance when only a pair of images from the target domain is available.

1 Introduction

Deformable image registration (DIR) is one of the key problems in medical image computing. It is a crucial step in numerous image analysis tasks, ranging from data aggregation for population analysis to atlas based anatomical segmentation. For more than three decades, the research community has made major efforts towards developing more accurate and efficient registration methods. DIR has been modelled through different approaches, ranging from diffusion equations [15] to probabilistic graphical models [8]. During the last years, we have witnessed the birth of new image registration methods learned from data. Since image data

© Springer Nature Switzerland AG 2018
Y. Shi et al. (Eds.): MLMI 2018, LNCS 11046, pp. 294–302, 2018.
https://doi.org/10.1007/978-3-030-00919-9_34

became massively available, and computational power grew powerful enough to process it, learning-based registration algorithms emerged as an alternative to traditional approaches based on iterative optimization.

CNN-Based Deformable Image Registration. Recently, several DIR methods based on deep learning have been proposed [1,7,14,16]. Most of them aim at learning a function (in the form of a CNN) to predict a spatial transformation mapping a *moving* image to a *fixed* image. These approaches can be categorised into supervised [14] and unsupervised [1,7,16] techniques based on how they utilise GT deformation fields. Note that, in the context of DIR, the term *unsupervised learning* refers to the case when no ground-truth annotations such as deformation fields are required for training. An alternative term that has been used in [7] to describe this approach is *self-supervised* DIR, given that learning is driven by image similarity metrics computed on the input data. In this work, we will use both terms interchangeably. Regarding supervised methods, since generating manual ground-truth annotations for DIR is an extremely hard and time consuming task, most supervised approaches resorted to using simulated annotations. The main limitation of such approaches is that their capture range is limited by the ground-truth annotations in the training datasets, which may not always be realistic.

On the contrary, unsupervised approaches like [1,7,16] do not inherit this limitation. These methods use a differentiable spatial transformer layer [4] to warp the source image during training, performing end-to-end optimization of a similarity metric between the deformed source and the target input images. The resulting CNN learns to predict (in a single forward pass) the transformation that maximizes such similarity. In this work, we follow a similar unsupervised approach and explore how it adapts to unseen scenarios where the images to be registered correspond to a domain different to that used at training time.

Domain Adaptation for CNN-based Deformable Image Registration. Different from CNN-based methods which learn from data, traditional image registration is usually performed through iterative optimization of a (dis)similarity measure. These methods are slower than CNN-based registration, but they are robust, can be used on unseen domains and work independently of the image resolution. Toolboxes like Elastix [6] for example, which use classical iterative image registration, have been widely applied to align different anatomical structures and image modalities[1]. In contrast, most of the aforementioned CNN-based image registration methods were validated only for specific domains such as brain MRI [1,7] and cardiac cine-MRI [16]. One of the fundamental questions that still needs to be addressed to enable the development of more robust and reusable CNN-based image registration toolboxes is how to adapt such models to new domains. The recent work [1] shows that, when dealing with multiple datasets of the same imaged anatomy (where the only difference among them is the machine used to capture the images or the acquisition parameters), registration models

---

[1] A complete list of configuration parameters for Elastix can be found in http://elastix. bigr.nl/wiki/index.php/Parameter_file_database.

tailored for a specific dataset outperforms more general models trained on all of them. This observation calls for a deeper adaptation study, focusing on more diverse datasets consisting of different anatomies and modalities. In this work, we show empirical evidence that such adaptation can be performed.

Contributions. We emphasize that the main contributions of this paper are not related to novel CNN-based architectures for image registration, but to addressing a more general question about the adaptability of such models. In that sense, our contributions are two-fold: (i) we present an explorative study of the performance of such models when they are trained, fine-tuned and tested on different organs/modalities and (ii) we show that a simple one-shot learning strategy can be used when the only available data is the pair of images to be registered.

2   Materials and Methods

2.1   Datasets and Clinical Context

For validation, we will focus on two clinically relevant applications of image registration with distinct domains, both in terms of anatomy and modality.

Cardiac Cine-MR Dataset: We employ a simplified version of the Sunnybrook Cardiac Dataset (SCD) [10][2]. It contains 45 cine-MR images (every image composed of 6 to 12 short-axis (SAX) 2D slices) captured at end-systole (ES) and end-diastole (ED) time points, amounting to a total of 416 2D images per cardiac phase. Image registration of 2D slices at different phases is crucial in many cardiac image analysis tasks, e.g. when generating strain fields to study left ventricular (LV) (dys)function [9]. After removing 27 slices because of lack of correspondence, we kept 256 pairs for training and 133 for testing (following the same test/train folds specified in the SegNetCMR site), where both images in every pair correspond to the same spatial location at ED and ES. Image resolution is 256×256, covering a field of view of $320\,\text{mm} \times 320\,\text{mm}$. The dataset includes expert annotations for the LV myocardium, which were used for quantitative evaluation. Image intensities were normalized to range [0,1].

Chest X-Ray Dataset: We used images from the chest X-ray dataset of the Japanese Society of Radiological Technology (JSRT) [13]. It includes 247 chest radiographs: 154 with one lung nodule and 93 healthy cases. We generated 247 pairs of images (with resolution 256×256) for registration (199 for training, 48 for testing, randomly split), by using the original image as fixed target and a left/right reversed version as moving image. In this context, DIR is used to warp the flipped image when applying a contralateral subtraction (C-Sub) technique [5], which consists in enhancing nodules in chest images by subtracting their reversed mirror version from the original. Since here we focus on deformable registration, images were previously aligned using affine registration [6]. At test time, we used expert annotations for left and right lungs (included in the dataset) for quantitative evaluation. Image intensities were normalized to range [0,1].

---

[2]publicly available at https://github.com/mshunshin/SegNetCMR.

2.2 Unsupervised CNN-Based Image Registration

Inspired by recent works on unsupervised CNN-based image registration [1,7,16], we employ a registration model consisting of two main components. The first one follows the U-Net architecture [11], taking the concatenated moving $\mathcal{M}$ and fixed $\mathcal{F}$ images as input and predicting a deformation field $\mathcal{D}_l = \mathcal{U}_l(\mathcal{M}, \mathcal{F}; \Theta_l)$, where $\mathcal{U}_l$ corresponds to a U-Net like CNN, Θ_l to the CNN parameters that have to be learned and l is the down-sampling factor applied to the input images. We perform down-sampling through an initial average-pooling layer in $\mathcal{D}_l$, where the pooling size is 2^l. Following [3], we reduce the model complexity by implementing skip connections via summations instead of the concatenation originally proposed by [11]. The second component is a differentiable spatial transformer module which warps the input moving image $\mathcal{M}$ using $\mathcal{D}_l$, producing a warped image $\mathcal{M} \circ \mathcal{D}_l$.

During training, the parameters Θ are learned using stochastic gradient descent (SGD) so that the warped moving image $\mathcal{M} \circ \mathcal{D}_l$ minimizes a particular dissimilarity measure with respect to $\mathcal{F}$. Since we are dealing with monomodal registration, the negative of the global normalized cross correlation $NCC(\mathcal{M} \circ \mathcal{D}_l, \mathcal{F})$ is adopted. NCC is known to perform well for monomodal cases and has been used in the context of CNN-based registration [1,7]. A regularization term imposing smoothness constraints is adopted to produce more anatomically plausible deformation fields. Following [7], we consider the total variation of the deformation field $TV(\mathcal{D}_l)$. Finally, an extra regularization term taking the L2 norm of $\mathcal{D}_l$ is included, resulting in the following loss function to be minimized during training:

$$\mathcal{L}(\mathcal{M}, \mathcal{T}, \mathcal{D}_l) = -NCC(\mathcal{M} \circ \mathcal{D}_l, \mathcal{F}) + \lambda_1 TV(\mathcal{D}_l) + \lambda_2 \frac{\|\mathcal{D}_l\|}{n}, \qquad (1)$$

where λ_1, λ_2 are weighting factors for the regularization terms and n is the number of pixels in the image.

2.3 Fine-Tuning and One-Shot Learning in the Context of Unsupervised CNN-Based Image Registration

Learning a discriminative classifier or other predictor in the presence of a shift between training and test distributions is known as domain adaptation [2]. In the context of DIR, such shift may be due to a change in the image modality, acquisition parameters or the organs being imaged. This is a rather common scenario for an image registration toolbox: users may download the software and use it to register a single pair of arbitrary images. In the case of iterative image registration algorithms like those implemented in Elastix, this is not a problem since the method will infer the transformation parameters by iteratively minimizing a similarity measure for the pair of images at hand. However, CNN-based DIR methods need to be trained before they can predict a deformation field. This is one of the main drawbacks of learning based image registration: models are trained on a *source* domain, and their performance decreases when being applied to images from a different *target* domain (see Sect. 3 for empirical evidence).

In this work, we focus on the case where the only sample available from the target domain is the actual pair of images to be registered. As stated before, this is a rather common scenario for people working in medical image computing, specially those developing toolboxes which could be used to register arbitrary images. In this scenario, we explore two alternatives:

1. **One-shot domain adaptation:** Here the pair of images to be registered is used to update a model pre-trained using images from a source domain (different to the target domain). Since we are in an unsupervised setting (in the sense that our method does not require image annotations at training time), nothing stops us from using the pair of test images for this update of the model parameters before registering them. We call this strategy *one-shot domain adaptation* by analogy with the concept of one-shot learning where the aim is to recognize categories based on very few training examples [12]. Such adaptation is performed by simply fine-tuning the pre-trained model.
2. **One-shot learning from scratch:** In this case, the CNN registration model is trained from scratch using only the pair of images to be registered and no pre-trained model. This is possible given the unsupervised nature of the approach. This scenario resembles the classic non-learning based iterative image registration algorithms, where the transformation parameters are learned from scratch by minimizing a dissimilarity measure on the pair of images to be registered. In our case, such parameters will be the CNN itself.

We also include results when fine-tuning a model pre-trained with images sampled from the target domain, using the pair of images to be registered. Clearly, this is not a case of domain adaptation, since the model has already been trained with images from the target domain. However, we include it to evaluate if fine-tuning an already good model following a one-shot strategy leads to even more accurate results. Finally, in terms of time restrictions, we consider two scenarios: (i) having real time constraints: the models are trained/fine-tuned for only 50 iterations (0.5 s in GPU) and (ii) no time constraints: the models are trained/fine-tuned until convergence using the pair of images to be registered. [3]

3   Results and Discussion

In this section we present the results for the alternative studies discussed in the previous section. We use the mean of absolute differences (MAD) between warped moving image and fixed target as an indicator of the quality of the registration since we are dealing with monomodal cases. Moreover, additional indicators reflecting complementary information (namely Dice coefficient (DSC)

---

[3] Fine-tuning for 50 iterations takes only 0.5 s on GPU. When training from scratch/fine-tuning until convergence, we update the model for 3000 iterations leading to about 30 s per registration case.

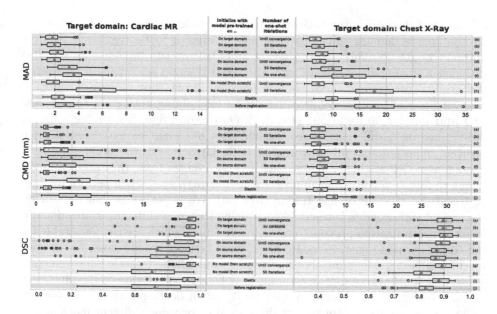

Fig. 1. Experimental validation when fine-tuning/training from scratch using a one-shot strategy. We report results for models pre-trained with images from the target domain (rows a, b, c), from the source domain (rows d, e, f) and without pre-training (rows g, h). See Sect. 3 for a complete analysis of these results.

and contour mean distance (CMD)) based on warped moving and fixed segmentations are also reported.[4] Results are presented in Fig. 1, considering the cardiac MR images as target domain and chest X-ray as source, and vice versa. We use down-sampling factor $l = 2$ in both cases, since it resulted to be the best performing level in our initial experiments.[5] Let us analyse Fig. 1 in detail.
- **Baselines:** For comparison, we include results before (row (j)) and after registration using the state-of-the-art Elastix toolbox [6] (row (i)).[6] At first sight, we can observe that models trained using images from the target domain (row (c)) achieve performance equivalent (and even better) to that of Elastix, significantly outperforming models trained on a different source domain (f). Note that in these experiments, training is performed from scratch as in previous works [1] (i.e., no one-shot strategy is applied).

---

[4] We used Python and Tensorflow for implementation. Experiments were run in a machine with CPU Intel Core i7-7700, 64GB of RAM and NVidia Titan XP GPU. In order to encourage reproducible research, the project source code and Elastix parameter files can be downloaded from: https://gitlab.com/eferrante/.

[5] The CNN-based models take 0.06s on GPU and 0.08 s on CPU to register a pair of images, while Elastix 2.47s. In all the experiments we used Adam optimization, with LR = 1e-4 and $\lambda_1 = \lambda_2 = 1e-6$.

[6] Elastix parameters were chosen by grid search using the training data and are available online in our project website.

- One-shot domain adaptation: In this case, we fine-tune a model pre-trained on the source domain using just the pair of images to be registered (from a different target domain)[7]. Note that, in order to simulate the one-shot scenario (i.e. just a single pair of images from the target domain is available), we restore the original pre-trained model before performing one-shot domain adaptation for every pair of images. We show results for fine-tuning until convergence (row (d)) and just for 50 iterations (row (e)). On the one side, fine-tuning a model pre-trained on a different source domain does not seem to have a systematic positive impact across all measures in both datasets. On the other side, fine-tuning a model originally trained with other images from the target domain seems to lead to a consistent improvement (row (a)), even when performing just 50 iterations of one-shot fine tuning (row (b)). We hypothesize that initializing the model with weights learned when training in a very different source domain leads the optimization process towards local minima which are not favourable for the target domain registration. However, when test images are closer to the ones used for training, doing one-shot fine-tuning results in systematic improvements. This suggests that one-shot fine-tuning may be a good solution to the multi-site domain adaptation problem reported by [1], when dealing with datasets of the same imaged anatomy captured at different sites or using different machines.

- One-shot learning from scratch: We train the model from scratch using only the pair of images to be registered (i.e. the model is initialized with random weights before registering every pair of images). We show results when training just for 50 iterations (row (h)) and until convergence (row (g)). Interestingly, one-shot learning from scratch (training until convergence) achieves results comparable to Elastix, and even at the level of those obtained when training with other images from the target domain. One could argue that doing one-shot learning from scratch is actually overfitting the model. However, this is not the case since we are following an unsupervised strategy in a one-shot scenario, obtaining a model that is performing well for the data of interest (i.e. the single pair of images from the target domain to be registered). Moreover, this model could be used as initialization to register similar images in the future.

4   Conclusions and Future Works

We present the first study on domain adaptation across different organs/modalities for unsupervised CNN-based DIR, focusing on the extreme case when a single pair of images from the target domain is available at test time. In this context, we evaluate the performance of a model pre-trained with data from a different source domain, observing a clear decrease in performance when used to register images from the target domain. As a potential solution, we propose one-shot domain adaptation, by fine-tuning the original model using the target pair of images, taking advantage of the unsupervised nature of proposed approach. Pre-training does not seem to help when dealing with images

---

[7] We experimented with fine-tuning the model in whole or in part, but we found that fine-tuning the complete model achieved better results in general.

from extremely different domains, but it achieves systematic improvement when fine-tuning a model pre-trained on similar images. This opens the door to future research where one-shot domain adaptation could alleviate problems when dealing with multi-site data. Last but not least, we show that one-shot learning for CNN-based DIR (trained from scratch using just the pair of images to be registered) achieves very good results, comparable to those produced by state of the art algorithms.

This work constitutes another step towards constructing more robust deep learning models for image registration. In the future, we plan to extend the validation to volumetric image registration and explore one-shot domain adaptation for multi-site datasets. Moreover, more sophisticated strategies focusing on learning features invariant to image domain could also be adopted.

Acknowledgements. EF is beneficiary of an AXA Research Grant. We thank NVIDIA Corporation for the donation of the Titan X GPU used for this project.

References

1. Balakrishnan, G., et al.: An unsupervised learning model for deformable medical image registration. Accepted at CVPR 2018 (2018)
2. Ganin, Y., Lempitsky, V.: Unsupervised domain adaptation by backpropagation. ICML (2015)
3. Guerrero, R., et al.: White matter hyperintensity and stroke lesion segmentation and differentiation using cnns. NeuroImage: Clin. **17**, 918–934 (2018)
4. Jaderberg, M., et al.: Spatial transformer networks. In: NIPS, pp. 2017–2025 (2015)
5. Kawaguchi, T., Harada, Y., Nagata, R., Miyake, H.: Image registration methods for contralateral subtraction of chest radiographs. In: IEE BMEI (2010)
6. Klein, S., Staring, M., Murphy, K., Viergever, M.A., Pluim, J.P.: Elastix: a toolbox for intensity-based medical image registration. IEEE TMI **29**(1), 196–205 (2010)
7. Li, H., Fan, Y.: Non-rigid image registration using self-supervised fully convolutional networks without training data. Accepted at ISBI 2018 (2018)
8. Paragios, N.: (hyper)-graphical models in biomedical image analysis. Med. Image Anal. **33**, 102–106 (2016)
9. Phatak, N.S.: Strain measurement in the left ventricle during systole with deformable image registration. Med. Image Anal. **13**(2), 354–361 (2009)
10. Radau, P., Lu, Y., Connelly, K., Paul, G., et al.: Evaluation framework for algorithms segmenting short axis cardiac MRI. MIDAS J. **49** (2009)
11. Ronneberger, O., Fischer, P., Brox, T.: U-net: convolutional networks for biomedical image segmentation. In: MICCAI, pp. 234–241. Springer, Cham (2015)
12. Salakhutdinov, R., Tenenbaum, J., Torralba, A.: One-shot learning with a hierarchical nonparametric Bayesian model. In: ICML Workshop Proceedings (2012)
13. Shiraishi, J.: Development of a digital image database for chest radiographs with and without a lung nodule: receiver operating characteristic analysis of radiologists' detection of pulmonary nodules. Am. J. Roentgenol. **174**(1), 71–74 (2000)
14. Sokooti, Hessam, de Vos, Bob, Berendsen, Floris, Lelieveldt, Boudewijn P.F., Išgum, Ivana, Staring, Marius: Nonrigid Image Registration Using Multi-scale 3D Convolutional Neural Networks. In: Descoteaux, Maxime, Maier-Hein, Lena, Franz, Alfred, Jannin, Pierre, Collins, D.Louis, Duchesne, Simon (eds.) MICCAI 2017.

LNCS, vol. 10433, pp. 232–239. Springer, Cham (2017). https://doi.org/10.1007/978-3-319-66182-7_27

15. Thirion, J.P.: Image matching as a diffusion process: an analogy with Maxwell's demons. Med. Image Anal. **2**(3), 243–260 (1998)

16. de Vos, Bob D., Berendsen, Floris F., Viergever, Max A., Staring, Marius, Išgum, Ivana: End-to-End Unsupervised Deformable Image Registration with a Convolutional Neural Network. In: Cardoso, M.Jorge, Arbel, Tal, Carneiro, Gustavo, Syeda-Mahmood, Tanveer, Tavares, João Manuel R.S., Moradi, Mehdi, Bradley, Andrew, Greenspan, Hayit, Papa, João Paulo, Madabhushi, Anant, Nascimento, Jacinto C., Cardoso, Jaime S., Belagiannis, Vasileios, Lu, Zhi (eds.) DLMIA/ML-CDS -2017. LNCS, vol. 10553, pp. 204–212. Springer, Cham (2017). https://doi.org/10.1007/978-3-319-67558-9_24

Early Diagnosis of Autism Disease
by Multi-channel CNNs

Guannan Li[1,2], Mingxia Liu[2], Quansen Sun[1(✉)], Dinggang Shen[2(✉)],
and Li Wang[2(✉)]

[1] School of Computer Science and Engineering, Nanjing University of Science
and Technology, Nanjing 210094, China
[2] Department of Radiology and Biomedical Research Imaging Center,
University of North Carolina at Chapel Hill, Chapel Hill, NC 27599, USA
{dgshen, li_wang}@med.unc.edu

Abstract. Currently there are still no early biomarkers to detect infants with risk of autism spectrum disorder (ASD), which is mainly diagnosed based on behavior observations at three or four years old. Since intervention efforts may miss a critical developmental window after 2 years old, it is significant to identify imaging-based biomarkers for early diagnosis of ASD. Although some methods using magnetic resonance imaging (MRI) for brain disease prediction have been proposed in the last decade, few of them were developed for predicting ASD in early age. Inspired by deep multi-instance learning, in this paper, we propose a patch-level data-expanding strategy for multi-channel convolutional neural networks to automatically identify infants with risk of ASD in early age. Experiments were conducted on the National Database for Autism Research (NDAR), with results showing that our proposed method can significantly improve the performance of early diagnosis of ASD.

Keywords: Autism · Convolutional neural network · Early diagnosis
Deep multi-instance learning

1 Introduction

Autism, or autism spectrum disorder (ASD), refers to a range of conditions characterized by challenges with social skills, repetitive behaviors, speech and nonverbal communication, as well as by unique strengths and differences. Globally, autism is estimated to affect 24.8 million people as of 2015 [1]. The diagnosis of ASD is mainly based on behaviors. Studies demonstrate that behavioral signs can begin to emerge as early as 6–12 months [2]. However, most professionals who specialize in diagnosing the disorder won't attempt to make a definite diagnosis until 2 or 3 years old [3]. As a result, the window of opportunity for effective intervention may have passed when the disorder is detected. Thus, it is of great importance to detect ASD earlier in life for better intervention.

Magnetic resonance (MR) examination allows researchers and clinicians to noninvasively examine brain anatomy. Structural MR examination is widely used to investigate brain morphology because of its high contrast sensitivity and spatial resolution

© Springer Nature Switzerland AG 2018
Y. Shi et al. (Eds.): MLMI 2018, LNCS 11046, pp. 303–309, 2018.
https://doi.org/10.1007/978-3-030-00919-9_35

[4]. Imaging plays an increasingly pivotal role in early diagnosis and intervention of ASD. Many neuroscience studies on children and young adults with ASD demonstrate abnormalities in the hippocampus [5], precentral gyrus [6], and anterior cingulate gyrus [7]. These researches demonstrate that it is highly feasible to detect ASD in early age.

In recent years, deep learning has demonstrated outstanding performances in a wide range of computer vision and image analysis applications. Many methods based on convolutional neural networks (CNNs) [8] are proposed for MRI analysis, e.g., classification of the Alzheimer's disease (AD). For example, Sarraf *et al.* [9] proposed a DeepAD for AD diagnosis, where the existing CNN architectures, LeNet [10] and GoogleNet [11], were used for MR brain scans on the slice level and subject level, respectively. But feature representations defined at whole-brain level may not be effective in characterizing early structural changes of the brain. Several patch-level (an intermediate scale between voxel level and region of interest (ROI)) features have been proposed to represent structural MR images for brain disease diagnosis. For example, a deep multi-instance learning framework for AD classification using MRI was proposed by Liu *et al.* [12], achieving promising results in AD diagnosis.

Compared with adult brains, the analysis of infant brains is more difficult due to the low tissue contrast caused by the largely immature myelination. Furthermore, the number of autistic subjects is usually very limited, making the task of computer-aided diagnosis of ASD more challenging.

Motivated by deep multi-instance learning [12], in this paper, we propose a patch-level data-expanding strategy in multi-channel CNN for prediction of ASD in early age. Figure 1 shows a schematic diagram of our method. We first preprocess MR images and then identify anatomical landmarks in a data-driven manner. In the patch extraction step, we utilize a patch-level data expanding strategy based on identified landmarks. In the last step, we use the multi-channel CNNs for ASD classification. Experimental results on 276 subjects with MRIs show that our method outperforms conventional methods in ASD classification.

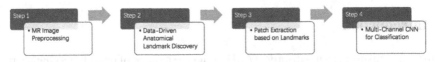

Fig. 1. Block diagram of the proposed scheme for automatic classification of ASD.

2   Materials and Methods

Data description. A total of 276 subjects gathered from National Database for Autism Research (NDAR) [13] were used in the study. More specifically, the dataset consists of 215 normal controls (NCs), 31 mild condition autism spectrum subjects, and 30 autistic subjects, as listed in Table 1. In the experiments, we regard the last two types as one group. All images were acquired at around 24 months of age on a Siemens 3T scanner, while subjects were naturally sleeping and fitted with ear protection, with their heads secured in a vacuum-fixation device. T1-weighted MR images were acquired with 160 sagittal slices using parameters: TR/TE = 2400/3.16 ms and voxel resolution = $1 \times 1 \times 1$ mm^3. T2-weighted MR images were obtained with 160 sagittal slices using parameters: TR/TE = 3200/499 ms and voxel resolution = $1 \times 1 \times 1$ mm^3.

Table 1. Description of 24-month subjects in the NADR datasets.

Category	Male/female
Autism	25/5
Autism spectrum	21/10
Normal control	133/82

MRI Pre-processing. We use in-house tools to perform skull stripping and histogram matching for T1 MR images. After skull stripping, we can estimate the whole brain volume for each subject. This pre-processing step is important for subsequent analysis steps.

Data-Driven Anatomical Landmark Identification. To extract informative patches from MRI for model training, we first identify discriminative ASD-related landmark locations using a data-driven landmark discovery algorithm [14]. The aim is to identify the landmarks with statistically significant group difference between ASD and NC subjects in local brain structures. The pipeline for defining ASD landmarks is shown in Fig. 2. Specifically, we first choose one T1-weighted image with high quality as a template. Then, a linear registration is used to locate the same location across all training images in the pre-processing step. Since the linearly-aligned images are not voxel-wisely comparable, nonlinear registration is further used for spatial normalization, thus corresponding relationship among voxels can be established. To identify local morphological patterns with statistically significant differences between groups, we use the histogram of oriented gradients (HOG) features as morphological patterns. Finally, the Hoteling's T2 statistic [15] is adopted for group comparison. Accordingly,

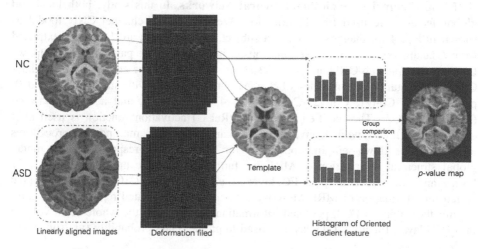

Fig. 2. The proposed pipeline for anatomical landmark definition.

each voxel in the template is assigned with a p-value. Any voxels in the template with p-values smaller than 0.001 are regarded as significantly different positions. To avoid redundancy, only local minimum (whose p-values are also smaller than 0.001) are defined as ASD landmarks in the template image.

Patch Extraction from MRI. By using the deformation field from nonlinear registration, we can get the corresponding patches in each linearly-aligned image. To address the issue of the limited number of autistic subjects, we propose a data expansion strategy on autistic subjects to have comparable number of samples as the number of NC subjects. As shown in Fig. 3(b), for each landmark, we randomly extract N (> 1) image patches as ASD training samples, but only 1 image patch as NC training sample (Fig. 3(c)). In the datasets, since the NC sample size is about 4 times larger than the ASD, we set $N = 4$ in the experiment.

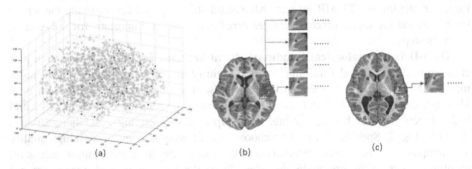

Fig. 3. Illustration of landmarks selection and patch extraction. The yellow color in **a** is the illustration of all identified anatomical landmarks, and the red points show the selected 50 landmarks which are chosen by both their p-values and spatial distances from other nearby points. **b** shows 4 randomly extracted patches around a landmark which are as ASD training samples, and **c** shows 1 randomly extracted patch which is used as NC training sample.

Multi-Channel Convolutional Neural Networks. In this study, both local and global features are used for classification. We use a multi-channel CNN model as shown in Fig. 4 for diagnosis. Given a subject, the input data are L patches extracted from L landmarks. To learn representations of individual image patch in one group, we first run multiple sub-CNN architectures. More specifically, we embed L parallel sub-CNN architectures with a series of 5 convolutional layers with stride size 1 and 0-padding (i.e., Conv1, Conv2, Conv3, Conv4, and Conv5), and a fully-connected (FC) layer (FC7). The rectified linear unit (ReLU) activation function is used after convolutional layers, while Conv2 and Conv4 are followed by max-pooling procedures to conduct the down-sampling operation for their outputs, respectively. To model global structural information of MRI, we further concatenate the outputs of L FC7 layers and add two additional FC layers (i.e., FC9, and FC10) to capture global structural information of MRI. Moreover, we use a concatenated representation comprising the output of FC8, personal information (gender) and the whole-brain volume into FC9 layer. Finally, FC11 layer is used to predict class probability (via soft-max).

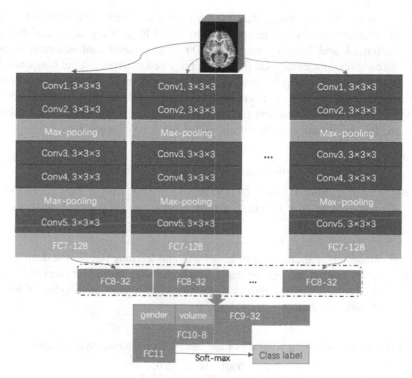

Fig. 4. Architecture of the proposed multi-channel CNN for ASD diagnosis. In each channel CNN, there is a sequence of convolutional (Conv) layers and fully connected (FC) layers.

3 Experiments and Results

In this section, we present our experimental results using the proposed data-expanding multi-channel CNNs (DE-MC) scheme. We also evaluate performance *with respect to* landmark number and learning rate. Ten-fold cross-validation was used in the experiment. In each fold, we selected 264 subjects, with 55 ASD training samples and 209 NC training samples for training, and used 6 ASD subjects and 6 NC subjects as testing samples. The patch size was set as 24 × 24 × 24. Since both T1w and T2w images are available, we concatenated the extracted T1w and T2w image patches as input to the multi-channel framework. The cross-entropy loss was used to train the network.

First, we compared our DE-MC method with 3D convolutional neural networks (3D CNN). The input of 3D CNN is the whole linearly aligned MR image and the network has 10 convolutional layers and 3 fully connection layers, and we have optimized all parameters for fair comparison. The performance of classification is evaluated by the overall classification accuracy (ACC), as shown in Table 2. We can see that, compared with 3D CNN, our method can get a much higher accuracy. In terms of overall accuracy, DE-MC achieves 24% improvement over 3D CNN. To evaluate the contributions of the proposed strategies, we further compare the DE-MC with its two variants: (1) multi-channel learning without patch-level data expansion (MC), and

(2) multi-channel learning using data expansion without additional information (i.e., gender information and whole-brain volume) (DE-MC$_2$). They all share the same $L = 50$ landmarks and learning rate $lr = 0.0001$. Compared multi-channel learning without patch-level data expansion (MC), the proposed method can get better result. It proves that the data expanding strategy can help get more useful information for classification and improve the performance. Compared with the proposed methods *with* and *without* additional information (i.e., gender information and whole-brain volume), we can see this additional information is useful for ASD diagnosis.

Table 2. Classification results achieved by different methods.

Method	3D CNN	DE-MC	MC	DE-MC$_2$
ACC	0.5234	**0.7624**	0.6231	0.7432

Hyper parameters, e.g., number of landmarks and learning rate, in the deep learning may significantly impact the performance, and hence they should be carefully chosen. Table 3 shows the results *with respect to* the use of different combination of learning rate and landmark number.

Table 3. Classification accuracy of our method with different hyperparameters.

L	lr 0.0001	0.001	0.01
30	0.6132	0.5244	0.4243
50	**0.7624**	0.6138	0.5471
100	0.7620	0.6249	0.5731
200	0.7431	0.6169	0.5708

4 Conclusion

In this paper, we proposed a patch-level data-expanding strategy to multi-channel CNN for early ASD diagnosis. In the patch extraction step, we utilized a patch-level data expanding strategy to balance the samples from NC and autistic groups, and the experiments show that this strategy is effective. The experiment results also showed that our proposed networks can achieve reasonable diagnosis accuracy. In our future work, we will further validate the proposed model on 6-month-old infant subjects with risk of ASD.

Acknowledgments. Data used in the preparation of this manuscript were obtained from the NIH-supported National Database for Autism Research (NDAR). NDAR is a collaborative informatics system created by the National Institutes of Health to provide a national resource to support and accelerate research in autism. This manuscript reflects the views of the authors and may not reflect the opinions or views of the NIH or of the Submitters submitting original data to NDAR.

This work was supported in part by National Institutes of Health grants MH109773, MH100217, MH070890, EB006733, EB008374, EB009634, AG041721, AG042599, MH088520, MH108914, MH107815, and MH113255.

References

1. Newschaffer, C.J., et al.: The epidemiology of autism spectrum disorders. Dev. Disab. Res. Rev. **8**, 151–161 (2002)
2. Filipek, P.A., et al.: The screening and diagnosis of autistic spectrum disorders. J. Autism Dev. Disorders **29**, 439–484 (1999)
3. Baird, G., Cass, H., Slonims, V.: Diagnosis of autism. BMJ Brit. Med. J. **327**, 488–493 (2003)
4. Chen, R., Jiao, Y., Herskovits, E.H.: Structural MRI in autism spectrum disorder. Pediatr. Res. **69**, 63R (2011)
5. Schumann, C.M., et al.: The amygdala is enlarged in children but not adolescents with autism; the hippocampus is enlarged at all ages. J. Neurosci. **24**, 6392 (2004)
6. Greimel, E., et al.: Changes in grey matter development in autism spectrum disorder. Brain Struct. Funct **218**, 929–942 (2013)
7. Thakkar, K.N., et al.: Response monitoring, repetitive behaviour and anterior cingulate abnormalities in autism spectrum disorders (ASD). Brain **131**, 2464–2478 (2008)
8. Ciresan, D.C., Meier, U., Masci, J., Maria Gambardella, L., Schmidhuber, J.: Flexible, high performance convolutional neural networks for image classification. In: IJCAI Proceedings-International Joint Conference on Artificial Intelligence, pp. 1237. Barcelona, Spain, (2011)
9. Sarraf, S., Tofighi, G.: DeepAD: Alzheimer's Disease Classification via Deep Convolutional Neural Networks using MRI and fMRI. bioRxiv 070441 (2016)
10. LeCun, Y.: LeNet-5, convolutional neural networks (2015). http://yann/.lecun.com/exdb/lenet20
11. Zhong, Z., Jin, L., Xie, Z.: High performance offline handwritten chinese character recognition using googlenet and directional feature maps. In: 13th International Conference on Document Analysis and Recognition (ICDAR), pp. 846–850. IEEE (2015)
12. Liu, M., Zhang, J., Adeli, E., Shen, D.: Landmark-based deep multi-instance learning for brain disease diagnosis. Med. Image Anal. **43**, 157–168 (2018)
13. Payakachat, N., Tilford, J.M., Ungar, W.J.: National Database for Autism Research (NDAR): Big data opportunities for health services research and health technology assessment. PharmacoEconomics **34**, 127–138 (2016)
14. Zhang, J., Gao, Y., Gao, Y., Munsell, B.C., Shen, D.: Detecting anatomical landmarks for fast Alzheimer's disease diagnosis. IEEE Trans. Med. Imaging **35**, 2524 (2016)
15. Mardia, K.: Assessment of multinormality and the robustness of Hotelling's T2 test. Appl. Stat., 163–171 (1975)

Longitudinal and Multi-modal Data Learning via Joint Embedding and Sparse Regression for Parkinson's Disease Diagnosis

Haijun Lei[1], Zhongwei Huang[1], Ahmed Elazab[2], Hancong Li[1],
and Baiying Lei[2(✉)]

[1] College of Computer Science and Software Engineering, Key Laboratory of
Service Computing and Applications, Guangdong Province Key Laboratory of
Popular High Performance Computers, Shenzhen University, Shenzhen 518060,
China
[2] School of Biomedical Engineering, National-Regional Key Technology
Engineering Laboratory for Medical Ultrasound, Guangdong Key Laboratory for
Biomedical Measurements and Ultrasound Imaging, Shenzhen University,
Shenzhen 518060, China
leiby@szu.edu.cn

Abstract. Parkinson's disease (PD) is a neurodegenerative progressive disease
that mainly affects the motor systems of patients. To slow this disease deterioration, robust and accurate diagnosis of PD is an effective way to alleviate
mental and physical sufferings of clinical intervention. In this paper, we propose
a new unsupervised feature selection method via joint embedding learning and
sparse regression using longitudinal multi-modal neuroimaging data. Specifically, the proposed method performs feature selection and local structure
learning, simultaneously, to adaptively determine the similarity matrix. Meanwhile, we constrain the similarity matrix to make it contains c connected
components for gaining the most accurate information of the neuroimaging data
structure. The baseline data is utilized to establish the feature selection model to
select the most discriminative features. Namely, we exploit baseline data to train
four regression models for the clinical scores prediction (depression, sleep,
olfaction, and cognition scores) and a classification model for the classification
of PD disease in the future time point. Extensive experiments are conducted to
demonstrate the effectiveness of the proposed method on the Parkinson's Progression Markers Initiative (PPMI) dataset. The experimental results demonstrate that, our proposed method can enhance the performance in clinical scores
prediction and class label identification in longitudinal data and outperforms the
state-of-art methods as well.

Keywords: Parkinson's disease · Unsupervised feature selection
Classification · Score prediction · Longitudinal data

© Springer Nature Switzerland AG 2018
Y. Shi et al. (Eds.): MLMI 2018, LNCS 11046, pp. 310–318, 2018.
https://doi.org/10.1007/978-3-030-00919-9_36

1 Introduction

Parkinson's disease (PD) is characterized as an intricate and ineluctable neurodegenerative disorder in the elderly. PD is primarily described by four motor symptoms (rigidity, bradykinesia, tremor, and postural instability) and four non-motor symptoms (depression, sleep, olfaction, and cognition disorders) [1]. These symptoms are mainly derived from the death of dopamine neurons in the substantia nigra [2]. Although the study of the cause of their deaths has made some preliminary progress, the cause of PD remains unknown. Meanwhile, existing studies did not find the phenomenon of dopaminergic deficit in some PD patients, especially, in the scans without evidence of dopamine deficit (SWEDDs). This situation has undoubtedly increased the challenges of PD diagnosis. Therefore, it is of great significance to establish a robust and accurate diagnostic model of the disease in longitudinal time points to slow the disease deterioration and alleviate mental and physical sufferings.

Since multiple modalities can provide more comprehensive information, the computer-aided PD diagnosis from multi-modal neuroimaging data has increasingly played vital role and attracted much attention [3]. Multimodal neuroimaging techniques used for PD diagnosis mainly include magnetic resonance imaging (MRI) and diffusion tensor imaging (DTI). However, for the multi-modal neuroimaging data, the feature dimension is relatively high, while the number of the subject is quite limited, which easily leads to overfitting issue and is difficult to generate a robust model. To address this shortcoming, feature selection is an effective way by discovering disease-related characteristics [4]. Feature selection mainly includes two methods: supervised and unsupervised. Most supervised feature selection methods can be either separate single task [5] or joint multi-task [6]. The latter methods are superior to the former ones in many aspects. Nevertheless, there are two main issues with joint multi-task feature methods. First, the selected features by these methods are mostly linearly correlated with multi-task targets but these methods ignore or weaken the learning importance of the structural characteristics of data itself. Second, joint multi-task feature selection methods require additional label and scores information for supervised learning. For unsupervised feature selection methods, they pay more attention to the learning of the data structure itself. Most unsupervised methods are either based upon filter methods [7], or embedded methods [8]. Embedded methods have good performance and have received much attention. Nevertheless, there are at least two issues with embedding methods. First, they compute the embedding and select features, respectively. Second, when computing the embedding, similarity matrix built with conventional method is usually not a good neighbor assignment. In other word, the optimal similarity matrix should have c connected components.

To relieve the impact of above problems, we propose a new unsupervised feature selection method via joint embedding learning and sparse regression using longitudinal multi-modal data. We highlight the contributions of this paper as follows:

1. A new unsupervised feature selection method is proposed. The method performs embedding learning and feature selection, simultaneously. It adaptively learns local manifold structure and thus can select discriminative features.

2. A reasonable constraint with exact connected components of similarity matrix equal to c is introduced to the method.
3. Extensive experiments are conducted to demonstrate the effectiveness of the proposed method on PPMI dataset. The experimental results demonstrate that our proposed method can enhance the performance in clinical scores prediction and class label identification and outperforms the state-of-art methods as well.

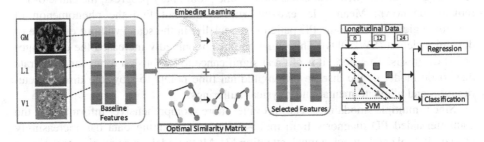

Fig. 1. Framework of proposed method via joint embedding learning and sparse regression

2   Related Work

Many supervised joint multi-task feature selection and unsupervised embedding feature selection methods were proposed in literature. The multi-modal multi-task (M3T) [3] trains a selection model to obtain a joint subset which consists of common relevant features using multi-task feature selection from each modality for multiple response variables. The multi-modal sparse learning (MMSL) [6] method simultaneously performs classification and clinical scores prediction based on an improved loss function that considers the relations among rows and the information among columns in response variables. Multi-Cluster Feature Selection (MCFS) [9] computes the embedding at first and then selects the features which can best preserve the clustering structure. Flexible manifold embedding (FME) [10] is a general framework adopted by many feature selection methods for dimensionality reduction. Robust spectral feature selection (RSFS) [11] simultaneously uses ℓ_1-norm and FME for robust feature selection. However, as previously mentioned, these methods have several problems. For example, supervised joint multi-task feature selection methods ignore or weaken the importance for learning the structural characteristics of data itself. Unsupervised embedding feature selection methods compute unreliable similarity matrix and make improper neighbor assignment.

3   Methodology

3.1   System Overview

The overall procedures for clinical scores prediction and class label classification are presented in Fig. 1. First, we extract features from gray matter (GM) of MRI, 1st eigenvalue (L1) and 1st eigenvector (V1) of DTI and linearly connect them. Then, we conduct feature selection based on joint embedding learning and sparse regression. Finally, we use support vector regression (SVR) and support vector classification (SVC) with sigmoid kernel to generate four regression models and a classification model. Specifically, we use the proposed method to choose the most discriminative features in baseline neuroimaging data and further train four regression models to predict the clinical scores in baseline data and a classification model to discriminate the clinical label in baseline, 12 months, and 24 months data.

3.2   Notations

In this study, uppercase boldface letters (e.g., $\mathbf{X}$) denote matrices, and lowercase boldface letters denote vectors. For a matrix $\mathbf{X} = [x_{ij}]$, where $\mathbf{x}^i$ denote its k-th row, the trace of matrix $\mathbf{X}$ is denoted as $\mathrm{tr}(\mathbf{X})$. The transpose of matrix $\mathbf{X}$ is denoted as $\mathbf{X}^{\mathbf{T}}$. The norm of matrix is defined as $\|\mathbf{X}\|$. We denote $\ell_{2,1}$-norm of a matrix $\mathbf{X}$ as $\|\mathbf{X}\|_{2,1} = \sum_k \|\mathbf{x}^k\|_2$.

3.3   Proposed Method

Let $\mathbf{Y} \in \mathbf{R}^{n \times m}$ and $\mathbf{S} \in \mathbf{R}^{n \times n}$ denote the low-dimensional manifold of the high-dimensional data $\mathbf{X} \in \mathbf{R}^{n \times d}$ and the similarity matrix, respectively, where $\mathbf{y}^i$ denote i-th sample of $\mathbf{Y}$, s_{ij} is an element of similarity matrix $\mathbf{S}$. In general, we compute $\mathbf{Y}$ by the following embedding function:

$$\min_{s^i 1 = 1, 0 \leq s_{ij} \leq 1} \sum_{i,j} \left(\|\mathbf{y}^i - \mathbf{y}^j\|_2^2 s_{ij} + \gamma s_{ij}^2 \right), \tag{1}$$

where γ is the regularization parameter to avoid the trivial solution. The method computes the embedding at first and then use regression coefficient to rank each feature. Separation of $\mathbf{Y}$ construction and feature selection causes the selected features to be highly dependent on the quality of the original data. However, neuroimaging data always contains many noise samples and features. To handle it, we simultaneously conduct feature selection and local structure learning, which is expressed as:

$$\min \sum_{i,j} \left(\|\mathbf{x}^i \mathbf{W} - \mathbf{x}^j \mathbf{W}\|_2^2 s_{ij} + \gamma s_{ij}^2 \right) + \lambda \|\mathbf{W}\|_{2,1}$$

$$s.t. \quad \mathbf{s}^i 1 = 1, \ 0 \leq s_{ij} \leq 1, \ \mathbf{W}^{\mathbf{T}} \mathbf{W} = \mathbf{I}, \tag{2}$$

where $\mathbf{W} \in \mathbf{R}^{d \times m}$ is the weight coefficient matrix and each column of $\mathbf{W}$ contains different weight coefficients of each feature. λ denotes weighting parameter that diminishes the weight as the feature as value of λ increases. In feature selection task, the dimension of multi-modal data is high, thus the covariance matrix of $\mathbf{X}$ easily becomes singular. Therefore, we adopt the constraint $\mathbf{W}^{\mathbf{T}} \mathbf{W} = \mathbf{I}$ to make the selected features discriminative after dimension reduction.

In addition, the optimal neighbor assignment means that similarity matrix has exact c connected components. However, the similarity matrix $\mathbf{S}$ gained by the solution of Eq. (2) is almost impossible to be in the above state. To tackle this issue, we need to make the rank of Laplacian matrix $\mathbf{L_S}$ of $\mathbf{S}$ equal to $n-c$, i.e. $rank(\mathbf{L_S}) = n - c$, and then we have

$$\min \sum_{i,j} \left(\|\mathbf{x}^i\mathbf{W} - \mathbf{x}^j\mathbf{W}\|_2^2 s_{ij} + \gamma s_{ij}^2 \right) + \lambda \|\mathbf{W}\|_{2,1}$$

$$s.t. \quad \mathbf{s}^i\mathbf{1} = 1, 0 \le s_{ij} \le 1, \mathbf{W}^T\mathbf{W} = \mathbf{I}, rank(\mathbf{L_S}) = n - c, \tag{3}$$

where $\mathbf{L_S}$ is equal to $\mathbf{D} - \frac{\mathbf{S}^T + \mathbf{S}}{2}$, the degree matrix $\mathbf{D}$ is a diagonal matrix and the i-th element in the diagonal equal to $\sum_j \frac{\mathbf{S}_{ij} + \mathbf{S}_{ji}}{2}$. Since the constraint $rank(\mathbf{L_S}) = n - c$ is also dependent on similarity matrix $\mathbf{S}$, it is difficult to solve Eq. (3). To handle it, let $\xi_i(\mathbf{L_S})$ denotes the i-th smallest eigenvalue of $\mathbf{L_S}$. Since $rank(\mathbf{L_S})$ is positive semi-definite, we have $\xi_i(\mathbf{L_S}) \ge 0$. Meanwhile, it can be easily proved that $rank(\mathbf{L_S}) = n - c$ which indicates $\sum_{i=1}^c \xi_i(\mathbf{L_S}) = 0$. Because the derivation of $\sum_{i=1}^c \xi_i(\mathbf{L_S})$ is difficult to handle, we exploit Ky Fan's Theorem [12] to obtain:

$$\sum_{i=1}^c \xi_i(\mathbf{L_S}) = \min_{\mathbf{P} \in \mathbb{R}^{n \times c}, \mathbf{P}^T\mathbf{P} = \mathbf{I}} \mathrm{Tr}(\mathbf{P}^T\mathbf{L_S}\mathbf{P}). \tag{4}$$

Thus, we can rewrite Eq. (3) as:

$$\min \sum_{i,j} \left(\|\mathbf{x}^i\mathbf{W} - \mathbf{x}^j\mathbf{W}\|_2^2 s_{ij} + \gamma s_{ij}^2 \right) + \lambda \|\mathbf{W}\|_{2,1} + \mu \mathrm{Tr}(\mathbf{P}^T\mathbf{L_S}\mathbf{P})$$

$$s.t. \quad \mathbf{s}^i\mathbf{1} = 1, 0 \le s_{ij} \le 1, \mathbf{W}^T\mathbf{W} = \mathbf{I}, \mathbf{P}^T\mathbf{P} = \mathbf{I}, \mathbf{P} \in \mathbb{R}^{n \times c}, \tag{5}$$

where μ is a hyperparameter that can be increased or decreased in each iteration when the connected components are smaller or greater than c, respectively.

4   Experiment

In this paper, all the subjects are collected from the PPMI dataset. There are 238 baseline subjects including 62 NC, 142 PD, and 34 SWEDD. There are 186 subjects including 54 NC, 123 PD, and 9 SWEDD subjects in 12 months. Meanwhile, there are 127 subjects including 7 NC, 88 PD, and 22 SWEDD in 24 months. The depression, sleep, smell, and cognition scores are evaluated by Geriatric Depression Scale (GDS), Epworth Sleepiness Scale (ESS), University of Pennsylvania Smell Identification Test (UPSIT), and Montreal Cognitive Assessment (MoCA), respectively.

4.1   Image Preprocessing

As for MRI data preprocessing, we first perform anterior commissure-posterior commissure (ACPC) reorientation and then use VBM tool [13] to extract GM from brain images. Finally, we register the segmented GM with the automated anatomical labeling (AAL) atlas [14] and then extract 116 features from GM using the registered AAL templates. As for DTI data preprocessing, we use FSL toolbox [15] to correct eddy current distortion and then calculate L1 and V1. Finally, we carry out ACPC reorientation on L1 and V1 data and use AAL to extract 116 dimensional features, respectively.

4.2   Experimental Setting

In our study, two future time points, both 12 months and 24 months data are used to evaluate the proposed method. Specifically, we conduct two binary classification experiments: NC vs. PD, and NC vs. SWEDD. Meanwhile, we consider four scores prediction and a label classification using a 10-fold cross-validation method to validate the performance of the proposed method using baseline data.

To estimate the classification performance, we utilize the quantitative measurements including accuracy (ACC), sensitivity (SEN), precision (PREC), and area under the receiver operating characteristic (ROC) curve (AUC). To validate the effectiveness of regression between the predicted and target clinical sores, we further calculate the correlation coefficient (CC)

We compare the present method with state-of-the-art methods including: (1) The Laplacian score (Lscore) with unsupervised feature selection [7]; (2) The RSFS simultaneously using ℓ_1-norm and FME for robust unsupervised feature selection [11]; (3) The M3T without regularization terms for supervised feature selection [3]; (4) The MMSL considering the relations among rows or the information among columns in response variables for supervised feature selection [6].

4.3   Classification Performance

Table 1 summarizes the classification performances of NC vs. PD, and NC vs. SWEDD in longitudinal multi-modality features. Overall, we can see that the proposed method is superior to the other method in all cases. Meanwhile, in the vertical direction, the established model by the proposed method achieves the steadiest performance, such as the accuracies of 81.45%, 83.05% and 97.14% for NC vs. PD, and the accuracies of 88.67%, 93.65% and 82.76% for NC vs. SWEDD, respectively.

Owing to not use labels and diagnostic information, unsupervised feature selection is more difficult than supervised feature selection. However, we can see that our method with unsupervised feature selection has better performance than M3T and MMSL methods with supervised feature selection. For example, in NC vs. PD, the proposed method has a higher accuracy (e.g., 81.45% vs. 79.40%) than M3T method using baseline data. In NC vs. SWEDD, the proposed method has a higher accuracy (e.g., 88.67% vs. 82.44%) than M3T method using baseline data. The reason is that the proposed method can effectively learn the inherent information of the data than these

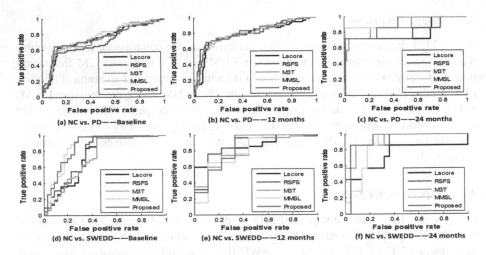

Fig. 2. ROC curves for longitudinal data using all method

Table 1. Classification performance of all methods. Boldface denotes the best performance.

Time	Method	NC vs. PD				NC vs. SWEDD			
		ACC	SEN	PREC	AUC	ACC	SEN	PREC	AUC
Baseline	Lscore	79.45	63.57	70.60	79.67	83.67	98.33	81.41	85.00
	RSFS	79.90	66.67	74.19	82.23	85.56	100.00	84.50	87.82
	M3T	79.40	62.62	75.21	80.82	82.44	100.00	80.98	84.90
	MMSL	80.88	67.62	**79.64**	82.80	87.56	100.00	86.85	**93.97**
	Proposed	**81.45**	**71.19**	79.54	**84.04**	**88.67**	100.00	**88.63**	92.98
12 m	Lscore	80.23	62.96	69.39	77.82	90.48	100.00	90.00	92.59
	RSFS	83.62	72.22	82.05	80.55	92.06	100.00	100.00	**98.56**
	M3T	80.23	64.81	68.63	79.39	90.48	100.00	92.86	95.47
	MMSL	81.36	**100.00**	**100.00**	80.68	92.06	100.00	96.08	97.53
	Proposed	**83.05**	85.19	80.65	**83.24**	**93.65**	100.00	**100.00**	98.35
24 m	Lscore	96.19	57.14	80.00	80.76	58.62	85.71	35.29	93.51
	RSFS	97.14	85.71	100.00	95.63	72.41	100.00	46.67	96.75
	M3T	94.29	71.43	57.14	91.40	65.65	100.00	41.18	95.45
	MMSL.	**98.10**	**100.00**	100.00	**96.21**	72.41	100.00	46.67	98.05
	Proposed	97.14	85.71	**100.00**	94.61	**82.76**	100.00	**58.33**	**100.00**

supervised methods that emphasize the largest linear-related multitasking targets but ignore the importance of the inherent information of the learning data itself. In addition, Fig. 2 shows various ROC curves, which further validate the good performance achieved by our proposed method.

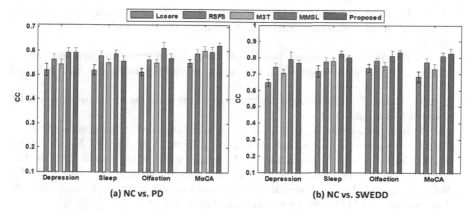

Fig. 3. Regression performance of the competing methods on the baseline data

4.4 Regression Performance

The values of CC are used to evaluate the regression performance, and results of CC are shown in Fig. 3. In the NC vs. PD, our proposed method has the best performance in prediction of depression and MoCA scores, which are 0.5920 (CC) and 0.6223 (CC). For sleep and olfaction scores, MMSL method achieves the best performance, which are 0.5887 (CC) and 0.6127 (CC).

In NC vs. SWEDD, our proposed method has the best performance in prediction of olfaction and MoCA scores, which are 0.8312 (CC) and 0.8256 (CC). For depression and sleep scores, MMSL method achieves the best performance, which are 0.7899 (CC) and 0.8236 (CC).

5 Conclusion

In this study, a new unsupervised feature selection method via joint embedding learning and sparse regression is proposed to simultaneously conduct two binary classifications and four clinical scores prediction for PD disease diagnosis using the longitudinal multi-modal neuroimaging data. Extensive experiments based on PPMI dataset demonstrate the performance of the proposed method outperforms its counterparts. In the meantime, for the classification performance in the vertical direction, the established model by our method has the steadiest performance.

References

1. Kalia, L.V., Lang, A.E.: Parkinson's disease. Lancet **386**, 896–912 (2015)
2. Lotharius, J., Brundin, P.: Pathogenesis of Parkinson's disease: dopamine, vesicles and [alpha]-synuclein. Nat. Rev. Neurosci. **3**, 932–942 (2002)

3. Zhang, D., Shen, D.: Multi-modal multi-task learning for joint prediction of multiple regression and classification variables in Alzheimer's disease. NeuroImage **59**, 895–907 (2012)
4. Nie, F., Zhu, W., Li, X.: Unsupervised feature selection with structured graph optimization. In: Proceedings of the Thirtieth AAAI Conference on Artificial Intelligence, pp. 1302–1308 (2016)
5. Zou, H., Hastie, T.: Regularization and variable selection via the elastic net. J. Roy. Stat. Soc. B **67**, 301–320 (2005)
6. Lei, H., Huang, Z., Zhang, J., Yang, Z., et al.: Joint detection and clinical score prediction in Parkinson's disease via multi-modal sparse learning. Expert. Syst. Appl. **80**, 284–296 (2017)
7. He, X., Cai, D., Niyogi, P.: Laplacian score for feature selection. In: Proceedings of the 18th International Conference on Neural Information Processing Systems, pp. 507–514 (2005)
8. Wang, S., Tang, J., Liu, H.: Embedded unsupervised feature selection. In: Proceedings of the Twenty-Ninth AAAI Conference on Artificial Intelligence, pp. 470–476 (2015)
9. Cai, D., Zhang, C., He, X.: Unsupervised feature selection for multi-cluster data. In: Proceedings of the 16th ACM SIGKDD International Conference on Knowledge Discovery and Data Mining, pp. 333–342 (2010)
10. Nie, F., Xu, D., Tsang, I.W.H., Zhang, C.: Flexible manifold embedding: a framework for semi-supervised and unsupervised dimension reduction. IEEE Trans. Image Process. **19**, 1921–1932 (2010)
11. Shi, L., Du, L., Shen, Y.D.: Robust spectral learning for unsupervised feature selection. In: 2014 IEEE International Conference on Data Mining, pp. 977–982 (2014)
12. Fan, K.: On a theorem of Weyl concerning eigenvalues of linear transformations I. Proc. Natl. Acad. Sci. U.S.A. **35**, 652–655 (1949)
13. Whitwell, J.L.: Voxel-based morphometry: an automated technique for assessing structural changes in the brain. J. Neurosci. **29**, 9661–9664 (2009)
14. Tzourio-Mazoyer, N., Landeau, B., Papathanassiou, D., Crivello, F., et al.: Automated anatomical labeling of activations in SPM using a macroscopic anatomical parcellation of the MNI MRI single-subject brain. NeuroImage **15**, 273–289 (2002)
15. Jenkinson, M., Beckmann, C.F., Behrens, T.E., Woolrich, M.W., Smith, S.M.: FSL. NeuroImage **62**, 782–790 (2012)

Prostate Cancer Classification on VERDICT DW-MRI Using Convolutional Neural Networks

Eleni Chiou[1,2]([✉]), Francesco Giganti[3,4], Elisenda Bonet-Carne[5], Shonit Punwani[5], Iasonas Kokkinos[1], and Eleftheria Panagiotaki[1,2]

[1] Department of Computer Science, UCL, London, UK
eleni.chiou.17@ucl.ac.uk
[2] Centre for Medical Image Computing, UCL, London, UK
[3] Department of Radiology, UCLH NHS Foundation Trust, London, UK
[4] Division of Surgery and Interventional Science, UCL, London, UK
[5] Division of Medicine, Centre for Medical Imaging, UCL, London, UK

Abstract. Currently, non-invasive imaging techniques such as magnetic resonance imaging (MRI) are emerging as powerful diagnostic tools for prostate cancer (PCa) characterization. This paper focuses on automated PCa classification on VERDICT (Vascular, Extracellular and Restricted Diffusion for Cytometry in Tumors) diffusion weighted (DW)-MRI, which is a non-invasive microstructural imaging technique that comprises a rich imaging protocol and a tissue computational model to map in vivo histological indices. The contribution of the paper is two fold. Firstly, we investigate the potential of automated, model-free PCa classification on raw VERDICT DW-MRI. Secondly, we attempt to adapt and evaluate novel fully convolutional neural networks (FCNNs) for PCa characterization. We present two neural network architectures that adapt U-Net and ResNet-18 to the PCa classification problem. We train the networks end-to-end on DW-MRI data and evaluate the diagnostic performance employing a 10-fold cross validation approach using data acquired from 103 patients. ResNet-18 outperforms U-Net with an average AUC of 86.7%. Our results show promise for the utilization of raw VERDICT DW-MRI data and FCNNs for automating the PCa diagnostic pathway.

Keywords: VERDICT MRI · Prostate cancer classification
Convolutional neural networks

1 Introduction

Prostate cancer (PCa) is the second most common cancer among men worldwide [1]. Early diagnosis and treatment are crucial to decrease the mortality rate in patients. Thus, the development of reliable and automated diagnostic tools is imperative. Currently, multi-parametric (mp)-magnetic resonance imaging (MRI), which consists of T2-weighted (T2W)-MRI, diffusion-weighted (DW)-MRI and dynamic contrast enhanced (DCE)-MRI, has become a useful tool for

© Springer Nature Switzerland AG 2018
Y. Shi et al. (Eds.): MLMI 2018, LNCS 11046, pp. 319–327, 2018.
https://doi.org/10.1007/978-3-030-00919-9_37

non-invasive PCa diagnosis. Moreover, VERDICT (Vascular, Extracellular and Restricted Diffusion for Cytometry in Tumors) DW-MRI, which is an advanced microstructural imaging technique for cancer characterization has currently been proposed as an additional, powerful diagnostic tool. However, radiological interpretation of different MRI sequences for PCa characterization remains a complex and time-consuming task.

Several methods for automated diagnosis of PCa on mp-MRI have been proposed to improve diagnostic accuracy and speed up the decision-making process. State-of-the-art methods use deep learning to classify and localize PCa on mp-MRI. For example, Kiraly et al. proposed a multi-channel image-to-image convolutional encoder-decoder to classify lesions achieving an area under the curve (AUC) of 83% [2]. Mehrtash et al. used a 3D convolutional neural network for automated detection of PCa on mp-MRI and reported an AUC of 80% [3]. However, these studies share a common limitation, i.e., they rely on mp-MRI data, which despite its merits has been shown to have low specificity [4].

DW-MRI has been demonstrated to be the most important component of mp-MRI compared to T2W-MRI and DCE-MRI due to its high sensitivity to microstructural changes related to cancer [5,6]. However, mp-MRI studies use DW-MRI in its simplest form by deriving the ADC map. This simplified model of water diffusion lacks biological specificity as it fails to discriminate the variety of histological changes that occur in cancer [7]. VERDICT DW-MRI improves on ADC maps by modelling directly the underlying microstructure [8,9]. More specifically, VERDICT combines an optimized DW-MRI acquisition protocol with a mathematical model to estimate and map microstructural features such as cell size, density, and vascular volume fraction, all of which change in cancer.

In this paper, we first aim to investigate the potential of model-free PCa characterization using the raw DW-MRI data from the VERDICT acquisition. Second, we attempt to adapt and evaluate fully convolutional neural networks (FCNNs) for automated characterization of PCa on VERDICT DW-MRI data.

2   Methods

2.1   VERDICT DW-MRI Data

In this study we use VERDICT DW-MRI data from 103 patients. VERDICT DW-MRI images (Fig. 1) were acquired with pulsed-gradient spin-echo sequence (PGSE) using an optimised imaging protocol for VERDICT prostate characterization with 5 b-values ($90, 500, 1500, 2000, 3000\,\mathrm{s/mm^2}$) in 3 orthogonal directions, on a 3T scanner (Achieva, Philips Healthcare, NL) [10]. Also, images with $b = 0\,\mathrm{s/mm^2}$ were acquired before each b-value acquisition. The DW-MRI sequence was acquired with a voxel size of $1.25 \times 1.25 \times 5\,\mathrm{mm^3}$, 5 mm slice thickness, 14 slices, a field of view of $220{\times}220\,\mathrm{mm^2}$ and the images were reconstructed to a $176{\times}176$ matrix size. The data was registered using rigid registration [11]. A dedicated radiologist highly experienced in prostate mp-MRI reporting (reporting more than 1000 scans per year) contoured malignant and benign lesions on the registered VERDICT DW-MRI using mp-MRI for guidance.

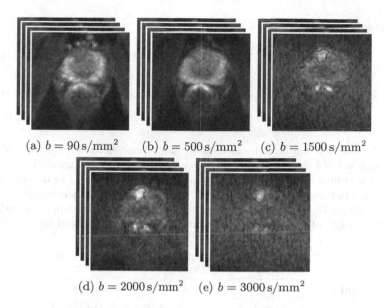

(a) $b = 90\,\mathrm{s/mm^2}$ (b) $b = 500\,\mathrm{s/mm^2}$ (c) $b = 1500\,\mathrm{s/mm^2}$

(d) $b = 2000\,\mathrm{s/mm^2}$ (e) $b = 3000\,\mathrm{s/mm^2}$

Fig. 1. VERDICT DW-MRI data acquired with 5 b-values in 3 orthogonal directions. Cancerous regions (noted in blue) are seen as a focus of high signal intensity on DW-MRI of $b = 2000, 3000\,\mathrm{s/mm^2}$ and as a focus of low signal intensity on the corresponding $b = 90\,\mathrm{s/mm^2}$ image.

2.2 Fully Convolutional Neural Networks

We formulate the problem as pixel-wise classification and use FCNNs trained end-to-end, on DW-MRI data. FCNNs have shown great success on pixel-wise classification tasks [12–14]. They adapt standard CNNs to the pixel-wise classification problem by converting fully connected layers to convolutional layers and adding upsampling layers to reach the original image resolution. They get as input the entire image and produce pixel-wise class probability maps. We implement and evaluate two encoder-decoder FCNNs. Encoder-decoder networks extract low resolution feature maps in the encoder module and gradually map them to full input resolution feature maps in the corresponding decoder module [13–15].

Objective Function. We consider two classes (malignant, benign/normal) and perform pixel-wise classification on predefined regions of interest (ROIs) on DW-MRI data. We define a label set $\mathcal{L} = \{0, 1, 2\}$, where 0 corresponds to benign/normal, 1 to malignant and 2 to ambiguous. Let $\mathbf{I} \in \mathbb{R}^{176 \times 176 \times 20}$ be a 20-channel DW-MRI image and $\mathbf{L} \in \mathcal{L}^{176 \times 176}$ the corresponding labelling. Also, let $\mathbf{P} \in [0, 1]^{176 \times 176}$ be the pixel-wise probability map indicating the probability of each pixel to belong to class 1. We train the networks using pixel-wise cross-entropy on pixels $j = \{j : l_j \neq 2,$ where l_j the label of pixel $j\}$. The cross-entropy loss is defined as

$$\text{CE} = -\sum_j l_j \log(p_j) + (1 - l_j) \log(1 - p_j), \tag{1}$$

where p_j is the probability of pixel j belonging to class 1 and l_j is the class label of pixel j.

Table 1. MRI-UNet. The encoder module includes 3 encoder blocks (encBlock). Each encBlock consists of a convolutional layer (conv) followed by batch normalization (BN), a rectified-linear unit (ReLU) and a max pooling operation (pool). The decoder module includes 3 decoder blocks (decBlock). Each decBlock consists of a convolutional layer followed by BN, a ReLU and a transposed convolution (convTransp). The last block (outBlock) consists of 2 convolutional layers. The last convolutional layer is followed by a pixel-wise softmax.

	Layer	Description
inBlock	input	64×64 DW-MRI images
encBlock1	conv1	3×3, 64, stride 1, BN, ReLU
	pool1	2×2 maxpooling, stride 2
encBlock2	conv2	3×3, 128, stride 1, BN, ReLU
	pool2	2×2 maxpooling, stride 2
encBlock3	conv3	3×3, 256, stride 1, BN, ReLU
	pool3	2×2 maxpooling, stride 2
decBlock1	conv4	3×3, 256, stride 1, BN, ReLU
	convTransp1	2×2, 256, stride 2
dencBlock2	conv5	3×3, 256, stride 1, BN, ReLU
	convTransp2	2×2, 128, stride 2
dencBlock3	conv6	3×3, 128, stride 1, BN, ReLU
	convTransp3	2×2, 64, stride 2
outBlock	conv7	3×3, 64, stride 1, BN, ReLU
	conv8	1×1, 2, stride 1, softmax

Network Architectures. The first network (MRI-UNet) (Table 1) is based on the U-Net architecture proposed in [13]. U-Net consists of an encoder module and a symmetric decoder module. MRI-UNet has fewer convolutional layers to avoid overfitting. The encoder module includes 3 encoder blocks (encBlock). Each encBlock consists of a convolutional layer followed by batch normalization (BN) [16], a rectified-linear unit (ReLU) [17] and a 2×2 max pooling operation with stride 2. Each convolutional layer performs 2D convolutions of the input maps with 3×3 kernels. The decoder module includes 3 decoder blocks (decBlock). Each decBlock consists of a convolutional layer followed by BN, a

Table 2. MRI-ResNet. The encoder module includes 3 encoder blocks (encBlock). Each encBlock consists of 2 convolutional layers (conv) each followed by batch normalization (BN) and a rectified-linear unit (ReLU). The decoder module includes 3 decoder blocks (decBlock). Each decBlock consists of a bilinear upsampling operation (bilUp) followed by 2 convolutional layers. The last convolutional layer is followed by a pixel-wise softmax.

	Layer	Description
inBlock	input	64 × 64 DW-MRI images
	conv1	7 × 7, 64, stride 2, BN, ReLU
encBlock1	conv2	3 × 3, 64, stride 1, BN, ReLU
	conv3	3 × 3, 64, stride 1, BN, ReLU
encBlock2	conv4	3 × 3, 128, stride 2, BN, ReLU
	conv5	3 × 3, 128, stride 1, BN, ReLU
encBlock3	conv6	3 × 3, 128, stride 2, BN, ReLU
	conv7	3 × 3, 128, stride 1, BN, ReLU
decBlock1	bilUp1	scale factor 2
	conv8	1 × 1, 128, stride 1, BN, ReLU
	conv9	3 × 3, 64, stride 1, BN, ReLU
decBlock2	bilUp2	scale factor 2
	conv10	1 × 1, 64, stride 1, BN, ReLU
	conv11	3 × 3, 64, stride 1, BN, ReLU
decBlock3	bilUp3	scale factor 2
	conv12	1 × 1, 64, stride 1, BN, ReLU
	conv13	3 × 3, 2, stride 1, BN, softmax

ReLU and a 2 × 2 transposed convolution with stride 2 to upsample low resolution feature maps. Concatenation of the upsampled feature maps with the corresponding encoder feature maps is performed before the convolutional layers. Each convolutional layer performs 2D convolutions of the input with 3 × 3 kernels. The last convolutional layer is followed by a pixel-wise softmax which provides class probability maps.

The second network (MRI-ResNet) has also an encoder-decoder structure (Table 2). The encoder module is similar to the ResNet-18 network proposed in [18]. We remove the max pooling layer in the beginning of the network and the global average pooling layer at the end of the network. Also, we replace the last fully-connected layer with a convolutional layer and decrease the number of convolutional layers. The encoder module includes 3 encBlock. Each encBlock consists of 2 convolutional layers each followed by BN and a ReLU. The decoder module is similar to the one proposed in [15] and has 3 decBlock. Each decBlock consists of a bilinear upsapmling operation followed by 2 convolutional layers. The low resolution feature maps are bilinear upsampled by a factor of 2 and then concatenated with the corresponding encoder feature maps. Then, a 1 × 1 convolutional layer followed by a 3×3 convolutional layer are applied to reduce the number of feature maps and refine the features. The last convolutional layer is followed by a pixel-wise softmax.

Training Settings. We implement both networks using Pytorch [19]. We employ a 10-fold cross validation (CV) approach to train and test the networks. We repeat each 10-fold CV 5 times. We train the networks for 200 epochs and select the model which has the smallest loss on a validation set (20% of the training set). We use stochastic gradient descent (SGD) with a mini-batch size of 32, a constant learning rate of 1e-5, a momentum of 0.9 and a weight decay of 1e-3.

Evaluation Metrics. We evaluate the binary pixel-wise classification using average sensitivity, specificity, AUC and precision. Sensitivity, specificity and precision are defined as

- sensitivity $= \frac{TP}{P}$, where TP is the number of true positive pixels and P is the number of positive pixels.
- specificity $= \frac{TN}{N}$, where TN is the number of true negative pixels and N is the number of negative pixels.
- precision $= \frac{TP}{FP+TP}$, where FP is the number of false positive pixels.

Table 3. Average AUC, sensitivity, specificity, precision of MRI-UNet and MRI-ResNet when evaluation is performed on (i) malignant and benign ROIs (malignant vs benign ROIs) and (ii) the entire image (malignant vs all).

Networks	Regions	AUC	Sensitivity	Specificity	Precision
MRI-UNet	Malignant vs benign ROIs	85.7%	75.7%	75.4%	86.2%
	malignant vs all	74.1%	75.6%	47.6%	2.0%
MRI-ResNet	Malignant vs benign ROIs	86.7%	71.8%	83.3%	90.0%
	Malignant vs all	71.9%	71.6%	57.1%	4.7%

Table 4. Average AUC, sensitivity, specificity, precision of MRI-UNet and MRI-ResNet when evaluation is performed on (i) malignant and benign ROIs (malignant vs benign ROIs) and (ii) the entire image (malignant vs all) when we use additional negative labelled ROIs.

Networks	Regions	AUC	Sensitivity	Specificity	Precision
MRI-UNet	Malignant vs benign ROIs	89.0%	82.9%	77.9%	88.8%
	Malignant vs all	94.2%	82.7%	91.2%	13.4%
MRI-ResNet	Malignant vs benign ROIs	87.6%	86.4%	72.6%	86.7%
	Malignant vs all	94.0%	86.4%	88.8%	11.2%

3   Results

We perform two different experiments and report the results.

1st Experiment. In the first experiment we train the networks on predefined malignant and benign/normal ROIs and ignore the rest of the pixels. Then, we evaluate the classification performance of the networks on (i) predefined malignant and benign/normal ROIs and (ii) the entire image (Table 3). In the second case regions which are not labelled as malignant are considered as benign/normal. Using MRI-ResNet results in slightly improved performance (AUC of 86.7%). Figure 2 shows the receiver operating characteristic (ROC) curves of MRI-UNet and MRI-ResNet when evaluation is performed on (i) predefined malignant and benign/normal ROIs and (ii) the entire image.

2nd Experiment. In the previous experiment the dataset is highly unbalanced since the number of malignant ROIs is higher than the number of benign/normal ROIs. To address this issue, we increase the number of negative labelled ROIs by randomly selecting and adding normal/background ROIs to the training set. Table 4 shows the classification performance of the networks when we increase the number of negative labelled ROIs. Using additional negative labelled ROIs improves AUC when classification is performed on the predefined regions or the entire image. Figure 3 shows the ROC curves of MRI-UNet and MRI-ResNet when evaluation is performed on (i) predefined malignant and benign ROIs and (ii) the entire image.

The results show that MRI-ResNet achieves an AUC of 86.7% in classifying benign and malignant ROIs. A recent study which uses an encoder-decoder network for classification of malignant and benign regions on the PROSTATEx dataset [20] reports a maximum AUC of 83.4% using mp-MRI data and a maximum AUC of 80.4% using the ADC map derived from the DW-MRI data [2]. Comparison of our results to the results of this study shows that VERDICT DW-MRI data combined with FCNNs give comparable performance and could be used as an alternative automated diagnostic tool for PCa classification. However, this comparison is limited due to the difference in the two datasets.

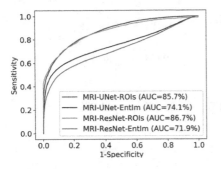

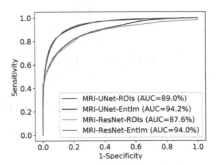

Fig. 2. 1st experiment. Receiver operating characteristic (ROC) curves of MRI-UNet and MRI-ResNet when evaluation is performed on (i) predefined malignant and benign ROIs and (ii) the entire image (EntIm).

Fig. 3. 2nd experiment. Receiver operating characteristic (ROC) curves of MRI-UNet and MRI-ResNet when evaluation is performed on (i) predefined malignant and benign ROIs and (ii) the entire image (EntIm).

4   Conclusion

We investigate the potential of model-free PCa classification on the raw VERDICT DW-MRI data using FCNNs. For this purpose, we adapt and evaluate two FCNN architectures. Previous studies are based on mp-MRI data to provide an automated solution for PCa classification. In this study, we use richer DW-MRI compared to DW-MRI from mp-MRI acquisitions, acquired for 5 b-values in 3 orthogonal directions to train and evaluate the FCNNs. MRI-ResNet behaves better than MRI-UNet achieving an AUC of 86.7% in classifying malignant and benign regions. The results indicate that VERDICT DW-MRI data combined with FCNNs show promise as an alternative diagnostic tool for PCa classification.

Future work will address the PCa classification problem in the entire image. The proposed networks are not suitable for PCa classification in the entire image due to foreground-background class imbalance characterizing the data. To address this issue we plan to include an additional step for prostate segmentation so as to limit the analysis on the prostate region. Finally, we plan to investigate techniques to provide visual explanations of decision from FCNNs models, which is crucial for medical diagnosis applications.

Acknowledgments. This research is funded by EPSRC grand EP/N021967/1. The Titan Xp used for this research was donated by the NVIDIA Corporation.

References

1. Torre, L.A., et al.: Global cancer statistics, 2012. CA Cancer J. Clin. **65**, 87–108 (2015)
2. Kiraly, A.P., et al.: Deep convolutional encoder-decoders for prostate cancer detection and classification. In: MICCAI (2017)
3. Mehrtash, A., et al.: Classification of clinical significance of MRI prostate findings using 3D convolutional neural networks. Proc. SPIE Int. Soc. Opt. Eng. (2017)
4. Ahmed, H.U., et al.: Diagnostic accuracy of multi-parametric MRI and TRUS biopsy in prostate cancer (PROMIS): a paired validating confirmatory study. Lancet **389**, 815–822 (2017)
5. Isebaert, S., et al.: Multiparametric MRI for prostate cancer localization in correlation to wholemount histopathology. J. Magn. Reson. Imaging **37**, 1392–1401 (2013)
6. Metzger, G.J., et al.: Detection of prostate cancer: Quantitative multiparametric MR imaging models developed using registered correlative histopathology. Radiology **279**, 805–816 (2016)
7. Bourne, R., et al.: Limitations and prospects for diffusion-weighted MRI of the prostate. Diagnostics **6**, 21 (2016)
8. Panagiotaki, E., et al.: Noninvasive quantification of solid tumor microstructure using VERDICT MRI. Cancer Res. **74**, 1902–1912 (2014)
9. Panagiotaki, E., et al.: Microstructural characterization of normal and malignant human prostate tissue with vascular, extracellular, and restricted diffusion for cytometry in tumours magnetic resonance imaging. Invest. Radiol. **50**, 218–227 (2015)
10. Panagiotaki, E., et al.: Optimised VERDICT MRI protocol for prostate cancer characterisation. In: ISMRM (2015)
11. Ourselin, S., et al.: Reconstructing a 3D structure from serial histological sections. Image Vis. Comput. **19**, 25–31 (2001)
12. Long, J., et al.: Fully convolutional networks for semantic segmentation. In: CVPR (2015)
13. Ronneberger, O., et al.: U-Net: Convolutional networks for biomedical image segmentation. In: MICCAI (2015)
14. Badrinarayanan, V.: Segnet: a deep convolutional encoder-decoder architecture for image segmentation. IEEE Trans. Pattern Anal. Mach. Intel. **39**, 2481–2495 (2017)
15. Chen, L.C., et al.: Encoder-decoder with atrous separable convolution for semantic image segmentation. ArXiv (2018)
16. Ioffe, S., et al.: Batch normalization: accelerating deep network training by reducing internal covariate shift. In: ICML (2015)
17. Nair, V., et al.: Rectified linear units improve restricted boltzmann machines. In: ICML (2010)
18. He, K., et al.: Deep residual learning for image recognition. In: CVPR (2016)
19. Paszke, A., et al.: Automatic differentiation in pytorch. In: Autodiff Workshop, NIPS (2017)
20. Litjens, G., et al.: Computer-aided detection of prostate cancer in MRI. IEEE Trans. Med. Imaging **33**, 1083–1092 (2014)

Detection of the Pharyngeal Phase in the Videofluoroscopic Swallowing Study Using Inflated 3D Convolutional Networks

Jong Taek Lee[1(✉)] and Eunhee Park[2,3]

[1] Electronics and Telecommunications Research Institute, Daegu,
South Korea
jongtaeklee@etri.re.kr
[2] Department of Rehabilitation Medicine,
Kyungpook National University Chilgok Hospital, Daegu, South Korea
[3] Department of Rehabilitation Medicine, School of Medicine,
Kyungpook National University, Daegu, South Korea

Abstract. Videofluoroscopic swallowing study (VFSS) is a standard diagnostic tool for dysphagia. Previous computer assisted analysis of VFSS required manual preparation to mark several anatomical structures and to select time intervals of interest such as a pharyngeal phase during swallowing. These processes were still costly and challenging for clinicians. In this study, we present a novel approach to detect the pharyngeal phase of swallowing through whole of VFSS video clips using Inflated 3D Convolutional Networks (I3D) without additional manual annotations.

Keywords: Action classification · Dysphagia · Inflated 3D convolutional networks · Videofluoroscopic swallowing study

1 Introduction

Dysphagia is a common symptom in older individuals [8] as well as several patients with central nervous system diseases, head and neck cancers, gastroesophageal disorders, and neuromuscular disorders [9]. Dysphagia can cause severe medical complications such as aspiration pneumonia, malnutrition, or death [9]. Therefore, accurate evaluation of swallowing function is essential to determine suitable therapeutic strategies for each individual.

The videofluoroscopic swallowing study (VFSS) is the gold standard test for diagnosis as dysphagia [12]. The subject ingests radiopaque foods or bolus via a fluoroscopy during the VFSS procedure. After the VFSS procedure, a clinician repeatedly inspects the recorded video in order to evaluate transit time of bolus, movement in anatomical structures, and presence of airway protection during swallowing process [12]. In recorded videofluoroscopic images, the swallowing

© Springer Nature Switzerland AG 2018
Y. Shi et al. (Eds.): MLMI 2018, LNCS 11046, pp. 328–336, 2018.
https://doi.org/10.1007/978-3-030-00919-9_38

process is composed of four complex and very short (around several seconds) phases as follows: the oral preparatory phase, the oral phase, the pharyngeal phase, and the esophageal phase (see Fig. 1). However, distinguishing swallowing phases and measuring structural or functional abnormalities of process through visual inspection is of a subjective nature for clinical interpretations.

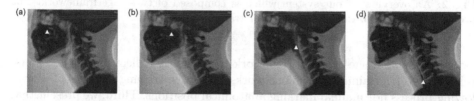

Fig. 1. Normal swallowing phase during a thick liquid bolus. (a) During the oral preparatory phase, a food is chewed and mixed with the saliva then formed into a bolus. (b) During the oral phase, the tongue pushes the bolus to the back of the mouth via an anterior to posterior squeezing motion. (c) During the pharyngeal phase, the airway is closed to prevent a transport of the bolus to the airway system. (d) Finally, during the esophageal phase, the bolus passes down the esophagus to the stomach. White triangles mean positions of the bolus at four different phases.

To quantify and measure parameters in the swallowing process from videofluoroscopic images, several software applications have been developed [1,3,5–7,10,11]. Traditional applications [3,7] provided a motion analysis of the anatomical points using a user-defined region-of-interest (ROI) from frame-to-frame. Recent quantitative analyses in VFSS tried to semi-automatically track the hyoid bone movement during swallowing [1,6,10,11]. However, these works have been labor-intensive as they required (1) selecting a specific interval of interest (*e.g.*, one pharyngeal phase), (2) defining the ROI (*e.g.*, hyoid bone) in single frame or every frame, and (3) calculating the coordination of anatomical landmarks in order to compensate for the subjects movement in each frame. Also, a clinician needed abundant time to be skilled for traditional image processing software (*e.g.*, Matlab).

In this study, we try to address such labor-intensive tasks for testing stage in analyzing VFSS images. The main reason for selection of an interval of interest, manual definition of the ROI, and registration of anatomical positions is that the entire VFSS video is extremely complicated. In this paper, we propose a novel system to detect a pharyngeal phase of swallowing through whole recorded videofluoroscopic images using inflated 3D ConvNets (I3D) [2]. The first stage detects pharyngeal phase candidates based on optical flow. Then, the I3D networks improves accuracy of the pharyngeal phase which nature is sophisticated and is conjugated with abrupt other motions (e.g head and neck movement).

Our contribution in this paper is threefold. First, we utilize unprecedented clinical dataset which indicated multiple levels of swallowing function from normal to severe dysphagia of 1,085 VFSS video clips in 144 subjects. Second,

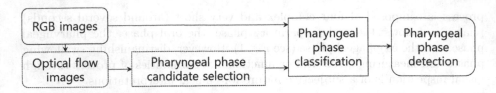

Fig. 2. An overview of our system which is composed of two-stage framework. The processes in dotted boxes are required for training the network.

we propose two-stage cascade framework to efficiently collect pharyngeal phase related clips for training the I3D networks without specifying intervals of a swallowing process nor manual marking anatomical positions. Third, we present that pre-trained I3D action classification network can be applied to classify pharyngeal phase on the VFSS video which is significantly different from general human actions [4].

2   Methodology

We propose a two-stage framework to detect the pharyngeal phase in the VFSS video instances (see Fig. 2). First, we detect intervals of frames having high optical flow values in Y component. The first stage is able to generate pharyngeal phase candidates with a small number of false negatives (88 out of 1,085 clips) because the bolus flow is distinguishable in optical flow map in a pharyngeal phase. However, this stage suffers from high false positives (1,680 out of 3,354 candidates) because a pharyngeal phase is often confused by patients' other actions such as coughing and preparation of swallowing as the pharyngeal phase. Therefore, we trained 3D convolutional networks to classify the interval of video frames with the label whether the interval is in a pharyngeal phase or not. For training, the first stage is mandatory as it reduces the amount of annotation tasks and generates balanced data. For testing, the first stage is optional, but it is useful for saving the detection process when optical flow is provided.

2.1   Dataset

The VFSS dataset was collected from 144 subjects who complained subjective difficulties of swallowing during diets and visited the inpatient and outpatient clinic of Department of Rehabilitation Medicine at Kyungpook National University Chilgok Hospital from March to December in 2017. This retrospective study was approved by the Institutional Review Board at the Kyungpook National University Chilgok Hospital. Clinical characteristics in subjects are described in Table 1.

A clinician performed the VFSS procedure according to the standard manual guideline [12]. The subject seated upright in front of a fluoroscopic equipment (Shimadzu RF-1000-150, 81 kv, 400 mA, 160 ms, Japan) while the camera recorded a lateral view of the head and neck area during VFSS procedures. Each subject performed swallowing of the following 8 substances which were mixed with diluted barium: 3, 6, and 9 mL of thick liquid (fruit pudding) and of thin liquid (milk), semi-solid (boiled rice), and solid (rice). Some subjects did not completely swallow all substances because they indicated severe aspiration or delayed swallowing reflex during the VFSS procedure.

Table 1. Clinical characteristics in subjects who were subjectively complained in difficulties of swallowing and examined in videofluoroscopic swallowing study

Characteristics	Number (percent)
Sex, female	44 (30.56%)
Age, years old	63.26 ± 16.37 (20–87)
Underlying medical conditions caused by dysphagia	
Central nerve system disorders (stroke, Parkinson's disease, etc.)	52 (36.11%)
Neuromuscular diseases	31 (21.52%)
Cancer	25 (17.36%)
Other conditions (aging, pneumonia, etc.)	36 (25.0%)

The collected dataset has 1,085 video clips, each of which contains one process of each patient with one type of substances. The duration of video clips is from 8 s to 3 min. Patients with severe dysphagia required a substantially large amount of time for swallowing. We sample frames at 15 frames per second.

2.2 Generating Pharyngeal Phase Candidates Using Optical Flow

Video analysis in machine learning needs to consider two challenges: large memory requirement and video length variation. For example, a hundred frame video requires 100 times of bigger memory than single image. Also, a long video can easily contains irrelevant frames to the pharyngeal phase. Therefore, we suggest a selection process to collect intervals of pharyngeal phase candidates by using optical flow.

The selection process is follows. (1) After converting the videos to grayscale, we apply a TV-L1 optical flow algorithm [13,14]. (2) Values are truncated to the range of −10 to 10, and divided by 10. (3) If the maximum of absolute values in Y component in the center region of the frame is larger than threshold (0.4 was applied in this paper), give a vote on the frame and its eight nearest frames. (4) After all voting is finished, find the highest number of the votes. (5) If the number of votes is greater than threshold (2.5 was applied in this paper) and the frame is not marked, then choose the frame and mark its surrounding 20 frames. (6) Repeat step 5 until we have no more than 5 chosen intervals.

After the selection process, 3,354 pharyngeal phase candidates are generated from 1,085 video clips. In 997 video clips, 1,674 candidates are correctly selected and there are no generated candidates in pharyngeal phase intervals from 88 video clips. Optical flow visualization of pharyngeal phase candidates shows the difficulty of optical flow analysis due to abrupt subjects' movements (see Fig. 3).

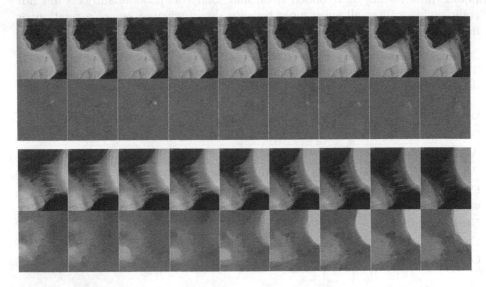

Fig. 3. Optical flow visualization of examples of the pharyngeal phase (top) and other actions (bottom, *e.g.*, head motions due to coughing) during ingesting thick liquid.

2.3 Training Inflated 3D Convolutional Networks Using RGB/Optical Flow/Joint

We experiment with I3D networks [2], which has 4 convolutional layers, 4 max-pooling layers, 9 inception modules, and 1 average-pooling layer. The models are pre-trained on ImageNet and Kinetics dataset [4]. We trained three I3D networks of different streams such as RGB only, optical flow only, and both of RGB and optical flow. The data of pharyngeal phase candidates is divided into two sets, 2,696 for training and 658 for testing.

The image is resized to 280×256 and at every training epoch, a 224×224 crop is randomly sampled near the center of the image. Our training used Adam optimizer with a mini-batch size of 6 and 0.1 initial learning rate. The training performance was saturated near 10K training iterations for one-stream I3D networks and near 30K for two-stream I3D networks. Two-stream I3D networks required the greater number of training iterations due to the high complexity of the network. Also, the processing time of one training step in two-stream I3D is three times longer than that in one-stream I3D. Therefore, the entire training process of two-stream I3Ds takes around ten times longer than that of one-stream I3Ds. Our implementation is derived from Tensorflow and 4 GPUs are used to perform training and testing.

Table 2. Accuracy rates of I3D networks using optical flow, RGB, and both

Method	# of training iterations	Accuracy rates
I3D-Flow	10 K	93.94%
I3D-RGB	10 K	95.91%
I3D-Joint	10 K	90.68%
I3D-Joint	30 K	95.64%

3   Experimental Results

We evaluated three I3D networks of single stream such as RGB (I3D-RGB) and optical flow (I3D-Flow) and two streams (I3D-Joint). The accuracy rate of the I3D-RGB was 2% higher than the I3D-Flow as shown in Table 2. The I3D-Joint showed only 90.68% accuracy rate when the network was trained by 10K iterations. When the I3D-Joint was trained by 30K iterations, the network showed 95.64% accuracy rate which is similar to the I3D-RGB. Although optical flow is very informative and provides distinctive directions, it can be also noisy due to patients' movement and video recording environments. Although two stream I3D networks showed better performance than single stream I3D networks in Kinetics, the performance difference between the I3D-RGB and I3D-Joint is negligible.

Figure 4 shows the Free Response Operating Characteristic (FROC) curve for the different streams (RGB and optical flow) of the network. They achieved a similar true positive rate (TPR) at around 0.03 false positives per clip (FPP), but the I3D-RGB achieved higher TPR at around 0.1 FPP.

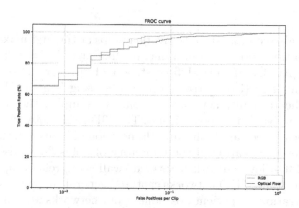

Fig. 4. Free response operating characteristic curve of the I3D-RGB and I3D-Flow. The I3D-RGB showed slightly better performance than the I3D-Flow.

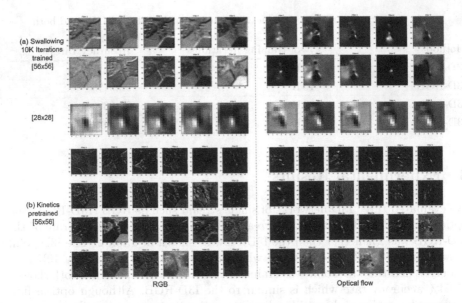

Fig. 5. Activation maps of sampled kernels of the I3D-RGB and I3D-Flow are on the left and on the right, respectively.

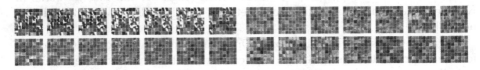

Fig. 6. Conv1 filter visualization of I3D-RGB (top left), I3D-Flow (top right), and I3D-Joint (bottom)

In Fig. 5, we also compared the activation maps at the first max-pooling layer in 56×56 resolution and the second max-pooling layer in 28×28 resolution of networks using RGB and optical flow stream of (a) our networks with 10K training iterations and (b) pre-trained networks using Kinetics dataset. Bright pixel values indicate highly activated region. We sampled the center frame in the sequence of activation map to display. The I3D-RGB networks captured the appearance of head, neck and bolus and the position of bolus. On the other hand, the I3D-Flow networks captured the trajectory of bolus flow. Also, both of the I3D-RGB and I3D-Flow networks captured swallowing related appearance and motion while pre-trained I3D networks captured general characteristics. Without any image registration for patient positioning, our networks were able to estimate the presence of bolus and its trajectory. The conv1 filter of the trained I3D-RGB, I3D-Flow, and I3D-Joint networks are shown in Fig. 6.

4 Conclusion

In this paper, we have presented a novel framework based on inflated 3D ConvNets to detect a pharyngeal phase during swallowing in VFSS. To the best of our knowledge, this is the first study to identify the pharyngeal phase of swallowing using the whole of VFSS video clips instead of using spatial or temporal segments with additional manual annotations. The algorithm is validated on large clinical dataset and achieves the state-of-the-art of human swallowing motion analysis. This study showed that a new framework could classify the pharyngeal phase of swallowing without any manual adjustments and should be a fundamental work for developing softwares of fully automatic analysis in VFSS.

References

1. Aung, M., Goulermas, J., Stanschus, S., Hamdy, S., Power, M.: Automated anatomical demarcation using an active shape model for videofluoroscopic analysis in swallowing. Med. Eng. Phys. **32**(10), 1170–1179 (2010)
2. Carreira, J., Zisserman, A.: Quo vadis, action recognition? a new model and the kinetics dataset. In: 2017 IEEE Conference on Computer Vision and Pattern Recognition (CVPR), pp. 4724–4733. IEEE (2017)
3. Dengel, G., Robbins, J., Rosenbek, J.C.: Image processing in swallowing and speech research. Dysphagia **6**(1), 30–39 (1991)
4. Kay, W., et al.: The kinetics human action video dataset. arXiv preprint arXiv:1705.06950 (2017)
5. Kellen, P.M., Becker, D.L., Reinhardt, J.M., Van Daele, D.J.: Computer-assisted assessment of hyoid bone motion from videofluoroscopic swallow studies. Dysphagia **25**(4), 298–306 (2010)
6. Lee, J.C., Nam, K.W., Jang, D.P., Paik, N.J., Ryu, J.S., Kim, I.Y.: A supporting platform for semi-automatic hyoid bone tracking and parameter extraction from videofluoroscopic images for the diagnosis of dysphagia patients. Dysphagia **32**(2), 315–326 (2017)
7. Logemann, J., Kahrilas, P., Begelman, J., Dodds, W., Pauloski, B.: Interactive computer program for biomechanical analysis of videoradiographic studies of swallowing. Am. J. Roentgenol. **153**(2), 277–280 (1989)
8. Logemann, J.A., Pauloski, B.R., Rademaker, A.W., Kahrilas, P.J.: Oropharyngeal swallow in younger and older women: videofluoroscopic analysis. J. Speech Lang. Hear. Res. **45**(3), 434–445 (2002)
9. Marik, P.E.: Aspiration pneumonitis and aspiration pneumonia. New Engl. J. Med. **344**(9), 665–671 (2001)
10. Molfenter, S.M., Steele, C.M.: Kinematic and temporal factors associated with penetration-aspiration in swallowing liquids. Dysphagia **29**(2), 269–276 (2014)
11. Noorwali, S.: Semi-automatic tracking of the hyoid bone and the epiglottis movements in digital videofluoroscopic images (2013)
12. Palmer, J.B., Kuhlemeier, K.V., Tippett, D.C., Lynch, C.: A protocol for the videofluorographic swallowing study. Dysphagia **8**(3), 209–214 (1993)
13. Pérez, J.S., Meinhardt-Llopis, E., Facciolo, G.: Tv-l1 optical flow estimation. Image Process. On Line **2013**, 137–150 (2013)

14. Zach, C., Pock, T., Bischof, H.: A Duality Based Approach for Realtime TV-L^1 Optical Flow. In: Hamprecht, Fred A., Schnörr, Christoph, Jähne, Bernd (eds.) DAGM 2007. LNCS, vol. 4713, pp. 214–223. Springer, Heidelberg (2007). https://doi.org/10.1007/978-3-540-74936-3_22

End-To-End Alzheimer's Disease Diagnosis and Biomarker Identification

Soheil Esmaeilzadeh[1], Dimitrios Ioannis Belivanis[1], Kilian M. Pohl[2], and Ehsan Adeli[1(✉)]

[1] Stanford University, Stanford, CA, USA
{soes,dbelivan,eadeli}@stanford.edu
[2] SRI International, Menlo Park, CA, USA
kilian.pohl@sri.com

Abstract. As shown in computer vision, the power of deep learning lies in automatically learning relevant and powerful features for any perdition task, which is made possible through end-to-end architectures. However, deep learning approaches applied for classifying medical images do not adhere to this architecture as they rely on several pre- and post-processing steps. This shortcoming can be explained by the relatively small number of available labeled subjects, the high dimensionality of neuroimaging data, and difficulties in interpreting the results of deep learning methods. In this paper, we propose a simple 3D Convolutional Neural Networks and exploit its model parameters to tailor the end-to-end architecture for the diagnosis of Alzheimer's disease (AD). Our model can diagnose AD with an accuracy of 94.1% on the popular ADNI dataset using only MRI data, which outperforms the previous state-of-the-art. Based on the learned model, we identify the disease biomarkers, the results of which were in accordance with the literature. We further transfer the learned model to diagnose mild cognitive impairment (MCI), the prodromal stage of AD, which yield better results compared to other methods.

1 Introduction

Alzheimer's disease is one of the most growing health issues, which devastated many lives, and the number of people with Alzheimer's dementia is predicted to be doubled within the next 20 years in the United States [2]. However, the basic understanding of the causes and mechanisms of the disease are yet to be explored. Currently, diagnosis is mainly performed by studying the individual's behavioral observations and medical history. Magnetic Resonance Imaging (MRI) is also used to analyze the brain morphometric patterns for identifying disease-specific imaging biomarkers.

This work was supported in part by NIH grants AA005965, AA017168, and MH11340-02, and benefited from the NIH Cloud Credits Model Pilot. The authors also thank the investigators within ADNI (http://adni.loni.ucla.edu).

Y. Shi et al. (Eds.): MLMI 2018, LNCS 11046, pp. 337–345, 2018.
https://doi.org/10.1007/978-3-030-00919-9_39

In recent years, numerous methods are introduced exploiting MRI data for distinguishing Alzheimer's Disease (AD) and its prodromal dementia stage, Mild Cognitive Impairment (MCI), from normal controls (NC). These approaches can be categorized in four main categories: Voxel-based methods [10], methods based on Regions-of-Interest (ROI) [6,7], patch-based methods [9], and approaches that leverage features from whole-image-levels (*i.e.*, without considering local structures within the MRIs) [13]. The voxel-based approaches are prone to overfitting [8] (due to high dimensionality input image) while ROI-based methods are confined to a coarse-scale limited number of ROIs [8] that may neglect crucial fine-scaled information secluded within or across different regions of the brain. Patch-based approaches often ignore global brain representations and focus solely on fixed-size rectangular (or cubic) image patches. In contrast, whole-image approaches cannot identify the subtle changes in fine brain structures. Leveraging a trade-off between the global and local representation of the brain can, therefore, contribute to a better understanding of the disease, while not overemphasizing on only one aspect.

With the recent developments of deep learning and Convolutional Neural Network (CNN) algorithms in computer vision studies, many such methods are developed for medical imaging applications. However, the majority of such previous works mainly focused on segmentation, registration, landmark or lesion detection [8]. For disease diagnosis, researchers have tried two-dimensional (2D) or three-dimensional (3D) patch-based models to train deep networks that diagnose diseases to a patch-level rather than subject-level. Only a few end-to-end deep learning methods (leveraging local and global MRI cues) are developed for the classification of neuroimages into different diagnostic groups [8,9], despite the power of deep learning owes to automatic feature learning made possible through end-to-end models. Not developing end-to-end models were mainly due to several limitations including: (1) not having enough labeled subjects in the datasets to train fully end-to-end models; (2) brain MRIs are 3D structures with high dimensionalities, which cause large computational costs; and (3) difficulties in interpretability of the results of end-to-end deep learning techniques from a neuroscience point-of-view. To resolve these challenges, instead of replicating standard deep learning architectures used in the computer vision domain, one requires explicit considerations and architectural designs. We conduct several experiments and tailor our architecture (through exploiting its numerous hyperparameters and architectural considerations) for classification of 3D MR images.

In this paper, we build a 3D Convolutional Neural Network (3D-CNN) and provide a simple method to interpret different regions of the brain and their association with the disease to identify AD biomarkers. Our method uses minimal preprocessing of MRIs (imposing minimum preprocessing artifacts) and utilizes a simple data augmentation strategy of downsampled MR images for training purposes. Unlike the vast majority of previous works, the proposed framework, thus, uses a voxel-based 3D-CNN to account for all voxels in the brain and capture the subtle *local* brain details in addition to better pronounced *global* specifics of MRIs. Using this detailed voxel-based representation of MRIs, we eliminate any a priori judgments for choosing ROIs or patches and take into account the whole brain. To avoid overfitting potentially caused by the large dimension of images, we carefully design our training model's architecture in a systematic way (not using standard computer vision architectures). We, then, propose a simple method to identify the MRI biomarkers of the disease by observing how confidently different regions of the brain contribute to the correct classification of the subjects. Finally, we propose a learning transfer strategy for MCI classification alongside the other two classes, in a three-class classification setting (AD, MCI, NC). Experiments on ADNI-1 dataset show superior results of our model compared to several baseline and prior works.

Table 1. ADNI-1 subjects demographic information.

Class	Sex	Count	Age					
			mean ± std	min	25%	50%	75%	max
AD	M	97	75.0 ± 7.9	55.2	70.8	75.3	80.4	91.0
	F	103	76.1 ± 7.4	56.5	71.1	77.0	82.3	87.9
MCI	M	265	75.4 ± 7.3	54.6	71.0	75.4	80.7	89.8
	F	146	73.6 ± 7.5	55.2	69.1	74.3	79.7	86.2
NC	M	112	76.1 ± 4.7	62.2	72.5	75.8	78.5	89.7
	F	118	75.8 ± 5.2	60.0	72.1	75.6	79.1	87.7

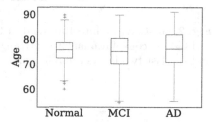

Fig. 1. Age distributions across groups.

2 Dataset and Preprocessing

In this study, the public Alzheimer's Disease Neuroimaging Initiative-1 (ADNI-1) [4] dataset is used, with all subjects having baseline brain T1-weighted structural MRI scans. The demographic information of the studied subjects is reported in Table 1. According to clinical criteria, such as Mini-Mental State Examination (MMSE) scores and Clinical Dementia Rating (CDR) (see http://adni.loni.usc. edu), subjects were diagnosed with AD or MCI conditions. There is a total of 841 subjects with baseline scans in the dataset, including 200 AD, 230 NC, and 411 MCI. Figure 1 shows the age distribution of different classes. Almost half of the subjects in each male/female category are in the MCI stage. Note that this stage is quite difficult to classify (from NC or AD) as it is a transition state and has similarities with both other classes. As can be seen, subjects are distributed proportionally similar across the three classes with respect to their age. Besides, both male and female groups have approximately similar portions of patients in each of the classes. Although the three classes are similar with respect to both age and gender distributions, we consider these two factors as input features to the model, as they can be confounding factors in MRI studies [1].

As a simple preprocessing step, the MR images of all subjects are skull-stripped, which includes removal of non-cerebral tissues like skull, scalp, and dura from brain images. To this end, we use the Brain Extraction Technique

(BET) proposed in [11]. This step reduces the size of images by a factor of two and hence slashes the amount of computational time spent for training the model.

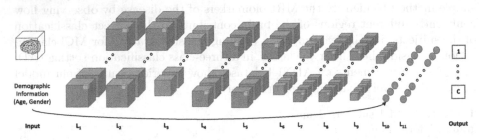

Fig. 2. 3D-CNN architecture used in this paper. The blue cubes (L_1, L_2, L_4, L_5, L_7, and L_8) are convolutional layers; Orange cubes (L_3, L_6, and L_9) are max-pooling layers; and the last two layers are fully connected (FC) layers.

3   3D-CNN Training and Evaluation

Architecture: For our end-to-end classification task, we build a three-dimensional Convolutional Neural Network (3D-CNN) using the TensorFlow framework. To evaluate the performance and to avoid overfitting, we consider two architectures: a complex architecture, as shown in Fig. 2, and a simplified version (with less number of filters, one less FC layer, and removing one Convolution (Conv.) layer at each stage). The complex architecture has $\mathcal{O}(10^5)$ trainable parameters, and the simple one has $\mathcal{O}(10^4)$ parameters. The fewer number of parameters helps the network avoid overfitting on a limited number of subjects.

The input MR images are re-sized to $116 \times 130 \times 83$ voxels. The first batch of Conv. layers ($L_{1,2}$) have $3^3 \times 32$ filter and the second ($L_{4,5}$) and the third ($L_{7,8}$) $3^3 \times 64$ and $3^3 \times 128$, respectively. The max-pooling layers (L_3, L_6, and L_9) are with sizes 2^3, 3^3, and 4^3, respectively. The fully connected (FC) layers have 512 (for L_{10}) and 256 (for L_{11}) nodes. The demographic variables of the subjects (age and gender) are added as two additional features in the first FC layer. We use a *rectified linear unit (ReLU)* as the activation function, and a cross-entropy cost function as the loss, which is minimized with the *Adam* optimizer. To optimize the architecture parameters and improve the trained model, we experiment by adding drop-out (D/O) and ℓ_2-regularization (Reg). Therefore, several hyperparameters are introduced to experiment on, including the β coefficient of the ℓ_2-regularization, the drop-out probability, and the size of input training batches, in addition to the learning rate, number of filters in the convolutional layers, and the number of neurons in the FC layers.

Data Augmentation: To train the model, we augment the data by flipping all subjects such that left and right hemispheres are swapped. This is a common strategy for data augmentation in the medical imaging as the neuroscientific studies suggest that the neurodegenerative disease (such as AD) impair the brain bilaterally [2].

Training Strategy: As can be seen in Fig. 2, the output layer defines c different classes. To better model the disease and identify its biomarkers, we first train the model on two classes ($c = 2$), *i.e.*, AD and NC. After training the classifier with two classes, we add a third class (*i.e.*, MCI) and fine-tune the weights to now classify the input into three categories. This is simply possible as we use a cross-entropy loss in the last layer of the network, which can be easily extended for multi-class cases. This fine-tuning strategy is actually conducting a transfer learning from the domain of the two-class learned model to the three-class case. We show in our experiments that, in the presence of limited sets of training data such as medical imaging applications, this transfer learning strategy leads to better results compared to training the three-class model from scratch. It is important to note that MCI is the intermediate stage between the cognitive decline of normal aging and the more pronounced decline of dementia (to some extent between AD and NC), and hence, first learning to separate AD from NC identifies the differences between the two classes. Then, adding the third class and fine-tuning the network transfers the learned knowledge to classify the middle condition, not jeopardizing the performance of AD Diagnosis.

Evaluation: We use the classification accuracy (Acc), F_2-score, precision (Pre) and recall (Rec) for evaluating the models. Having true positive, true negative, false positive, and false negative denoted by TP, TN, FP, and FN, respectively, precision and recall are computed as $Pre = TP/(TP + FP)$, $Rec = TP/(TP + FN)$. and then the F_2-score is defined by weighing recall higher than precision (*i.e.*, placing more emphasis on false negatives, which is important for disease diagnosis): $F_2 = (5 \times Pre \times Rec)/(4 \times Pre + Rec)$.

4 Experiment Results

To evaluate the model, at each iteration of 10-fold cross-validation, we randomly split the dataset into three sets of training (80%), validation (10%), and testing (10%). Starting from the training model shown in Fig. 2 (the *complex* architecture), we simplified the network, as described before, to avoid early overfitting. Besides, we investigated the effect of ℓ_2-regularization of kernels and biases in the Conv. layers, as well as the FC layers with the regularization hyperparameter searched in the set {0.01, 0.05, 0.1, 0.5, 1.0}. Regularization coefficient 0.5 for the kernels and 1.0 for the biases are found to result in the best validation F_2-score. We also tested the drop-out strategy in the last two FC layers in the training process, controlling the drop-out extent by the value of keep-rate. We tested regularized simple and complex model architectures with different keep-rate values for the FC layers ranging from 0.15 to 0.85 and found that keep-rates of 0.15 and 0.25 for the first and second FC layers lead to the best validation-set accuracy in the complex model and keep-rate of 0.4 gives the best validation-set accuracy in the simple model.

Table 2. Ablation tests: testing performance comparison of different models (last row is our model). The comparison includes the Accuracy (Acc), F_2 score, Precision (Pre), and Recall (Rec) of all methods (Reg: Regularization, D/O: Drop-Out, Aug: Augmentation).

Model	Simple				Complex			
	Acc%	F_2	Pre	Rec	Acc%	F_2	Pre	Rec
3D-CNN	68.7	0.71	0.68	0.72	66.5	0.69	0.67	0.70
3D-CNN+Reg	77.6	0.77	0.74	0.78	77.4	0.75	0.72	0.76
3D-CNN+Reg+D/O	83.1	0.811	0.78	0.82	79.7	0.82	0.79	0.84
3D-CNN+Reg+D/O+Aug (Ours)	**94.1**	**0.93**	**0.92**	**0.94**	88.3	0.89	0.88	0.91

Table 3. Comparisons with prior works for AD diagnosis.

Method	Modalities	Acc%	Sen	Spe
[12]	MRI+PET	85.7	0.99	0.54
[3]	MRI	90.8	N/A	N/A
[10]	MRI	91.1	0.88	0.93
[5]	MRI	93.9	0.94	0.93
Ours	MRI	94.1	0.94	0.91

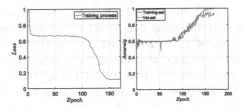

Fig. 3. (Left) training loss and (Right) training-validation accuracies with respect to the number of epochs for our 3D-CNN.

AD *vs* NC Classification Results (Two-Class Case): Table 2 shows the results of our model on the testing set in comparison with respect to ablation tests (removing components from the model and monitor how the performance changes). To test the significance of the classification results, we test our models using a Fisher exact test, in which our simple and complex models led to a p-value of less than 0.001. This indicates that the classifiers are significantly better than chance. As it can be seen, augmenting the size of the dataset led to improvement in the testing F_2 score, increasing it by 12.2% from its value of 81.1% in the non-augmented case. Another interesting observation is that the simple network outperforms the complex one, as it is less prone to overfitting.

Figure 3 shows the training and validations accuracy and loss function values with respect to the number of epochs for the best model (*i.e.*, the one with validation-set F_2 score of 0.933). The learning process is terminated when the accuracy of the training set reaches near 1.0. Furthermore, the drop in the loss function curve after a middle stage plateau, where it reaches a saddle point, can be attributed to the hyperparameter tuning inherent to the *Adam* optimizer during the training process. The model converges to a steady optimum without overfitting to the training data and hence yields reliable testing accuracies.

Comparisons with Prior Works: Table 3 compares the results of our AD *vs.* NC classification with prior works in terms of accuracy, sensitivity (Sen), and Specificity (Spe) as reported in the respective references. Although the experimental setup in these references is slightly different, this table shows that our end-to-end classification model can classify the subjects more accurately. The improved accuracy can be attributed to the end-to-end manner of classifying the data, which helps to learn better features for the specific task of AD diagnosis and hence yield better results compared to other works.

Identification of AD Biomarkers: To identify the regions of the brain that cause AD, we simply perform an image occlusion analysis on our best model (*i.e.*, 3D-CNN+Reg+D/O+Aug) by sliding a box of $1 \times 1 \times 1$ zero-valued voxels along the whole MR image of AD patients that were correctly labeled as AD by our trained model. The importance of each voxel, hence, can be characterized as the relative confidence of the samples being classified as AD. The resulting heat map is shown in Fig. 4, in which the color map indicates the relative importance of each voxel. The red areas decrease the confidence of the model, suggesting that they are areas that are of critical importance in diagnosing AD. The red regions in Fig. 4 coincides with the hippocampus, amygdala, thalamus, and ventricles of the brain, which have been reported to be responsible for short-term memory and early stages of AD [2,3,7,10].

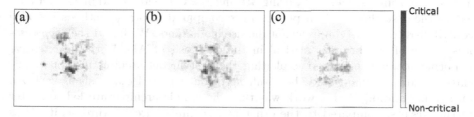

Fig. 4. Relative importance of different voxels associated with AD diagnosis.

Table 4. Testing performance for three-class Alzheimer classification.

Method	Simple				Complex			
	Acc%	F_2	Pre	Rec	Acc%	F_2	Pre	Rec
3D-CNN+D/O+Reg+with learning transfer	**61.1**	**0.62**	**0.59**	**0.63**	57.2	0.59	0.55	0.61
3D-CNN+D/O+Reg+w/o learning transfer	0.54	53.4	0.49	0.55	48.3	0.50	0.45	0.52

Learning Transfer (Three-Class Classification): We use the best model for the binary classification of AD *vs.* NC in Table 2 and fine-tune it to develop a learning transfer strategy for classification MCI subjects. Doing so, we build a three-class classifier to classify NC *vs.* MCI *vs.* AD. To this end, the output layer of our model changes to $c = 3$ instead of the previous $c = 2$ classes. We keep the previously learned weights in the network and fine-tune the network by exposing it to the sample from the MCI class. Table 4 shows the results of training with learning transfer strategy, in comparison with the method that trains based on three classes from scratch. As it can be seen, our model results in 61.1% accuracy, while if we train the model from scratch with all three classes, the model results in worse accuracies. This is due to the difficulty of the MCI class to distinguish from AD or NC. When training based on all three classes at once, the model gets stuck in local optima easier and overfit to the training data. On the other hand, the learning transfer strategy helps first learning the easy problem (*i.e.*, AD *vs.* NC) and then transfer the knowledge to the domain of the harder class (*i.e.*, MCI). Interestingly, our three-class classification results are better than the results of other works for the three-class AD, MCI, and NC classification. For instance, Liu *et al.* [10] obtained a 51.8% accuracy, compared to which, our results are better by a large margin (*i.e.*, 9.3%). Again, this improvement can be attributed to the end-to-end design of our model and the learning transfer strategy.

5   Conclusion

In this paper, we developed a 3D-CNN model to diagnose Alzheimer's disease and its prodromal stage, MCI, using MR images. Our end-to-end model not only led to the best classification performance compared to other methods but also contributed to identifying relevant disease biomarkers. We found the *hippocampus* region of the brain is critical in the diagnosis of AD. With an extensive hyperparameter tuning and exploiting the best model architecture for binary classification, we fine-tuned the resulting model for MCI diagnosis as well. An interesting finding of this work was that the simple architecture led to better testing results, compared to the other more complex architecture, as it is less prone to overfitting to the training data.

References

1. Adeli, E., Kwon, D., Pohl, K.M.: Multi-label transduction for identification of disease comorbidity patterns. In: MICCAI (2018)
2. Association, Alzheimer's: 2017 Alzheimer's Disease Facts and Figures. Alzheimers Dement **13**, 325–373 (2017)
3. Hosseini-Asl, E., Keynton, R., El-Baz, A.: Alzheimer's disease diagnostics by adaptation of 3D convolutional network. In: 2016 IEEE International Conference on Image Processing (ICIP), pp. 126–130. IEEE (2016)
4. Jack, C.R., et al.: The alzheimer's disease neuroimaging initiative (ADNI): MRI methods. J. Magn. Resonance Imaging **27**(4), 685–691 (2008)
5. Khajehnejad, M., Saatlou, F.H., Zade, H.M.: Alzheimer's disease early diagnosis using manifold-based semi-supervised learning. Brain Sci. **7**(8), 109 (2017)
6. Klöppel, S., et al.: Automatic classification of MR scans in Alzheimer's disease. Brain **131**(3), 681–689 (2008)
7. Laakso, M., et al.: Hippocampal volumes in Alzheimer's disease, Parkinson's disease with and without dementia, and in vascular dementia an MRI study. Neurology **46**(3), 678–681 (1996)

8. Litjens, G., et al.: A survey on deep learning in medical image analysis. Med. Image Anal. **42**, 60–88 (2017)
9. Liu, M., Zhang, J., Adeli, E., Shen, D.: Deep multi-task multi-channel learning for joint classification and regression of brain status. In: MICCAI (2017)
10. Liu, M., Zhang, J., Adeli, E., Shen, D.: Landmark-based deep multi-instance learning for brain disease diagnosis. Med. Image Anal. **43**, 157–168 (2018)
11. Smith, S.M.: Fast robust automated brain extraction. Hum. Brain Mapp. (2002)
12. Suk, H.I., Lee, S.W., Shen, D.: Hierarchical feature representation and multimodal fusion with deep learning for AD/MCI diagnosis. NeuroImage **101**, 569–582 (2014)
13. Wolz, R., Aljabar, P., Hajnal, J.V., Lötjönen, J., Rueckert, D.: Nonlinear dimensionality reduction combining MR imaging with non-imaging information. Med. Image Anal. **16**(4), 819–830 (2012)

Small Organ Segmentation
in Whole-Body MRI Using a Two-Stage
FCN and Weighting Schemes

Vanya V. Valindria[1]($\boxtimes$), Ioannis Lavdas[2], Juan Cerrolaza[1], Eric O. Aboagye[2],
Andrea G. Rockall[2], Daniel Rueckert[1], and Ben Glocker[1]

[1] Biomedical Image Analysis Group, Department of Computing, London, UK
v.valindria15@imperial.ac.uk
[2] Comprehensive Cancer Imaging Centre, Department of Surgery and Cancer,
Imperial College London, London, UK

Abstract. Accurate and robust segmentation of small organs in whole-body MRI is difficult due to anatomical variation and class imbalance. Recent deep network based approaches have demonstrated promising performance on abdominal multi-organ segmentations. However, the performance on small organs is still suboptimal as these occupy only small regions of the whole-body volumes with unclear boundaries and variable shapes. A coarse-to-fine, hierarchical strategy is a common approach to alleviate this problem, however, this might miss useful contextual information. We propose a two-stage approach with weighting schemes based on auto-context and spatial atlas priors. Our experiments show that the proposed approach can boost the segmentation accuracy of multiple small organs in whole-body MRI scans.

1 Introduction

Multi-organ segmentation in abdominal and whole-body scans is challenging as there are various organs and structures the need to be captured simultaneously. The size, shape and appearance of abdominal organs vary considerably between patients, but also the relative positions change to some degree. Small organs are less often investigated compared to major organs, although small organs are of interest for diagnosis and clinical applications such as cancer screening. Machine learning methods have been used to segment multiple organs in abdominal images [7]. However, small organs are still underrepresented and show lower accuracies compared to the large ones with less shape variability (e.g., lungs, heart, spine). Small object segmentation is generally more challenging due to large class imbalance between object and background samples. For example, the ratio of small organs in whole-body MRI in our data is less than 0.007% of the overall volume. We focus on bladder, sacrum, rectum, clavicles, pancreas, gallbladder, and adrenal gland. The complexity of background intensity and weak boundaries often make it more difficult to segment small organs.

© Springer Nature Switzerland AG 2018
Y. Shi et al. (Eds.): MLMI 2018, LNCS 11046, pp. 346–354, 2018.
https://doi.org/10.1007/978-3-030-00919-9_40

Most of the multi-organ segmentation work is applied to CT for which data seems more widely available. We focus on MRI, as there are still fewer works on this modality while whole-body MRI has become an important diagnostic tool for cancer screening. Early works of multi-organ abdominal segmentation include multi-atlas label fusion [1] and statistical shape models [3]. Multi-atlas techniques register images from a reference database to each new image and fuse multiple atlases to obtain the final segmentation. More recent work has made use of deep learning, for example, architectures for multi-organ segmentation, such as the dense V-network [5]. Weighted U-Net with weight proportion for foreground and background has been used to address the class imbalance problem [11].

In the medical domain, a coarse-to-fine approach has been applied for small structures, such as lesion segmentation in the pancreas [17] and liver [4]. Combination of multi-atlas and CNN techniques were used in [6], where localization of region of interest using a multi-atlas approach is combined with voxel-wise binary classification using CNNs. A more advanced iterative coarse-to-fine approach has been proposed by [18], which uses a smaller input region for a more accurate segmentation from multi-view coarse segmentations. However, finer segmentation consists of iterative refinement of at least 10 iterations, which can be time consuming.

Pancreas is the most studied small organ in previous works, as it is an abdominal organ of great importance with high anatomical variability. An earlier work on pancreas segmentation by [12] combined regional CNNs with superpixels at multiple scales. Later, [13] integrated semantic mid level cues (organ interior and boundary maps) via spatial aggregation and [2] applied long short-term memory (LSTM), to address the contextual learning and pancreas segmentation consistency problem. A novel approach with self-attention gating in CNNs was introduced in [9] for a more specific local region segmentation. As an end-to-end approach, they showed an improvement in pancreas segmentation, compared to standard FCNs, dense dilated FCNs [5], holistically nested FCNs [13], and standard U-Net. To alleviate the missing contextual information in the common two-stage approach, a recurrent saliency transformation network was proposed to relate the coarse and fine stages [16]. This saliency transformation module repeatedly transforms the segmentation probability map from previous iterations as spatial priors. However, performance can be lower than the coarse segmentation results because of the unsatisfying convergence over iterations.

Our contributions are as follows: (1) Previous works focus on CT segmentation and a single organ [2,5,9,12,13], while we study segmentation of multiple small organs on whole-body MRI including structures such as bones rarely considered. (2) This work is based on a coarse-to-fine framework [2,15,18] but goes one step further by incorporating weighting schemes and a specialized ROI selection. Weighting helps with class imbalance. For fine-scale segmentation, we apply auto-context with spatial information obtained from atlases so that coarse-and-fine-scaled networks are optimized jointly.

2   Materials and Methods

2.1   Materials

In-house whole-body MRI data was obtained from 48 healthy volunteers using the protocol described in [8]. Segmentations include 11 abdominal organs (heart, right lung, left lung, liver, adrenal gland, gall bladder, right kidney, left kidney, spleen, pancreas, and bladder) and 7 bones (spine, right clavicle, left clavicle, pelvis, humerus, sacrum). For our experiments, we only use T2w sequences, which we were resampled to a size (112, 80, 256) with isotropic 4 mm spacing.

2.2   Two-Stage Network: A Coarse-to-Fine Approach

Our aim is to segment multiple small organs from MRI scans, which occupy only a very small part of an MRI volume. We apply a two-stage network, which has been shown to be successful in an organ segmentation task [2,12,18]. CNN-based methods produce less accurate results when detecting small organs, particularly because the network is confused by the complicated context in the background and other organs. A coarse-scale is first used to locate the organ of interest for a subsequent fine-scale organ segmentation.

The two-stage strategy effectively reduces the complexity of the background while enhancing the discriminative information of a small organ. We train a coarse-scale segmentation to deal with the multi-organ segmentation on the whole-body scan. Then, at the fine-scale segmentation, we only focus with the ROI selection according to the coarse segmentation. For each stage, we trained a separate network. Similarly in testing stage, the coarse-scale network was first used to obtain the rough position of multiple small organs. Then, fine-scale networks were employed for binary segmentation for each of the small organs.

To counter the class imbalance of the small organs, we use a weighted-FCN [11] in both segmentation scales (coarse and fine). For coarse segmentation we use a weighted-FCN for multi-class segmentation with different weights set for each class. Small weights were set for bigger organs (such as livers, lungs, etc.) and large weights were applied for small organs, according to the relative size to the whole body volumes. This per-class-weight proportion was chosen via experimentation and the statistics of each organ proportion in the database.

ROI Selection In whole-body scans, each organ is located in a specific region. Therefore, context and spatial information is crucial for organ segmentation. After organ localisation from the coarse-scale segmentation, we found that in some cases, the FCN fails to locate small organs, leading to a much wider ROI for the fine-scale segmentation. Therefore, we need to induce spatial priors in order to guide the second stage network with a better ROI. A multi-atlas technique was chosen for producing spatial priors, because with multi-atlas segmentation, although the segmentation accuracy is lower than CNN-based accuracy, it mostly generates good organ localisation [7]. As shown in Fig. 1, the bladder segmentation result of multi-atlas is focused in one specific location instead of

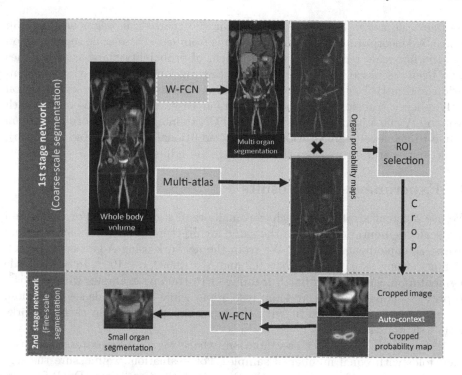

Fig. 1. Overview. First stage: Coarse-scale segmentation with multi-organ segmentation with weighted-FCN, where we obtain the segmentation results and probability map for each organ. Second stage: Fine-scale binary segmentation per organ. The input consists of a cropped volume and a probability map from coarse segmentation.

having multiple predictions scattered in other areas (shown in FCN probability maps).

In the multi-atlas approach, each atlas image is registered to the target and then fused using the methods described in [1]. We chose the PBAF (patch-based segmentation with augmented features) label fusion technique, as compared to other methods, this provides better accuracy for small organs. While [6] used a multi-atlas approach for organ localisation at first step before binary segmentation via CNNs, we only incorporate it after the coarse-scale segmentation. Here, the probability maps of coarse-segmentation is multiplied with the one from the multi-atlas approach (as a spatial prior for false-positive reduction, so that the fidelity of the final probability map is improved) to produce the 3D bounding box for fine-scale segmentation, see Fig. 1 top for details. We denoted this part of spatial prior incorporation as combined multi-atlas.

Auto-Context We utilize the classical approach of auto-context [14] into our framework to fuse and to integrate the information from different stages with the context. The problem of coarse-to-fine segmentation is that sometimes the cropped ROI within the bounding box has less sufficient spatial context, making the fine-scale networks more confused than the coarse-scale segmentation [13]. Hence, we incorporate the probability maps from the coarse-scale segmentation into the fine-scale segmentation. The benefit of probability maps as visual cues have been discussed in [13] as a spatial aggregation from multi-view segmentation and in [16] as an updated input for an iterative fine-scale segmentation with saliency transformation network. In our case, a simple auto-context with probability maps incorporation helps the FCN to integrate the information from coarse-to-fine level segmentation. By using additional input (see Fig. 1 bottom), uncertainties and errors from the first stage are adjusted.

3   Experiments and Results

We use different strategies to achieve small organ segmentation. For coarse and fine scale segmentation, we use the same architecture of an FCN with residual layers, as implemented in [10]. We train the network using Adam optimisation with a learning rate of 0.001, $\beta_1 = 0.9$ and $\beta_2 = 0.999$, $\epsilon = 10^{-5}$. In coarse-scale segmentation, we use mini-batch training of 16 training examples with size 64^3, to provide enough context at 4 mm resolution, while in fine-scale segmentation, the example size are 8^3 to fit with the input images. We train each networks with 10 K iterations.

We perform two-fold cross-validation, where we split the dataset into two fixed folds with equal number of samples. For evaluation, we measure the segmentation accuracy by computing the Dice Similarity Coefficient (DSC) for each subject.

First stage of the network was trained for multi-organ (18 classes, including large organs) on the entire 3D whole-body ROI. However, for our study, we were only interested in small organs as large organs, such as heart, liver, lungs, and spine - have achieved satisfactory results (with above 0.9 DSC). Our complete benchmarks for different strategies applied in small organ segmentation are shown in Table 1. Although the overall results on 18 organs for multi-atlas segmentation are lower (DSC: 0.486) than baseline FCN (DSC: 0.516) (without weights, auto-context, two-stage network and combined multi-atlas), the accuracy for small organs improved.

We then investigate the role of introducing different weights when taking training samples from different classes on coarse-scale multi-organ segmentation. As we give larger weights on small organs, we can reduce the effect of class imbalance [11]. This weighted-FCN gives significant improvement over small organs compared to the baseline FCN, with overall small organ accuracies increase from 0.244 to 0.483 DSC.

To evaluate the spatial prior in combined multi-atlas, we multiply the probability maps from the weighted-FCN with the multi-atlas prediction. Table 1 shows that it slightly improves the accuracy for small organ segmentation, especially adrenal gland (DSC: 0.203). However, some organs, such as both clavicles are worse because of the lower accuracy on multi-atlas segmentation. The probability maps given by multi-atlas are tighter, so that the segmentation misses some parts of the region of interested.

Table 1. Different strategies on segmentation of small organs, using the baseline FCN, weighted-FCN (W), auto-context (AC), two-stage networks (2SN), and combined multi-atlas (CMA) for ROI selection. Improvements in overall small organ segmentation accuracy (reported in DSCs) was achieved with our proposed approach.

Approaches				Adrenal gland	Gall bladder	Pancreas	Bladder	R. Clavicle	L. Clavicle	Rectum	Sacrum	Avg.
Multi-atlas				0.044	0.298	0.377	0.680	0.135	0.163	0.429	0.466	0.324
FCN												
W	AC	2SN	CMA									
✗	✗	✗	✗	0.006	0.330	0.373	0.401	0.055	0.080	0.346	0.361	0.244
✓	✗	✗	✗	0.097	0.443	0.465	0.689	0.462	0.484	0.526	0.701	0.483
✓	✗	✗	✓	**0.203**	0.436	0.519	0.717	0.381	0.397	0.549	0.693	0.487
✗	✓	✓	✗	0.046	0.375	0.455	0.594	0.274	0.379	0.393	0.490	0.376
✓	✓	✓	✗	0.133	0.507	**0.612**	0.729	0.519	0.535	0.591	0.721	0.543
✓	✓	✓	✓	0.146	**0.532**	0.567	**0.754**	**0.541**	**0.547**	**0.658**	**0.735**	**0.560**

To verify that the two-stage network can segment small organs more accurately, we run the state-of-the-art method [17], which takes input from baseline FCN segmentation to crop the ROI for fine-scale segmentation. Compared to the small organ segmentation accuracies produced by the FCN baseline (DSC: 0.244), we observe an improvement of about 50%. This result shows the advantage of using a two-stage network on small organ segmentation.

We then employ a two-stage scheme using the weighted-FCN with auto-context and the probability map from the weighted-FCN prediction as an additional input to the network. With this strategy, we get much higher accuracy on all organs (see Table 1). Weightings, auto-context, and region cropping are shown to boost the performance of small organ segmentation.

To add the spatial prior, we crop the ROI for fine-scale segmentation for organ-specific bounding box, according to the Sect. 2.2. As detailed in Table 1, adding spatial priors is useful in almost all small organs, except the pancreas because of its poor tissue contrast and shape variability. For adrenal gland, too, we find that the results of direct multiplication between coarse-scale segmentation and spatial prior gives better results. Multi-atlas prior information gives better localisation for adrenal gland, which is the smallest organ in our task (only occupied about 0.0001% of the whole volume). Overall, the addition of auto-context and spatial priors to two-stage weighted-FCN gives the best results on small organ segmentation (DSC: 0.560), as detailed in Table 1.

4   Discussion and Conclusion

The challenge in small organ segmentation is our main motivation in this work. A standard CNN-based approach gives good performance on larger organs, but still fails to accurately segment small organs. We found that by setting different weights on training examples per class could boost the performance of small organ segmentation. The class imbalance problem is countered by a multi-class weighted-FCN. As the target is often very small, we need to focus on a local input region. The two-stage network scheme seems to help the small organ segmentation. However, lack of contextual information and spatial knowledge sometimes make the network confused. Hence, we apply a simple auto-context, which uses the coarse-scale probability map to carry useful context information for fine-scale segmentation.

Some examples of small organ fine-scale segmentation are shown in Fig. 2. We can see that the two-stage weighted-FCN with auto-context and combination with multi-atlas produce better results in small organ segmentation. False positives are reduced and the ROIs are more focused to the specific organ. Our experiments show that the proposed approach outperforms the baseline (standard FCN and previous state-of-the art) on multiple small organs segmentations. This work shows a promising result for small organ and bone segmentation in whole-body MRI.

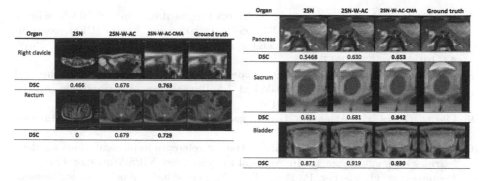

Fig. 2. Fine-scale segmentation of small organs. Two-stage network (2SN) with weighting (W), auto-context (AC), and combined spatial prior from multi-atlas (CMA) can improve small organ segmentation results.

Acknowledgments. V. Valindria is supported by the Indonesia Endowment for Education (LPDP)- Indonesian Presidential PhD Scholarship programme. B. Glocker received funding from the European Research Council (ERC) under the EU's Horizon 2020 research and innovation programme (grant agreement No 757173, project MIRA, ERC-2017-STG).

The MRI data has been collected as part of the MALIBO project funded by the Efficacy and Mechanism Evaluation (EME) Programme, an MRC and NIHR partnership (EME project 13/122/01). The views expressed in this publication are those of the authors and not necessarily those of the MRC, NHS, NIHR or the Department of Health.

References

1. Bai, W., et al.: A probabilistic patch-based label fusion model for multi-atlas segmentation with registration refinement: application to cardiac MR images. IEEE Trans. Med. Imaging **32**(7), 1302–1315 (2013)
2. Cai, J., Lu, L., Xie, Y., Xing, F., Yang, L.: Improving deep pancreas segmentation in CT and MRI images via recurrent neural contextual learning and direct loss function. arXiv preprint arXiv:1707.04912 (2017)
3. Cerrolaza, J.J., Summers, R.M., Linguraru, M.G.: Soft multi-organ shape models via generalized PCA: a general framework. In: Ourselin, S., Joskowicz, L., Sabuncu, M.R., Unal, G., Wells, W. (eds.) MICCAI 2016. LNCS, vol. 9902, pp. 219–228. Springer, Cham (2016). https://doi.org/10.1007/978-3-319-46726-9_26
4. Christ, P.F., et al.: Automatic liver and lesion segmentation in CT using cascaded fully convolutional neural networks and 3D conditional random fields. In: Ourselin, S., Joskowicz, L., Sabuncu, M.R., Unal, G., Wells, W. (eds.) MICCAI 2016. LNCS, vol. 9901, pp. 415–423. Springer, Cham (2016). https://doi.org/10.1007/978-3-319-46723-8_48
5. Gibson, E., et al.: Automatic multi-organ segmentation on abdominal CT with dense V-networks. IEEE Trans. Med. Imaging (2018)
6. Larsson, M., Zhang, Y., Kahl, F.: Robust abdominal organ segmentation using regional CNNs. In: Scandinavian Conference on Image Analysis, pp. 41–52 (2017)

7. Lavdas, I., et al.: Fully automatic, multiorgan segmentation in normal whole body magnetic resonance imaging (MRI), using classification forests (CFs), convolutional neural networks (CNNs), and a multi-atlas (MA) approach. Med. Phys. **44**(10), 5210–5220 (2017)

8. Lavdas, I., et al.: Apparent diffusion coefficient of normal abdominal organs and bone marrow from whole-body DWI at 1.5 T: the effect of sex and age. Am. J. Roentgenol. **205**(2), 242–250 (2015)

9. Oktay, O., et al.: Attention U-net: learning where to look for the pancreas. arXiv:1804.03999 (2018)

10. Pawlowski, N., et al.: DLTK: state of the art reference implementations for deep learning on medical images. In: Medical Imaging meet NIPS Workshop (2017)

11. Ronneberger, O., Fischer, P., Brox, T.: U-Net: convolutional networks for biomedical image segmentation. In: Navab, N., Hornegger, J., Wells, W.M., Frangi, A.F. (eds.) MICCAI 2015. LNCS, vol. 9351, pp. 234–241. Springer, Cham (2015). https://doi.org/10.1007/978-3-319-24574-4_28

12. Roth, H.R., et al.: DeepOrgan: multi-level deep convolutional networks for automated pancreas segmentation. In: Navab, N., Hornegger, J., Wells, W.M., Frangi, A.F. (eds.) MICCAI 2015. LNCS, vol. 9349, pp. 556–564. Springer, Cham (2015). https://doi.org/10.1007/978-3-319-24553-9_68

13. Roth, H.R., Lu, L., Farag, A., Sohn, A., Summers, R.M.: Spatial aggregation of holistically-nested networks for automated Pancreas segmentation. In: Ourselin, S., Joskowicz, L., Sabuncu, M.R., Unal, G., Wells, W. (eds.) MICCAI 2016. LNCS, vol. 9901, pp. 451–459. Springer, Cham (2016). https://doi.org/10.1007/978-3-319-46723-8_52

14. Tu, Z., Bai, X.: Auto-context and its application to high-level vision tasks and 3D brain image segmentation. IEEE PAMI **32**(10), 1744–1757 (2010)

15. Yu, F., Koltun, V.: Multi-scale context aggregation by dilated convolutions. In: ICLR (2016)

16. Yu, Q., Xie, L., Wang, Y., Zhou, Y., Fishman, E.K., Yuille, A.L., et al.: Recurrent saliency transformation network: incorporating multi-stage visual cues for small organ segmentation. In: CVPR (2018)

17. Zhou, Y., Xie, L., Fishman, E.K., Yuille, A.L.: Deep supervision for pancreatic cyst segmentation in abdominal CT scans. In: MICCAI (2017)

18. Zhou, Y., Xie, L., Shen, W., Wang, Y., Fishman, E.K., Yuille, A.L., et al.: A fixed-point model for Pancreas segmentation in abdominal CT scans. In: MICCAI (2017)

Masseter Segmentation from Computed Tomography Using Feature-Enhanced Nested Residual Neural Network

Haifang Qin[1], Yuru Pei[1(✉)], Yuke Guo[2], Gengyu Ma[3], Tianmin Xu[4],
and Hongbin Zha[1]

[1] Key Laboratory of Machine Perception (MOE),
Department of Machine Intelligence, Peking University, Beijing, China
peiyuru@cis.pku.edu.cn
[2] Luoyang Institute of Science and Technology, Luoyang, China
[3] uSens Inc., San Jose, CA, USA
[4] School of Stomatology, Peking University, Beijing, China

Abstract. Masticatory muscles are of significant aesthetic and functional importance to craniofacial developments. Automatic segmentation is a crucial step for shape and functional analysis of muscles. In this paper, we propose an automatic masseter segmentation framework using a deep neural network with coupled feature learning and label prediction pathways. The volumetric features are learned using the unsupervised convolutional auto-encoder and integrated with multi-level features in the label prediction pathway to augment features for segmentation. The label prediction pathway is built upon the nested residual network which is feasible for information propagation and fast convergence. The proposed method realizes the voxel-wise label inference of masseter muscles from the clinically captured computed tomography (CT) images. In the experiments, the proposed method outperforms the compared state-of-the-arts, achieving a mean Dice similarity coefficient (DSC) of $93 \pm 1.2\%$ for the segmentation of masseter muscles.

1 Introduction

Masticatory muscles play an essential role in the morphological development of craniofacial structures [13]. The clinical and experimental studies support that the bite force of the mandibular muscles partly determines the form of the face and the underlying bones. A comprehensive insight into the masticatory muscles is a prerequisite to the treatments planning and the etiology analysis of malocclusion and mandible deformation. Volumetric CT images provide the 3D geometries of masseter muscles. Automatic segmentation of patient-specific masseter muscles from volumetric CT images, relieving efforts in manual and interactive labeling [12], is desirable in clinical orthodontics. However, the automatic segmentation of masseter muscles is still a challenging issue considering the imaging noise and artifacts, the boundary confusions with surrounding soft tissues, and the inhomogeneous interiors.

© Springer Nature Switzerland AG 2018
Y. Shi et al. (Eds.): MLMI 2018, LNCS 11046, pp. 355–362, 2018.
https://doi.org/10.1007/978-3-030-00919-9_41

There are a number of investigations published on the automatic muscle segmentation, including the deformable shape model [14], the Markov random field [5], the watershed [6], and level-set-based [4] methods. The deformable simplex mesh [14] and the shape-based interpolation [7] are used to create the patient-specific masseter muscles. The Markov random field model [5] has been used in muscle segmentation, in which the deliberately-designed unary and smoothness terms are required to infer the foreground probabilities. A gradient vector flow [11] and level-set-based methods [4] are used to segment facial soft-tissues from CT and MRI images. The level-set-based method is known to rely on the initial values and prone to the error accumulation. Existing methods struggle to handle soft edges and inhomogeneous interiors of muscles using 3D shape priors [14] or interactive labeling [12]. The 3D nonrigid deformable shape [14] and the statistical shape model [5] facilitate the muscle segmentation in the reduced parameter space. However, the mesh deformation and online adaptation are time-consuming and prone to a local minimum.

Recently, the convolutional neural network (CNN) becomes the mainstream in the computer vision community and is used for medical image segmentation [9,15]. The pre-trained AlexNet coupled with a PCA head is used to infer muscle boundaries of MRI [3]. Nie et al. [8] integrated the 3D u-net-based coarse segmentation and a context-guided CNN-based fine-grained segmentation for cranio-maxillofacial structures from MRI. Shortcut connections are prevalent in the CNN to fuse the multi-scale abstracted features for label prediction [1,10,16]. Mixed long-jump and local residual connections are used in the CNN for 3D volumetric image segmentation [16]. Aside from the popular short-cut connections based feature fusion, a more powerful feature is desirable to handle the muscle segmentation considering the inhomogeneous masseter interiors and the confusions with surrounding soft tissues.

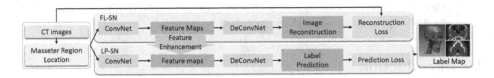

Fig. 1. System framework.

To address these challenges, we propose a deep learning-based framework with two separate sub-networks addressing volumetric feature learning and discrete label map prediction respectively (Fig. 1). Particularity, regarding the label prediction subnet (LP-SN), we adopt a fully convolutional neural network with nested residual connections for the end-to-end masseter segmentation from CT images. Aside from the feature fusion using nested short-cut connections, we introduce a feature learning subnet (FL-SN) using the convolutional auto-encoder (CAE). The volumetric CAE duplicates the mainstream structures of the LP-SN. The multi-level structural feature volumes from the CAE, which are crucial to the image reconstructions, are leveraged as additional information for the robust label prediction. Both the FL-SN and the LP-SN are composed of the symmetric convolutional network (ConvNet) and the de-convolutional network (DeConvNet) for feature extraction and reconstruction/prediction tasks respectively. A multi-level concatenation scheme is used to integrate the crucial structural features of image reconstruction to the label prediction pathway. The integration augments the volumetric features and especially avoids the labeling ambiguity due to inhomogeneous masseter interiors and surrounding soft tissues.

2 Methods

The proposed method is conducted on 3D volumetric CT images. A preprocessing step is performed to give candidate regions of masseter muscles. They are then fed to the feature learning and label prediction sub-networks for feature abstraction and masseter segmentation respectively. The output voxel-wise potential map is used to derive the masseter boundaries.

2.1 Masseter Region Location

In the preprocessing stage, a regression random forest [2] is used to detect the candidate region of the left and right masseters to remove the disruption of various contents in the background regions. The labeled CT images associated with bounding boxes, parameterized as a six-dimensional distance vector to the bounding planes, are used to train the regression forest. We sample voxels every 2 cm and employ the mean intensity feature over two cuboidal volumetric regions [2]. In the testing stage, the voxels sampled in the same pattern as the training stage are fed to the regression forest. The predicted distance vector with the largest probability is used to locate the bounding box of the masseter muscle. In our experiments, two regression forests are used to find the bounding boxes of the left and the right masseter muscles respectively.

2.2 Feature-Enhanced Nested Residual Neural Network

The proposed framework is composed of two duplicated sub-networks for feature learning and label prediction. As shown in Fig. 1, the FL-SN shares the same architecture with the LP-SN. The multilevel feature volumes with comprehensive structural information obtained by the FL-SN are integrated with the LP-SN to leverage the structural information in the muscle segmentation. The combined loss function considers both the image reconstruction in the FL-SN and the label prediction in the LP-SN.

Feature Learning Sub-Network. The FL-SN is used to obtain the feature volumes with comprehensive structural information for image reconstruction and voxel-wise segmentation map prediction. We use the unsupervised CAE network. The FL-SN has two symmetric pathways: the front-end compression pathway for feature extraction and the back-end decompression pathway for CT image reconstruction. The front-end compression pathway is composed of four convolutional blocks (CB) including two duplicated $3 \times 3 \times 3$ convolutional layers with a stride of one and one pooling layer with a factor of 2. The rectified linear unit layer (RELU) follows each convolutional layer. The decompression pathway is composed of four deconvolutional blocks (DB). The DB consists of one convolutional layer with a stride of 1/2 for upsampling feature volumes and a duplicated convolutional layer with a stride of 1 and a receptive field of $3 \times 3 \times 3$.

Label Prediction Sub-Network. We explicitly learn the voxel-wise image labeling model using the feature-enforced nested residual connections. The LP-SN is developed from the 3D u-net [1] with symmetric feature abstraction and label prediction pathways. Aside from the shortcut connections between convolutional blocks of the same resolutions, the cross-scale residual connections are added between the CBs and the DBs of different resolutions (see Fig. 2), resulting to a nested residual network for information propagation and fast convergence. An additional convolutional layer is introduced to fuse the feature volumes from two sub-networks. The proposed framework exploits the integrated feature volumes from both the FL-SN and the LP-SN to predict labels of masseter muscles.

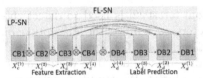

	Input Size	Output Size		Input Size	Output Size
CB1	1, 64x128x96	16, 32x64x48	DB4	64, 4x8x6	64, 8x16x12
CB2	16, 32x64x48	32, 16x32x24	DB3	64, 8x16x12	32, 16x32x24
CB3	32, 16x32x24	64, 8x16x12	DB2	32, 16x32x24 8, 32x64x48
CB4	64, 8x16x12	64, 4x8x6	DB1	8, 32x64x48	2, 64x128x96

Fig. 2. The architecture and specifications of the LP-SN.

Formulation. The training data $\{(V_i, S_i) | i = 1, \ldots, N\}$ are composed of the volumes V of masseter muscles located by the regression forest from CT images (Sect. 2.1) and the corresponding binary label maps S. The sub-volume V of the masseter muscle is normalized to $[0, 1]$. $S \in \{0, 1\}$ denotes the labels of the foreground masseter muscles. The proposed feature-enhanced nested residual network is learned from these data. The output label map X_o is defined by the sigmoid function as follows:

$$X_o = sigm(X_d^{(1)}), \text{ and} \tag{1}$$

$$X_d^{(l)} = X_c^{(l)} \otimes X_f^{(l)} + g(X_d^{(l+1)}, W_d^{(l+1)}) + \underbrace{\sum_{i=l+1}^{L} g(X_c^{(i)} \otimes X_f^{(i)}, W_r^{(i)})}_{H^{(l)}}, \tag{2}$$

where g is a convolution operator followed by the ReLU. W_d and W_r denote the weight and bias parameters of the back-end DBs in the label prediction pathway and the cross-level short-cut connections. X_c, X_d, and X_f denote the feature volumes obtained in front-end feature extraction, the back-end label prediction pathways of the LP-SN, and the front-end encoder of the FL-SN respectively. L denotes the number of CBs and set to 4 in our experiments. Both the DBs and the accumulated cross-level connections from the front-end feature abstraction pathway contribute to the final output. Note that the feature volumes are enhanced by their counterparts in the FL-SN. The feature volumes from two sub-networks are fused using an additional convolution denoted as $\otimes$. The feature volumes $X_d^{(l)}$ of the l-th DB is defined using the residual function $H^{(l)}$ (Eq. 2). The final loss function $\mathcal{L}$ is defined as an integration of the image reconstruction loss of the FL-SN and the label prediction loss of the LP-SN.

$$\mathcal{L} = \|X_o - V\|^2 - \sum_{x_i \in X_o,\, s_i \in S} (s_i \ln x_i + (1 - s_i) \ln(1 - x_i)). \tag{3}$$

Training. The proposed network is utilized for the end-to-end segmentation of masseter muscles from CT images. Different from the subvolume clipping and sliding, the voxel-wise labels are obtained simultaneously. In the first stage, the stochastic gradient descent (SGD) solver of the Caffe toolbox is used to optimize the parameters of the FL-SN. In the second stage, the mainstream structure of the LP-SN is initialized by the parameters of the FL-SN. The voxel-wise cross-entropy loss function measures the distance between the predicted and the ground truth segmentation labels. The parameters of the LP-SN and the FL-SN are optimized jointly using the SGD solver of the Caffe toolbox.

Online Inference. In the online testing, the left and right masseter regions are located using the regression forest (Sect. 2.1). The resulted sub-volumes are re-scaled to be of the same resolution of the training data and fed to the FL-SN and the LP-SN. The output label map indicates the voxel-wise probability belonging to masseter muscles. The final segmentation map is obtained by thresholding.

3   Experiments

The proposed method is tested on 50 clinically captured head CT images. The CT image is of a resolution of $512 \times 512 \times 200$. The voxel size is $0.4 \times 0.4 \times 1.25$ mm^3. The candidate region of the masseter is cropped (Sect. 2.1) and re-scaled to a resolution of $64 \times 128 \times 96$. The ground truth label maps of the masseter muscles are interactively defined using the software ITK-Snap. The data augmentation is performed using the nonrigid volumetric image deformation. We randomly sample 2000 points in the subspace spanned by the displacement fields of the CT images in the training dataset. The volumetric images associated with the label maps of the masseter muscles are determined by sampling in the subspace and used to train the network. The automatic masseter segmentation is evaluated by the Dice similarity coefficients (DSC) and the mean surface deviations (MSD). The four-fold cross-validation is performed. In the training stage, the augmented volumetric images of the training dataset are used to train the network. We compare with variants of CNN-based segmentation methods, including the 3DCNN without residual connections [9], the u-net [1], the mixed residual network (MRN) [16], and the nest residual networks (NRN) without feature enhancements [10]. In our experiments, all label prediction networks have the same mainstream structures, including four convolutional and four deconvolutional blocks.

Results. Concerning the volumetric segmentation of masseter muscles, Fig. 3 (a) and (b) show two views of the left and right masseter muscles obtained by the proposed method and the underlying skull. Six sampled slices with overlapped label maps of the masseter muscles are shown side by side (Fig. 3 (c)). The extracted contours using the proposed method are consistent with the CT images regarding the contour completeness and accuracies. Note that we use one neural network based regression model for both the left and right masseter muscles. We mirrorize the sub-volumes of the masseter muscle along the sagittal plane in both the training and the testing stages. The mean DSCs obtained by the 3DCNN [9], the u-net [1], the MRN [16], and the NRN [10] are 0.86, 0.87, and 0.89, and 0.91, in contrast, a value of 0.93 is achieved by the proposed method (Fig. 4(d)). The automatically extracted masseter contours on two sampled slices are shown side by side in Fig. 4 (a, b). The masseter contours extracted using the proposed method with feature enhancements are more reliable than compared approaches, especially in the discrimination from the surrounding soft tissues.

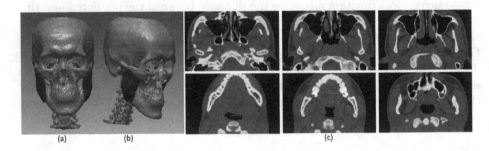

Fig. 3. (a) and (b) are two viewpoints of surface meshes of the left and right masseter muscles obtained by the proposed method and the underlying skull. (c) Six sampled slices with overlapped label maps extracted using the proposed method.

Regarding the surface meshes extracted from the label maps, the MSDs obtained by the 3DCNN [9], the u-net [1], the MRN [16], and the NRN [10] are 0.45 mm, 0.34 mm, 0.32 mm, and 0.30 mm, in contrast, a value of 0.25 mm is achieved by the proposed method (Fig. 4(e)). The proposed method outperforms the compared variants of 3DCNNs regarding both the DSC and the MSD in experiments. Figure 4 (c) visualizes the distance between masseter surfaces extracted by the automatic segmentation methods and the ground truth. The proposed approach is feasible to minimize the gap between the resulted surface and ground truth. The masseter surface obtained by the proposed method is consistent with the ground truth compared with other methods regarding the surface completeness and reliability.

We compare the learning behavior of the proposed method, the MRN [16], the NRN [10], the u-net [1], and the 3DCNN [9] methods on the testing data (Fig. 4

(f)). The proposed method converges with the segmentation losses decreasing faster than the compared approaches.

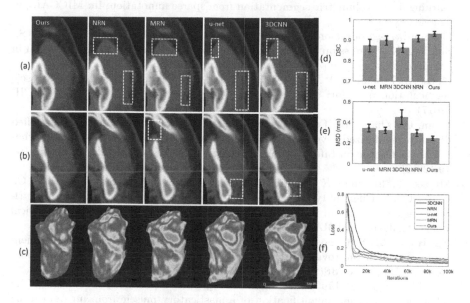

Fig. 4. (a) and (b) are sampled slices with labels using the proposed method, the NRN [10], the MRN [16], the u-net [1], and the 3DCNN [9] methods (from left to right) with errors blocked. (c) Visualization of distances between masseter surfaces extracted using the proposed method, the NRN [10], the MRN [16], the u-net [1], and the 3DCNN [9] methods (from left to right) and the ground truth. (d) The DSC and (e) the MSD of the masseter segmentation. (f) Comparison of learning curves.

4   Discussion and Conclusion

In this paper, we propose a feature-enhanced nested residual network for end-to-end segmentation of masseter muscles. Aside from the common short-cut connection-based feature fusion, we introduce the feature learning sub-network for the volumetric features with the comprehensive structural information specific for the CT image reconstruction. The proposed method is feasible to handle the soft edges and image artifacts of the CT images without additional image preprocessing. The proposed method realizes a mean DSC of 0.93, and the MSD of 0.25 mm in the masseter segmentation from CT images, achieving performance improvements over the compared approaches in both the contour reliability and the surface completeness.

Acknowledgments. This work was supported by NSFC 61272342.

References

1. Cicek, z., Abdulkadir, A., Lienkamp, S.S., Brox, T., Ronneberger, O.: 3d u-net: learning dense volumetric segmentation from sparse annotation. In: MICCAI, pp. 424–432
2. Criminisi, A., Robertson, D., Konukoglu, E., Shotton, J., Pathak, S., White, S., Siddiqui, K.: Regression forests for efficient anatomy detection and localization in computed tomography scans. Med. Image Anal. **17**(8), 1293–1303 (2013)
3. Ghosh, S., Boulanger, P., Acton, S.T., Blemker, S.S., Ray, N.: Automated 3d muscle segmentation from mri data using convolutional neural network. In: IEEE ICIP (2017)
4. Guan, Q., Zhang, B., Long, H., Hu, H., Zhuang, X., Hu, Y., et al.: A modified distance regularized level set evolution for masseter segmentation. In: International Conference on Information Technology in Medicine and Education, pp. 16–19 (2017)
5. Majeed, T., Fundana, K., Lüthi, M., Kiriyanthan, S., Beinemann, J., Cattin, P.C., et al.: Using a flexibility constrained 3d statistical shape model for robust mrf-based segmentation. In: IEEE Workshop on Mathematical Methods in Biomedical Image Analysis (MMBIA), pp. 57–64. IEEE (2012)
6. Ng, H.P., Ong, S.H., Foong, K.W., Goh, P.S., Nowinski, W.L.: Masseter segmentation using an improved watershed algorithm with unsupervised classification. Comput. Biol. Med. **38**(2), 171–184 (2008)
7. Ng, H.P., Ong, S.H., Liu, J., Huang, S., Foong, K.W.C., Goh, P.S., Nowinski, W.L.: 3d segmentation and quantification of a masticatory muscle from mr data using patient-specific models and matching distributions. J. Digit. Imaging **22**(5), 449 (2009)
8. Nie, D., et al.: Segmentation of craniomaxillofacial bony structures from mri with a 3d deep-learning based cascade framework. In: International Workshop on Machine Learning in Medical Imaging, pp. 266–273 (2017)
9. Noh, H., Hong, S., Han, B.: Learning deconvolution network for semantic segmentation. In: IEEE International Conference on Computer Vision,. pp. 1520–1528 (2015)
10. Pei, Y., et al.: Multi-scale volumetric convnet with nested residual connections for segmentation of anterior cranial base. In: MLMI (2017)
11. Piau, N.H.: Segmentation of human muscles of mastication from magnetic resonance images. Basic Res. J. Agric. Sci. Rev. **180**(2), 1167–1175 (2008)
12. Ray, N., Mukherjee, S., Nakka, K.K., Acton, S.T., Blanker, S.S.: 3d-to-2d mapping for user interactive segmentation of human leg muscles from mri data. In: Signal and Information Processing, pp. 50–54 (2015)
13. Sellatunis, T., Pokhojaev, A., Sarig, R., OHiggins, P., May, H.: Human mandibular shape is associated with masticatory muscle force. Sci. Rep. **8**(1), 6042 (2018)
14. Yan, G., Ullrich, S., Grottke, O., Rossaint, R., Kuhlen, T., Deserno, T.M., et al.: Scene-based segmentation of multiple muscles from mri in mitk. Bildverarbeitung fr die Medizin (2011)
15. Yao, J., Kovacs, W., Hsieh, N., Liu, C.Y., Summers, R.M.: Holistic segmentation of intermuscular adipose tissues on thigh mri. In: MICCAI, pp. 737–745 (2017)
16. Yu, L., Yang, X., Chen, H., Qin, J., Heng, P.A.: Volumetric convnets with mixed residual connections for automated prostate segmentation from 3d mr images. In: AAAI (2017)

Iterative Interaction Training for Segmentation Editing Networks

Gustav Bredell[(✉)], Christine Tanner, and Ender Konukoglu

Computer Vision Laboratory, ETH Zurich, Zurich, Switzerland
gbredell@student.ethz.ch

Abstract. Automatic segmentation has great potential to facilitate morphological measurements while simultaneously increasing efficiency. Nevertheless often users want to edit the segmentation to their own needs and will need different tools for this. There has been methods developed to edit segmentations of automatic methods based on the user input, primarily for binary segmentations. Here however, we present an unique training strategy for convolutional neural networks (CNNs) trained on top of an automatic method to enable interactive segmentation editing that is not limited to binary segmentation. By utilizing a robot-user during training, we closely mimic realistic use cases to achieve optimal editing performance. In addition, we show that an increase of the iterative interactions during the training process up to ten improves the segmentation editing performance substantially. Furthermore, we compare our segmentation editing CNN (interCNN) to state-of-the-art interactive segmentation algorithms and show a superior or on par performance.

1 Introduction

Segmentation is one of the main medical image analysis tasks that when automated substantially facilitates morphological measurements and increase efficiency in treatment planning [11,17,18]. With the introduction of machine learning and especially convolutional neural networks (CNNs) the performance of automatic segmentation approaches improved greatly [7]. Recent studies showed that CNN-based approaches were able to achieve inter- and intra-expert performance in certain segmentation tasks, for example prostate segmentation in Magnetic Resonance Images (MRIs) as shown in [4,8]. Although these approaches achieve impressive performance on average, when considering an individual image, there are often parts of the segmentation users would like to change and improve to fit their needs. The need for edits and improvement is even larger when the test image differs slightly from the training dataset, for example due to scanner differences, and more errors are expected.

To address the need for editing, interactive segmentation algorithms have been proposed such as GrabCut, GeoS or Random Walker [3,5,14] that allow operators to modify segmentations. Even though accurate results have been shown with these methods, the interaction can be time consuming as large number of interactions might be necessary. In particular, updates aiming to correct

© Springer Nature Switzerland AG 2018
Y. Shi et al. (Eds.): MLMI 2018, LNCS 11046, pp. 363–370, 2018.
https://doi.org/10.1007/978-3-030-00919-9_42

segmentation in one region can lead to inaccuracies in another region, consequently requiring further interactions.

In recent years, studies such as [1,9,19] proposed CNNs for interactive segmentations and showed better results compared to traditional methods. These initial works focused on segmenting objects in medical images from scratch using simple user interactions, and mostly in the form of binary segmentations. More recently, authors in [20] proposed a CNN-based method for editing segmentations predicted by an automatic algorithm, one of the most important steps in translating automatic segmentations in practice, and showed the benefits for binary segmentations. In the same work, authors assumed multiple scribbles to be made at a single time and the editing network was trained to take into account all the edits, initial prediction and the image to generate an updated segmentation. This training strategy may not be ideal since it does not take into account the fact that a user may be interacting with the tool over several iterations, each time providing scribbles based on the result of the last update.

In this work, we present a different strategy for training a CNN that interactively edits segmentations. As in [20], we assume the editing CNN is an auxiliary tool that supports a base segmentation algorithm and is optimized to take into account user edits and improve segmentation accuracy. Different than [20], we investigate training in an iterative interaction fashion on simulated user inputs and we also focus on multi-label segmentation problems as well as binary ones. We assess the potential of the proposed training strategy on the prostate data of the NCI-ISBI 2013 challenge and show the value of iterative interaction training. Moreover, we empirically compare networks for editing segmentations with a state-of-the-art fully interactive segmentation algorithm that segments the image from scratch using user-made scribbles.

2   Methods

Interactive segmentation editing networks, which we refer to as *interCNN*, are trained on top of a base segmentation algorithm, specifically to interpret user inputs and make appropriate adjustments to the predictions of the base algorithm. During test time, an interCNN sees the image, initial predictions of the base algorithm and user edits in the form of scribbles, and combines all to create a new segmentation, see Fig. 1. In case the new segmentation needs more edits, an interCNN can be applied in an iterative fashion until the segmentation is satisfactory by accepting additional scribbles and taking the image and its own predictions as inputs. Training of an interCNN can be done in two ways. First, as done in [20], given the segmentation of the base network, a set of scribbles are provided and the interCNN is trained to update the segmentation the best way possible by using all the scribbles, image and the base network's segmentation. Ideally, human users should provide the scribbles during the training, however, this is clearly infeasible and a robot user is often utilized to provide the scribbles and has been shown to perform well.

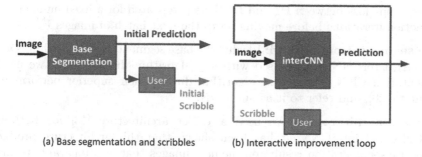

Fig. 1. Illustration of interactive segmentation editing networks. (a) generation of initial prediction with base segmentation and first user input, (b) interactive improvement loop with proposed interCNN. Here, we use a CNN for the base segmentation algorithm for demonstration but other methods can be used. interCNN can be applied iteratively until the segmentation is satisfactory. During training, to make it feasible, the user is replaced by a robot user that places scribbles based on the discrepancy between ground truth and predicted segmentations for the training images.

Algorithm 1: training interCNN for B batch and K interaction iterations

---

Input : images $\mathbf{I}^b$, ground-truth labels $\mathbf{L}^b$
Output: interCNN weights $\mathbf{W}_K$, predictions $\mathbf{P}_K^b$

1 **for** $b \in \{1, 2, ..., B\}$ **do**
2 $\quad$ $\mathbf{P}_0^b \leftarrow$ autoCNN$(\mathbf{I}^b)$
3 $\quad$ $\mathbf{S}_0^b \leftarrow$ random-user$(\mathbf{P}_0^b, \mathbf{L}^b)$
4 $\quad$ **for** $k \in \{1, ..., K\}$ **do**
5 $\quad\quad$ $\mathbf{P}_k^b \leftarrow$ interCNN$(\mathbf{I}^b, \mathbf{P}_{k-1}^b, \mathbf{S}_{k-1}^b)$
6 $\quad\quad$ $\mathbf{S}_k^b \leftarrow$ random-user$(\mathbf{P}_k^b, \mathbf{L}^b)$
7 $\quad\quad$ backpropagate cross-entropy$(\mathbf{P}_k^b, \mathbf{L}^b)$ loss to update $\mathbf{W}_k$
8 $\quad$ **end**
9 **end**

Iterative interaction training: The alternative training strategy, which we propose here, is to replicate the testing procedure and integrate iterative interactions to optimize the network. An overview of this strategy is presented as a pseudocode in Algorithm 1. Images in the training set $(\mathbf{I}^b)$ are fed batch-wise into the base algorithm to create initial predictions $(\mathbf{P}_0^b)$. Scribbles $(\mathbf{S}_k^b)$ are produced by a robot user based on the discrepancy between $\mathbf{P}_k^b$ and the ground truth segmentations $(\mathbf{L}^b)$. $\mathbf{S}_k^b$ has an image format in which the user-selected wrongly classified pixels are marked according to their correct class and all other pixels are set to max$(\mathbf{L}^b) + 1$. The initial scribbles $\mathbf{S}_0^b$, along with $\mathbf{P}_0^b$ and $\mathbf{I}^b$ are subsequently fed into interCNN to get an updated prediction $(\mathbf{P}_1^b)$. Based on $\mathbf{P}_1^b$ new scribbles are produced by the robot user $(\mathbf{S}_1^b)$ and are fed into the interCNN in the next iteration $(k+1)$ together with $\mathbf{I}^b$ and $\mathbf{P}_1^b$. During interaction iteration k the weights of interCNN $(\mathbf{W}_k)$ are updated with backpropagation based on the cross-entropy loss between $\mathbf{P}_k^b$ and $\mathbf{L}^b$. This is repeated for a fixed number of K interaction iterations before moving on to the next batch of images $\mathbf{I}^{b+1}$.

Base segmentation method: Ideally, the base segmentation algorithm is arbitrary. An interCNN can be used with any algorithm. In this work, we used a segmentation CNN as the base algorithm due to their superior performance, similar to [20], and refer to it as autoCNN.

Network architecture: We used a U-Net architecture [13] for both the autoCNN and interCNN. It has been shown that this architecture produces automatic segmentation results on medical images that is comparable to more complex architectures [16,21]. Our implementation consists of 4 down- and 4 up-convolutional layers. Each down-convolutional layer is also connected to its respective up-convolutional layer through skip-connections. The final prediction of the U-Net is obtained by a softmax layer. The input consisted of 320×320 pixel patches. Most U-Net networks take the image as the only input. interCNN, however, takes three inputs: image, prediction and scribble mask.

For the base segmentation model autoCNN, we also used the same U-Net architecture but with only the image as the input. For both interCNN and autoCNN, we used drop-out and batch normalization during training [6,15].

We note that more complex networks can also be used both for autoCNN and interCNN. Here, we use a relatively simple architecture since our focus is on the training strategy rather than the architecture.

Robot user: The robot user we utilized for training the network is based on the model introduced by Nickisch et al. [10]. Here a random-user model is used. At each iteration a scribble is produced for every class in the image by comparing the prediction to the ground truth. First, all incorrectly classified pixel are identified. Subsequently, a pixel from the incorrectly classified pixels is chosen randomly for each class separately. In a next step, a region of 9×9 pixels is placed around each randomly chosen pixel and all the pixels in this region belonging to the class the scribble is currently made for are saved as the scribble for the respective class. This process is repeated for all classes in each iteration. The scribbles from all classes are then added together to obtain the final scribble mask for the respective iteration. The randomness in choosing the scribbles prevents the interCNN from over-fitting to a specific strategy that the user may not reproduce during test time, for instance always choosing the center of gravity of the difference set.

Implementation details: We used PyTorch [12] and Python to implement our U-net and robot user, respectively. The training took place on the in-house GPU cluster mainly consisting of GeForce GTX TITAN X with 12GB memory. The Adam optimization algorithm was used for training. The batch size was fixed to 4 images, learning rate to 0.0001 and the maximal number of iterations was 140'000. The images were normalized by taking the median of the training images and dividing all images by this value. To prevent over-fitting, data augmentation was used during training. For each batch, cropping, rotation or flipping was applied to all the images within the batch with a probability of 0.5.

3 Experiments and Results

Materials: We used the prostate dataset of the NCI-ISBI 2013 challenge [2]. The dataset consists of T2-weighted MRIs of the prostate acquired with a 3.0 T scanner. In total the dataset includes 60 patient volumes, each containing 15–20 slices. Of the 60 patients only 29 had multi-class ground truth segmentations, where the central gland and the peripheral zone were labeled. We focused our experiments on these 29 subjects to present results in multi-class segmentation.

We randomly divided the patients into 4 groups G1–G4. G1 contained 15 patients and was used as training data for the base segmentation algorithm, autoCNN. G2 consisted of 8 patients and was used as validation data for autoCNN. For training interCNN, both G1 and G2 were used. Training inter-CNN with G2 is crucial, since often the base method already performs very well on its training data, so interCNN would not encounter large incorrect classifications if only trained with G1. One patient, G3, was used as validation data to select the best performing interCNN. G4 constituted the test data and consisted of 5 patients.

For the benchmarking against other approaches, which were all focused on binary segmentation, we kept the same groups, but transformed the multi-class labels to binary by fusing the central gland and peripheral zone.

Evaluation: We employed the random robot-user for assessing test performance for the sake of efficiency. This neglects potential user errors but it does not simulate an ideal user nor favours a particular behaviour due to the randomness.

The segmentation performance was quantified using the Dice score (DSC): $DSC = \frac{2|S_g \cap S_p|}{|S_g| + |S_p|}$ where S_g is the ground truth and S_p is the predicted segmentation, and $|\cdot|$ denotes the number of pixels. We simulated that the user was interactively editing the proposed segmentations of each test image up to 20 times. We calculated the Dice score after every simulated user interaction to see how the segmentation results are influenced by the number of user inputs.

Computation speed: The interCNN produced an updated prediction per interactive iteration with a mean time of $3.9 \, ms \pm 0.2 \, ms$, thus enabling real-time use. GrabCut needs 1.2s per update (openCV implementation). Hence a substantial increase in update speed is obtained with interCNN over GrabCut.

Iteration training parameter: As shown in Algorithm 1, the proposed training strategy is to train interCNN for a fixed K number of iterations per batch. Meaning the predictions of every batch of images are iteratively updated together with their respective scribbles and fed back into interCNN for K number of consecutive iterations before moving on to the next batch. To inspect the influence of number of iterations during training, we varied K from 1 to 15.

The results for the two prostate structures are shown in Fig. 2. It can be seen that the Dice score improvement is substantially lower if iteration parameter K is set to 1 or 5, compared to a K of 10 and higher. Even though there is an initial improvement of the Dice score with a low K, the improvement slows down at later interaction iterations. One possible explanation for this observation

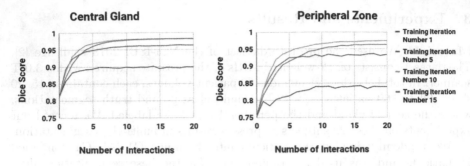

Fig. 2. Segmentation performance for interCNN trained with 1 to 15 iterations (K) for (left) central gland and (right) peripheral zone.

could be that the interCNN is mostly confronted with large incorrectly classified areas during training for low iteration parameters and learns to make large segmentation adjustments which is not required or beneficial at later stages.

Comparison to interactive segmentation from scratch: To evaluate the value of segmentation editing compared to state-of-the-art interactive segmentation from scratch, we looked at two recently proposed approaches.

UI-Net: The method is based on a CNN taking scribbles and the image as input to update its segmentation [1]. No automatic segmentation takes place, but rather initial scribbles are provided by the user. In contrast to [1], the initial scribbles were chosen randomly and not by erosion and dilation. As CNN we used the same U-Net architecture as for interCNN.

BIFSeg: This method is based on fine-tuning the last-layer of a CNN to update segmentations based on user inputs [19]. The algorithm starts by asking the user to draw a bounding-box around the object of interest. An initial segmentation is then computed and the scribbles of the user in the following iterations are used to fine-tune the last layer of the CNN that predicted the initial segmentation. We used their open-source code to benchmark against, which is claimed to also work on objects not seen during training.

In Fig. 3 the results of the comparison to interCNN with 10 training iterations can be seen. As both of the methods we compare to require user interaction, their Dice scores only start at iteration one. For BIFSeg this initial input is the bounding-box annotation. We investigated how the Dice score changed for all these methods over the course of 20 user interactions. It can be observed that interCNN, which edits existing segmentations, required substantially fewer user interactions than BIFSeg to reach a high Dice score (5 vs. 20). The performance of UI-Net, on the other hand, was very similar to the proposed method for this dataset, but it also used the full training dataset as it was trained from scratch.

The iterative improvement of the base segmentation by interCNN is illustrated on a representative test example in Fig. 4.

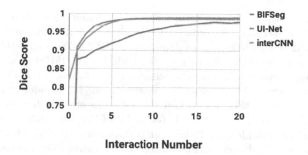

Interaction Number

Fig. 3. Segmentation performance of proposed method (interCNN) in comparison to state-of-the-art methods for increasing number of user interactions (1–20).

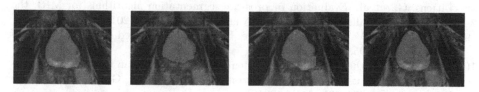

Fig. 4. Visual examples: segmentation overlays for (left→right) ground truth, autoCNN (DSC:0.84), and interCNN after interaction 1 (DSC:0.93) and 5 (DSC:0.98).

4   Conclusions

We proposed an iterative interaction training strategy for efficient segmentation editing with networks. Compared to non-iterative training, the proposed strategy yielded higher segmentation accuracy. The difference was the highest when the iteration parameter for training was at ten and higher. The proposed strategy allows the CNN to learn to correct small and large errors. Finally, we compared our method to alternatives that perform interactive segmentation from scratch. We observed that interCNN when trained with the proposed strategy yielded results on par with the state-of-the-art methods. The advantage of segmentation editing networks, such as interCNN, compared to interaction segmentation from scratch is that they do not need user interaction to initialize segmentation.

Acknowledgments. We thank the Swiss Data Science Center (project C17-04 deep-MICROIA) for funding and acknowledge NVIDIA for GPU support.

References

1. Amrehn, M., et al.: UI-Net: Interactive artificial neural networks for iterative image segmentation based on a user model. arXiv:1709.03450 (2017)
2. Bloch, N., Madabhushi, A., Huisman, H., et al.: NCI-ISBI 2013 challenge: automated segmentation of prostate structures. The Cancer Imaging Archive (2015)

3. Criminisi, A., Sharp, T., Blake, A.: GeoS: geodesic image segmentation. In: Forsyth, D., Torr, P., Zisserman, A. (eds.) ECCV 2008. LNCS, vol. 5302, pp. 99–112. Springer, Heidelberg (2008). https://doi.org/10.1007/978-3-540-88682-2_9

4. van Ginneken, B., Kerkstra, S., Litjens, G., Toth, R.: PROMISE12 challenge results (2018). https://promise12.grand-challenge.org/evaluation/results/

5. Grady, L., Schiwietz, T., Aharon, S., Westermann, R.: Random walks for interactive organ segmentation in two and three dimensions: implementation and validation. In: Duncan, J.S., Gerig, G. (eds.) MICCAI 2005. LNCS, vol. 3750, pp. 773–780. Springer, Heidelberg (2005). https://doi.org/10.1007/11566489_95

6. Ioffe, S., Szegedy, C.: Batch normalization: Accelerating deep network training by reducing internal covariate shift. arXiv:1502.03167 (2015)

7. Litjens, G., et al.: A survey on deep learning in medical image analysis. Med. Image Anal. **42**, 60–88 (2017)

8. Litjens, G., et al.: Evaluation of prostate segmentation algorithms for MRI: the PROMISE12 challenge. Med. Image Anal. **18**(2), 359–373 (2014)

9. Mahadevan, S., Voigtlaender, P., Leibe, B.: Iteratively trained interactive segmentation. arXiv:1805.04398 (2018)

10. Nickisch, H., Rother, C., Kohli, P., Rhemann, C.: Learning an interactive segmentation system. In: Indian Conference on Computer Vision, Graphics and Image Processing, pp. 274–281. ACM (2010)

11. Pasquier, D., Lacornerie, T., Vermandel, M., Rousseau, J., Lartigau, E., Betrouni, N., et al.: Automatic segmentation of pelvic structures from magnetic resonance images for prostate cancer radiotherapy. Int. J. Radiat. Oncol. **68**(2), 592–600 (2007)

12. Paszke, A., et al.: Automatic differentiation in pytorch. In: NIPS-W (2017)

13. Ronneberger, O., Fischer, P., Brox, T.: U-Net: convolutional networks for biomedical image segmentation. In: Navab, N., Hornegger, J., Wells, W.M., Frangi, A.F. (eds.) MICCAI 2015. LNCS, vol. 9351, pp. 234–241. Springer, Cham (2015). https://doi.org/10.1007/978-3-319-24574-4_28

14. Rother, C., Kolmogorov, V., Blake, A.: GrabCut: interactive foreground extraction using iterated graph cuts. In: ACM Transactions on Graphics (TOG), vol. 23, pp. 309–314. ACM (2004)

15. Srivastava, N., Hinton, G., Krizhevsky, A., Sutskever, I., Salakhutdinov, R.: Dropout: a simple way to prevent neural networks from overfitting. J. Mach. Learn. Res. **15**(1), 1929–1958 (2014)

16. Tian, Z., Liu, L., Zhang, Z., Fei, B.: PSNet: prostate segmentation on MRI based on a convolutional neural network. J. Med. Imaging **5**(2), 021208 (2018)

17. Toth, R., et al.: Accurate prostate volume estimation using multifeature active shape models on T2-weighted MRI. Acad. Radiol. **18**(6), 745–754 (2011)

18. Vos, P., Barentsz, J., Karssemeijer, N., Huisman, H.: Automatic computer-aided detection of prostate cancer based on multiparametric magnetic resonance image analysis. Phys. Med. Biol. **57**(6), 1527 (2012)

19. Wang, G., Li, W., Zuluaga, M.A., Pratt, R., Patel, P.A., Aertsen, M., et al.: Interactive medical image segmentation using deep learning with image-specific fine-tuning. IEEE Trans. Med. Imaging (2018)

20. Wang, G., et al.: DeepIGeoS: a deep interactive geodesic framework for medical image segmentation. IEEE Trans. Pattern Anal. (2018)

21. Zhu, Q., Du, B., Turkbey, B., Choyke, P.L., Yan, P.: Deeply-supervised CNN for prostate segmentation. In: International Joint Conference on Neural Networks, pp. 178–184. IEEE (2017)

Temporal Consistent 2D-3D Registration of Lateral Cephalograms and Cone-Beam Computed Tomography Images

Yungeng Zhang[1], Yuru Pei[1(✉)], Haifang Qin[1], Yuke Guo[2], Gengyu Ma[3], Tianmin Xu[4], and Hongbin Zha[1]

[1] Key Laboratory of Machine Perception (MOE), Department of Machine Intelligence, Peking University, Beijing, China
peiyuru@cis.pku.edu.cn
[2] Luoyang Institute of Science and Technology, Luoyang, China
[3] uSens Inc., San Jose, CA, USA
[4] School of Stomatology, Peking University, Beijing, China

Abstract. Craniofacial growths and developments play an important role in treatment planning of orthopedics and orthodontics. Traditional growth studies are mainly on longitudinal growth datasets of 2D lateral cephalometric radiographs (LCR). In this paper, we propose a temporal consistent 2D-3D registration technique enabling 3D growth measurements of craniofacial structures. We initialize the independent 2D-3D registration by the convolutional neural network (CNN)-based regression, which produces the dense displacement field of the cone-beam computed tomography (CBCT) image when given the LCR. The temporal constraints of the growth-stable structures are used to refine the 2D-3D registration. Instead of traditional independent 2D-3D registration, we jointly solve the nonrigid displacement fields of a series of input LCRs captured at different ages. The hierarchical pyramid of the digitally reconstructed radiographs (DRR) is introduced to fasten the convergence. The proposed method has been applied to the growth dataset in clinical orthodontics. The resulted 2D-3D registration is consistent with both the input LCRs concerning the structural contours and the 3D volumetric images regarding the growth-stable structures.

1 Introduction

Craniofacial growths and developments are of great importance to the dentofacial orthopedic and orthodontic treatments. The maxillary and mandibular growth is a crucial factor of treatment planning, especially for the adolescents undergoing growth accelerations. The yearly longitudinal growth datasets of lateral cephalometric radiographs (LCR) have been collected in clinical orthodontics for craniofacial growth analysis [1]. The linear and angular measurements of craniofacial structures in the vertical and sagittal dimensions are used for growth analysis and prediction. However, it is hard to measure and visualize the 3D

Y. Shi et al. (Eds.): MLMI 2018, LNCS 11046, pp. 371–379, 2018.
https://doi.org/10.1007/978-3-030-00919-9_43

structural growth from the 2D LCRs. The 2D-3D registration bridges the 2D radiographs and the 3D volumetric images [2]. Instead of the 2D-3D registration of one stand-alone radiograph, a temporal consistent 2D-3D registration of a series of radiographs captured at different ages is desirable to measure the person-specific 3D growth and the statistical analysis of the growth dataset.

The 2D-3D registration has been addressed in the medical imaging community for decades [2]. The intensity-based 2D-3D registration [7,11,14] tries to minimize the difference between the DRR projections of deformed volumetric images and the target radiographs. The parameter space of the nonrigid 2D-3D registration is extremely large considering the dense voxel-wise displacements of the volumetric image. There are several approaches to reduce the parameter space, such as the image interpolation [13] and the subspace projection [10]. The B-spline-based interpolation is used to estimate the dense displacement field by the tri-linear interpolation of control parameters [8]. The statistical model employs the principal component analysis (PCA) to estimate the dense displacement field by limited orthogonal components. The traditional parameter solving relies on the iterative optimization to incrementally deform the reference volume to make it consistent with the input radiograph. The online computational complexity is primarily due to enormous estimations of the DRR images. In recent years, a pre-trained regression model is introduced to downsize the online computational complexity. The partial least squares regression (PLSR) [12], the random forest [5], and the convolutional neural network (CNN) [3] have been used to build the regression models. The above regression models are learned from generated pairs of radiographs and volumetric images without explicitly addressing the temporal consistencies regarding the growth and developments.

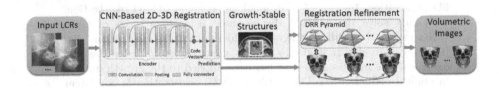

Fig. 1. System framework.

In this paper, we propose a temporal-consistent 2D-3D registration method to estimate the 3D volumetric images from the LCRs in the craniofacial growth dataset (Fig. 1). We parameterize the 3D volumetric image by projecting the dense displacement fields to the low-dimensional linear subspace. When given a series of homogeneous LCRs captured at different ages, we initialize the corresponding volumetric images using the CNN-based regression. The temporal constraint is introduced using the growth-stable structure of the anterior cranial base (ACB). The volumetric deformation parameters embedded in the subspace are refined given the temporal constraints. We introduce the DRR pyramid for the online parameter solving, in which the low-resolution DRRs are used for coarse registration, and high-resolution DRRs for further fine registration. The proposed method has been applied to the growth dataset [1] for the temporal consistent reconstruction and visualization of 3D craniofacial growths. To the best of our knowledge, it is the first attempt to analyze the 3D growth from the growth and development dataset of LCRs in clinical orthodontics.

2   Method

The input is a collection of LCRs $\mathcal{I} = \{I_1, \ldots, I_K\}$ captured at different ages of the same subject with normal occlusion. The goal is to jointly estimate 3D volumetric images $\mathcal{V} = \{V_1, \ldots, V_K\}$ corresponding to the input LCRs. The reconstructed volumetric images are required to be consistent with the LCRs in the sense of the DRR projection. Moreover, considering the homogeneous nature of the input LCRs, the corresponding volumetric images are required to be temporal consistent by retaining the growth-stable structures.

Preprocessing. The input LCRs are aligned in the preprocessing. The stable structure of the ACB determines the overall superimposition (see Fig. 4(c)). Such superimposition is often used to measure the maxillary, mandibular, and fiducial point changes in the study of craniofacial growths and developments. The existing automatic parsing and landmark location system, such as the active shape model [9], can be used to locate the tracing of LCRs for the alignments.

Volumetric Image Representation. In order to reduce the parameter space of the volumetric deformation, we combine the cubic B-spline-based interpolation and the PCA techniques. The cubic B-splines are used to define the deformation, $M = \sum_{i=0}^{3} \sum_{j=0}^{3} \sum_{k=0}^{3} B_i(u) B_j(v) B_k(w) G$. B and G denote the base functions and the control grid of B-splines respectively. The nonrigid deformation is recovered from the displacement vectors at the control grid G by the cubic interpolation. When given a training image dataset $\mathcal{V}_s = \{V_i | i = 1, \ldots, N\}$ and a reference volume V_r, a group of nonrigid deformations from V_r are represented by the displacement vectors t on the reference control grid G_r. We build a statistical deformation model of the displacement vectors. The average image $\bar{V}$ of the dataset is estimated based on the average deformation field, and $\bar{V} = f(V_r, M(\frac{1}{N} \sum_{i=1}^{N} t_i))$. The function $f(V_r, t)$ applies the displacement field determined by t to V_r for nonrigid image warping. The deformation field related to the average image $\bar{V}$ is updated, $t'_i = (1 - \frac{1}{N}) t_i - \frac{1}{N} \sum_{j=1, j \neq i}^{N} t_j$. We apply the PCA to the displacement vector t'_i. The low dimensional subspace coordinate α and the associated projection matrix P are used to represent the volumetric image, and $V = f(\bar{V}, M(\alpha P))$.

2.1   CNN-Based 2D-3D Registration

We perform the initial 2D-3D registration using the deep neural network-based regression. The framework is based on the VGG-face model [4] including 13 convolutional and 5 pooling layers. Specifically, we add the long-jump residual connections between intermediate convolutional layers and the fully connected layer for the multi-scale feature fusion (see Fig. 1). The down-sampling of feature maps from the intermediate layers are performed by convolutions with strides of 2^k, $k = 1, \ldots, 4$. The concatenation of feature maps is performed by an additional convolutional layer, where the stack of features maps with the size of $z^2 \times l$ is convolved using a kernel of $1 \times 1 \times l/2$. l is set to the number of input feature maps. The input of the network is an LCR cropped and scaled to 200×200 pixels. The training data including the paired radiographs and volumetric images are generated by random sampling in the subspace of the displacements fields as in [6]. The loss function is defined by the L_2 distance between the predicted and the ground truth subspace coordinates associated with the volumetric images.

2.2 Temporal Consistent 2D-3D Registration

We jointly estimate 3D volumetric images of a series of LCRs captured at different ages. Given the initial 2D-3D registration of the LCR and the volumetric images, we refine the registration by introducing temporal constraints. Since there exist structures reaching the full growth at a very early age, we use such growth-stable structure of the ACB for the temporal consistency of resulted volumetric images. The objective function is defined as $E(\alpha) = E_c + \gamma E_r$. The first data term $E_c(\alpha) = \sum_i^K d^2_{MI}(I_i, I'_i)$, where I'_i denotes the DRR of the deformed volumetric image $f(\bar{V}, M(\alpha_i P))$. The function d_{MI} returns the image distance using the mutual information (MI)-based metric. The constant γ is set to 10^{-7} in our experiments. The resulted volumetric images are consistent with the input LCR images regarding the DRR projections by minimizing E_c.

The second pairwise regularization term E_r is used to guarantee the consistency of volumetric images at different ages by minimizing the shape differences of stable structures.

$$E_r(\alpha) = \sum_{i,j=1}^{K} s_{ij} \| U \circ (M(\alpha_i P) - M(\alpha_j P)) \|^2 + \mu \sum_{i=1}^{K} \|\alpha_i\|_1^2, \tag{1}$$

where α_i denotes the deformation parameters of the i-th LCR. s denotes the similarity of the input LCRs, $s_{ij} = \exp(-d^2_{MI}(I_i, I_j))$. U is a mask represented by a matrix of the same size as the reference volume V_r. We use the stable structure of the ACB in our system. The entry U_i is set to 1 when the corresponding voxel is inside the stable structure, and 0 otherwise. We regularize the deformation parameters in the subspace by minimizing $\|\alpha\|_1$. The constant μ is set at 10^4 in our experiments. The Gauss-Newton method is used to solve the optimization problem. The initial values are set at $\alpha^{(0)}$ obtained by the initial CNN-based registration (Sect. 2.1). The residual function F is defined as follows:

$$F(\alpha_i) = \begin{pmatrix} d_{MI}(I_i, I'_i) \\ \sqrt{s_{i,j}}[U \circ (M(\alpha_i P) - M(\alpha_j P))] \\ \|\alpha_i\|_1 \end{pmatrix}. \tag{2}$$

In each iteration, the subspace coordinate is updated by the newly estimated $\delta\alpha$, and $\delta\alpha = (J'J)^{-1}J'F(\alpha)$. J denotes the Jacobian matric of F with the partial derivative $\frac{\partial F}{\partial \alpha_i}$ defined as follows:

$$\frac{\partial F}{\partial \alpha_i} = \begin{pmatrix} \sum_{a,b}\left(1 + \log \frac{p_{II'}}{p_{I'}}\right)\frac{1}{N_I}\sum_x \varphi(a - \bar{I}_i(x))\frac{\partial \varphi(b - \bar{I}'_i(x,\alpha_i))}{\partial \alpha_i} \\ \frac{\sqrt{s_{i,j}}[U\circ(M((\alpha_i+\delta\alpha_i)P)-M(\alpha_iP))]}{\delta a_i} \\ sign(\alpha_i) \end{pmatrix}, \quad (3)$$

where $p_{I'}$ and $p_{II'}$ denote the probability distribution and joint probability distribution functions of I and I'. N_I denotes the number of pixels of the LCR. $\bar{I}(x)$ denotes the discretized image according to the number of histogram bins. a and b denote the intensity values of histogram bins with respect to the image I and I'. φ is a Kroneckers function. $\varphi(x) = 1$ when $x = 0$, and $\varphi(x) = 0$ otherwise.

DRR Pyramid. The DRR by volumetric rendering is known to be time-consuming with a complexity depending on the image size. In our system, we employ the DRR pyramid to accelerate the evaluation of the energy function. A Gaussian image hierarchy is built for the LCRs with a factor of 3. The bottom layer of the hierarchy is the original image. The image is down-sampled by a Gaussian smoothing operator. The optimization starts with the highest level of the pyramid. When it comes to the original resolution, limited iterations are enough for convergence.

3 Experiments

To demonstrate the validity of the proposed method, we perform the temporal consistent 2D-3D registration on 30 groups of LCRs in the longitudinal population dataset [1]. The LCRs are captured from 30 adolescents including 14 boys and 16 girls between 9 and 15 years of ages with normal occlusion. The input LCRs are cropped and re-scaled to 200×200 pixels. No ground truth volumetric images are available in the longitudinal growth dataset.

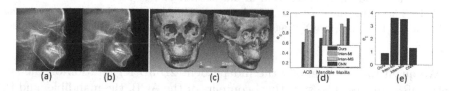

Fig. 2. The overlapping of structural contours of the ACB, the mandible, and the maxilla between the DRR of the estimated volumetric volumes and the ground truth (a) before and (b) after the 2D-3D registration (yellow-reference, red-target, blue-deformed reference). (c) Two viewpoints of the visualization of the MSDs between the estimated volumetric image and the ground truth. (d) e_c and (e) e_t of the proposed method, the Inten-MS, the Inten-MI [14], and the CNN [4]-based method.

The training data of the CNN used in the initial 2D-3D registration (Sect. 2.1) are generated from a volumetric image dataset with 120 CBCT images. The CBCT images are re-scaled to a resolution of $200 \times 200 \times 190$ with a voxel size of $1 \times 1 \times 1\ mm^3$. The generated DRR image is with a resolution of 200×200. The nonrigid deformation-based data augmentation is performed similar to [6].

Qualitative Assessment. The proposed 2D-3D registration is evaluated by the mean contour deviation of the ACB, the maxilla, and the mandible. $e_c = \frac{1}{n_c} \sum_{i=1}^{n_c} \|x_i - x_i^{gt}\|$. x_i and x_i^{gt} denote n_c evenly sampled points on the structural contours of the generated DRRs and the input LCRs. In our system, we employ the B-spline-based nonrigid deformation and evaluate the volumetric images using the deviations at the control grid, $e_t = \frac{1}{n_t} \sum_{i=1}^{n_t} \|t_i - t_i^{gt}\|$. t and t^{gt} denote the estimated and the ground truth displacement vectors at n_t control points. We also measure the mean surface deviation (MSD) of the 3D stable structure of the ACB before and after the 2D-3D registration. We compare with the intensity-based 2D-3D registration using the mean squared metric (MS) (Inten-MS) and the MI metric (Inter-MI) [14], and the CNN-based regression model [4].

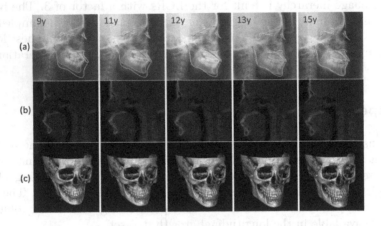

Fig. 3. (a) The overlapping of structural contours of the ACB, the mandible, and the maxilla before and after registration of one subject aging between 9 and 15 years of ages. (b) The semi-transparent sagittal cross-sectional overlappings between 9 years (red) and 11–15 years (gray) of ages. (c) The visualization of estimated 3D volumes.

We quantitatively evaluate the independent 2D-3D registration on the synthetic DRR images. The structural contours of the ACB, the mandible, and the maxilla of estimated volumetric images are consistent with the input LCRs as shown in Fig. 2 (a, b). The overlappings of the skull surfaces clearly show that the 2D-3D registration reduces the gap between the estimated volumetric image and the ground truth (Fig. 2(c)). Figure 2(d, e) show the comparison with the Inten-MS and Inten-MI [14], and the CNN [4]-based methods in terms of e_c and e_t. The proposed method outperforms the compared approaches in terms of contour consistencies and nonrigid volumetric deformation.

Regarding the joint 2D-3D registration of a series of LCRs of the same subject at different ages, we assess both the contour and the growth-stable structure consistencies as shown in Fig. 3 and Fig. 4. The structural contours of the ACB, the mandible, and the maxilla of the DRR from the estimated volumetric image are consistent with the input LCRs as shown in Fig. 3(a). The overlappings of estimated 3D volumetric images clearly show the 3D maxillary, mandibular growths (see Fig. 3(b)). We visualize 3D skulls of one subject aging from 9 to 15 years of ages. The overlappings of stable structures of the ACB before and after temporal-consistent registration are shown in Fig. 4(a, b). The MSDs of the ACB decrease from 0.78 mm to 0.12 mm when given the temporal constraints.

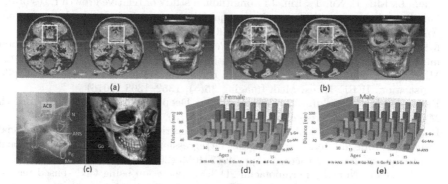

Fig. 4. Overlapping of skull surface meshes before and after the temporal consistent registration of two age pairs, i.e., (a) 9–11 years of ages and (b) 13–15 years of ages. From left to right: overlapping before the temporal consistent registration, two viewpoints of overlappings after the temporal consistent registration. The ACB regions are white blocked. (c) Landmarks used in the growth measurements. Craniofacial growth between 9 and 15 years of ages of (d) the female and (e) the male.

The estimated 3D volumetric images corresponding to the input LCRs enable the measurements of 3D growths as shown in Fig. 4 (c–e). Instead of traditional linear measurements on the 2D LCRs [1], we measure the distances of N-ANS, N-S, Go-Me, Go-Pg, S-Go, and N-Me in the 3D space. Note that the 3D measurement is more intuitive without considering the depth losing in the LCRs. The 3D volumes not only enable vertical and sagittal measurements similar to LCRs but the oblique measurements, such as Go-Me.

4   Conclusion

In this paper, we propose a novel temporal consistent 2D-3D registration method for joint estimation of volumetric images related to the LCRs. Aside from the stand-alone 2D-3D registration of one LCR, the proposed method imposes the temporal constraints to maintain the 3D growth-stable structures of the ACB.

Our framework takes advantage of the CNN-based regression and the DRR pyramid for efficient registration. The proposed method is applied to a longitudinal growth dataset of LCRs, resulting to volumetric images consistent with both the 2D LCR regarding structural contours and the 3D growth-stable structures. The experiments demonstrate the potential of the proposed temporal consistent 2D-3D registration for the craniofacial growth measurements in the 3D space.

Acknowledgment. This work was supported by NSFC 61272342.

References

1. Chen, L., Liu, J., Xu, T., Lin, J.: Longitudinal study of relative growth rates of the maxilla and the mandible according to quantitative cervical vertebral maturation. Am. J. Orthod. Dentofac. Orthop. **137**(6), 736.e1–736.e8 (2010)
2. Markelj, P., Tomaževič, D., Likar, B., Pernuš, F.: A review of 3d/2d registration methods for image-guided interventions. Med. Image Anal. **16**(3), 642–661 (2012)
3. Miao, S., Wang, Z.J., Liao, R.: A cnn regression approach for real-time 2d/3d registration. IEEE Trans. Med. Imaging **35**(5), 1352–1363 (2016)
4. Parkhi, O.M., Vedaldi, A., Zisserman, A.: Deep face recognition. In: British Machine Vision Conference, pp. 41.1–41.12 (2015)
5. Pei, Y., Dai, F., Xu, T., Zha, H., Ma, G.: Volumetric reconstruction of craniofacial structures from 2d lateral cephalograms by regression forest. In: IEEE International Conference on Image Processing, pp. 4052–4056 (2016)
6. Pei, Y., et al.: Non-rigid craniofacial 2D-3D registration using CNN-based regression. In: Cardoso, M.J., Arbel, T., Carneiro, G., Syeda-Mahmood, T., Tavares, J.M.R.S., Moradi, M., Bradley, A., Greenspan, H., Papa, J.P., Madabhushi, A., Nascimento, J.C., Cardoso, J.S., Belagiannis, V., Lu, Z. (eds.) DLMIA/ML-CDS -2017. LNCS, vol. 10553, pp. 117–125. Springer, Cham (2017). https://doi.org/10. 1007/978-3-319-67558-9_14
7. Perona, P., Shiota, T., Malik, J.: Anisotropic diffusion. In: Geometry-Driven Diffusion in Computer Vision, pp. 73–92 (1994)
8. Yu, W., Tannast, M., Zheng, G.: Non-rigid free-form 2d–3d registration using a b-spline-based statistical deformation model. Pattern Recognit. **63**, 689–699 (2017)
9. Yue, W., Yin, D., Li, C., Wang, G., Xu, T.: Automated 2-d cephalometric analysis on x-ray images by a model-based approach. IEEE Trans. Biomed. Eng. **53**(8), 1615–1623 (2006)
10. Zheng, G.: Statistically deformable 2d/3d registration for accurate determination of post-operative cup orientation from single standard x-ray radiograph. In: Medical Image Computing and Computer-Assisted Intervention–MICCAI 2009, pp. 820–827 (2009)
11. Zheng, G.: Effective incorporating spatial information in a mutual information based 3d–2d registration of a ct volume to x-ray images. Comput. Med. Imaging Graphics **34**(7), 553–562 (2010)
12. Zheng, G.: 3d volumetric intensity reconsturction from 2d x-ray images using partial least squares regression. In: IEEE International Symposium on Biomedical Imaging, pp. 1268–1271 (2013)
13. Zheng, G., Gollmer, S., Schumann, S., Dong, X., Feilkas, T., Ballester, M.A.G.: A 2d/3d correspondence building method for reconstruction of a patient-specific 3d bone surface model using point distribution models and calibrated x-ray images. Med. Image Anal. **13**(6), 883–899 (2009)

14. Zollei, L., Grimson, E., Norbash, A., Wells, W.: 2d–3d rigid registration of x-ray fluoroscopy and ct images using mutual information and sparsely sampled histogram estimators. In: IEEE Conference on Computer Vision and Pattern Recognition (2001)

Computation of Total Kidney Volume from CT Images in Autosomal Dominant Polycystic Kidney Disease Using Multi-task 3D Convolutional Neural Networks

Deepak Keshwani[✉], Yoshiro Kitamura, and Yuanzhong Li

Imaging Technology Center, Fujifilm Corporation, Tokyo, Japan
deepak.keshwani@fujifilm.com

Abstract. Autosomal dominant polycystic kidney disease (ADPKD) characterized by progressive growth of renal cysts is the most prevalent and potentially lethal monogenic renal disease, affecting one in every 500–1000 people. Total Kidney Volume (TKV) and its growth computed from Computed Tomography images has been accepted as an essential prognostic marker for renal function loss. Due to large variation in shape and size of kidney in ADPKD, existing methods to compute TKV (i.e. to segment ADKP) including those based on 2D convolutional neural networks are not accurate enough to be directly useful in clinical practice. In this work, we propose multi-task 3D Convolutional Neural Networks to segment ADPK and achieve a mean DICE score of 0.95 and mean absolute percentage TKV error of 3.86%. Additionally, to solve the challenge of class imbalance, we propose to simply bootstrap cross entropy loss and compare results with recently prevalent dice loss in medical image segmentation community.

Keywords: Autosomal dominant polycystic kidney disease (ADKPD)
Multi-task learning · 3D fully convolutional network (3D FCN)

1 Introduction

Autosomal dominant polycystic kidney disease is a hereditary systemic disorder which is characterized by progressive development and growth of bilateral renal cysts filled with fluid [1]. ADPKD effected kidneys can grow as much as 10–15 times in size before complete renal function is lost. It is one of the leading causes of end-stage renal diseases resulting in dialysis or kidney transplantation in majority of the patients. In United States alone, number of patients effected by ADPKD is estimated to be 500,000 [3]. Recently, drugs based on new compound Tolvaptan can slow the rate of cyst growth in ADPKD patients [2]. As per the guidelines, use of the drug is recommended after evaluating the age, stage of ADPKD and whether the disease is progressing rapidly. Rapid progression is defined by total kidney volume (TKV) increase of over 5% per year, where TKV is the combined volume of both left and right kidney. It means that TKV should be measured within 5% precision from Computed Tomography (CT) or Magnetic Resonance (MR) images to be useful in clinical practice. In this

© Springer Nature Switzerland AG 2018
Y. Shi et al. (Eds.): MLMI 2018, LNCS 11046, pp. 380–388, 2018.
https://doi.org/10.1007/978-3-030-00919-9_44

work, we target computing TKV from CT images but the methodology is extendable to MR images as well.

Automatic segmentation of ADPK is very challenging due to large changes in its size, shape and position in the abdomen. Figure 1 shows the difference between contrast enhanced normal kidney and ADPK. A normal kidney roughly measures few hundred milliliters each while an ADPK can measure anywhere from several hundred up to several thousand milliliters. ADPK lose renal function disabling them from filtering contrast agents inserted in blood stream. Thus, kidneys in most ADPKD patients is non-contrast enhanced making the segmentation task even more challenging. Finally, many ADPKD patients develop hepatic cysts which come in contact with renal cysts as shown in Fig. 1. Distinguishing them is the most challenging part in ADPK segmentation, difficult even for a human observer.

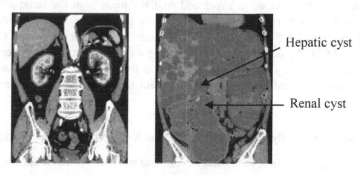

Fig. 1. Comparison of normal kidney and ADPK. Left: Contrast enhanced normal kidney, right: non-contrast enhanced ADPK.

A recently proposed automated method to segment ADPK from CT images use 2D fully convolutional neural networks and reports a mean dice score of 0.86 and mean absolute TKV error of over 10% [4]. But as already mentioned that even 5% TKV change can be clinically important. In this work, we improve the ADPK segmentation accuracy to an extent that it can be directly useful for clinical practice with following contributions:

(1) We propose a multi-task 3D Fully Convolutional Neural Network (FCN) for ADPK segmentation. The multi-task approach utilizes not only ADPK dataset (abdomen CT images and kidney mask pairs) but also Liver dataset (abdomen CT images and liver mask pairs) for learning ADPK segmentation task. This approach not only surpass existing 2D FCN approach [4] by large margin but also shows improvement over single task 3D FCN approach which learns only from ADPK dataset. Learning from multiple segmentation datasets to boost performance is an interesting solution to data scarcity in medical imaging domain.

(2) We propose that by simply bootstrapping cross entropy loss can the resolve class imbalance issue rather than using intricate dice loss recently popular for medical image segmentation tasks.

2   Materials and Methods

2.1   Dataset and Preprocessing

ADPK dataset: This dataset is taken from an existing study performed by clinical experts in which they analyze various semi-automated methods to compute TKV from CT images in ADPKD affected patients [1]. The dataset contains a total of 203 abdominal CT image and kidney mask pairs, mostly non-contrast enhanced with various slice thickness ranging from 0.5 to 5 mm. Due to small size of the dataset, rather than preparing a separate test set, we perform 3-fold cross validation.

Liver dataset: This dataset contains 176 contrast and non-contrast enhanced abdominal CT images with corresponding liver masks, all utilized for training. Most scans in the dataset contain tumorous liver, and only a single image contains hepatic cyst. Note that no two images in Liver and ADKP dataset is of the same patient.

Preprocessing: Due to memory limitations, the input images are rescaled to uniform voxel spacing of 1.5 mm. Also, rather than setting an entire abdomen CT image as input to 3D FCN, the images are cropped along z direction (axial) to generate crops roughly of size z = 144, y = 250, x = 250. This is true both for the Liver and ADPK dataset. Rotation and scaling is applied as a data augmentation technique to avoid overfitting.

2.2   Multi-task 3D Fully Convolutional Network for ADPK Segmentation

ADPK shows large variation in its shape, size and position in the abdomen, thus the network should be trained using large and diverse dataset. But, one of the major challenges in medical domain is difficulty in obtaining large datasets validated by clinical experts. This is both due to regulatory hurdles and time consuming 3D labelling task. In our case, the dataset contains 203 3D images and mask pairs, of which a quarter is used for validation. To counter data scarcity challenge, our idea is to use not only ADPK dataset but also datasets of other organs to increase the segmentation accuracy of ADPK. To be specific, we propose a multi-task 3D FCN architecture as shown in Fig. 2 to learn from both the Liver and ADPK dataset.

3D FCN have already shown good performance on anatomy segmentation tasks [5, 6]. Popular 3D FCN architectures like VNet [6] are characterized by a contracting encoder part to extract global features from input image and decoder part to produce full resolution output. In our proposed architecture, encoder layer weights are shared between ADPK and Liver segmentation tasks, with unique decoder part for each task. This is different from recently proposed multi-task multi-modality learning approach using a single encoder-decoder architecture [7]. One of the important reason to split the network at decoder level is due to inconsistent background class definition in the two datasets. In the ADPK dataset, background class encompasses liver region, while in the Liver dataset it encompasses kidney region. Using a single encoder decoder architecture prohibits use of such inconsistent datasets. Figure 2 illustrates the detailed network architecture. When each segmentation task is looked at individually, our network architecture is based on 3D UNet. Although relative to 3D UNet, we increase the depth of our network to have a cumulative receptive field roughly the same size as that of

ADPK. In the encoder part, each "conv block" consists of two $3 \times 3 \times 3$ convolutional filters each followed by a batch normalization and ReLU unit. The conv block is followed by a $2 \times 2 \times 2$ max pooling layer. In the decoder part, each "deconv block" consists of an upconvolution of stride 2 in each dimension. At the end of each decoder network is a $1 \times 1 \times 1$ convolution layer to reduce the number of channels to the number of classes in each segmentation task. Finally, we also fuse high resolution feature maps from encoder network to the decoder network using long skip connections, same as 3D UNet architecture. When training, the network is provided with two input images, one from each liver and ADPK dataset.

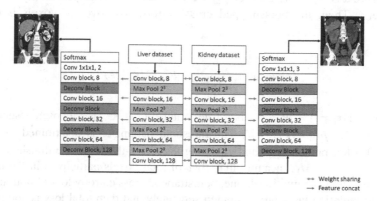

Fig. 2. Multi-task 3D FCN: The central towers show shared encoder part of the network whose outputs goes into two separate decoders to generate liver and ADPK segmentation masks.

2.3 Bootstrapping Cross Entropy Loss

Class imbalance is a major issue in medical image segmentation, more so when the input is 3D. In this case, the background to kidney voxels ratio is roughly 50:1 which makes conventional cross entropy loss optimization heavily biased towards the background class. To tackle this problem, dice loss has been proposed recently which results in accurate foreground segmentation than simply using weighted cross entropy loss [6]. Let C be the number of classes and let $p_{i,c}$ and $g_{i,c}$ be the prediction and ground truth probabilities belonging to class $c \in \{1,...,C\}$ at voxel $i \in \{1,...,N\}$. Then multi-class dice loss is defined in Eq. 1.

$$L_{dice} = -\frac{1}{C} \sum_c^C \frac{2 * \sum_i^N p_{i,c} g_{i,c}}{\sum_i^N p_{i,c} + \sum_i^N g_{i,c}} \tag{1}$$

In practice though, multi-class dice loss can be unstable. For example, when input image does not contain kidney region ($\sum_i^N g_{i,kidney} = 0$), making loss corresponding to kidney class zero ($\sum_i^N p_{i,kidney} g_{i,kidney} = 0$), even though false positives may exist

$(\sum\limits_{i}^{N} p_{i,kidney} \neq 0)$. Since, we crop the abdomen CT scan image along z dimension, it often happens that the kidney region is not present in the input crop. Additionally, while dice loss does solve the issue of inter-class imbalance to some extent, it does not take into account intra-class imbalance. In this work we propose bootstrapping of cross entropy loss for solving both inter and intra class imbalance following from an existing work in the domain of RGB image segmentation [8]. The idea behind bootstrapping is to backpropagate cross entropy loss not from all but a subset of voxels with posterior probability less than threshold value. Let $y_1, \ldots y_N \in \{1, \ldots, C\}$ be the target class labels for voxels $1, \ldots . N$, and let $p_{i,j}$ be the posterior class probability of class j and voxel i. Then, the bootstrapped cross entropy loss over K voxels is defined in Eq. 2.

$$L_{bootstrap} = -\frac{1}{K} \sum_{i=1}^{N} 1\left[p_{i,y_i} < t_K\right] \log p_{i,y_i} \qquad (2)$$

Where $1[x] = 1$ iff x is true and $t_K \in \mathbb{R}$ is chosen such that $\left|\{i \in \{1, \ldots . N\} : p_{i,y_i} < t_K\}\right| = K$. The threshold parameter is determined by sorting the predicted log probabilities and choosing the $K + 1$-th one as the threshold. In this work, we set $K = 0.1N$, meaning that 10% of total voxels participate in the training. Since our problem is a multi-task one, bootstrapped cross entropy loss of both liver and ADKP segmentation tasks are computed separately and then total loss is computed as the mean of two.

3   Experiments and Training

2D FCN: The existing work on ADPK segmentation use 2D FCN on a dataset that is not available publically [4]. So we implement 2D FCN approach as mentioned in the literature on our dataset and report the results. This experiment forms the baseline to which we compare the methods proposed in this work.

   3D FCN: A standard 3D FCN based on 3D UNet architecture is implemented which learns from ADPK dataset. The architecture is shown in Fig. 2, except that only ADPK part of the network is used for training.

   Multi-task 3D FCN: We perform multi-task learning using network architecture as shown in Fig. 2 and compare the results with single task learning.

   Multi-task 3D FCN and bootstrapping of cross entropy loss: Above mentioned 3D FCN and multi-task 3D FCN use dice loss function for optimization. To analyze bootstrapping as a solution to class imbalance, in this experiment we training the multi-task network by minimizing bootstrapped cross entropy loss.

   We optimize both dice loss and bootstrapped cross entropy loss using Adam optimizer with a base learning rate of 0.001. All the experiments are run for approximately 100 epochs of ADPK dataset. For multi-task network, one epoch is counted as parsing through entire ADPK and Liver dataset.

4   Results

We summarize the mean dice score of left and right kidney in percentage for each experiment in Table 1. Valid A, B and C represent validation sets used for 3-fold cross validation.

Table 1. Comparison of mean left and right kidney dice score in percentage for various experiments

Method	Loss	Valid A	Valid B	Valid C
2D FCN [4]	Dice	82.7%	84.8%	85.2%
3D FCN	Dice	94.2%	93.6%	94.4%
Multi-task 3D FCN	Dice	94.5%	**94.6%**	**94.8%**
Multi-task 3D FCN	Bootstrap cross entropy	**94.9%**	94.4%	**94.8%**

Qualitatively, the results are summarized in Fig. 3 where each row represents a different case from ADPK dataset. It is clear that 3D FCN in itself improves the segmentation accuracy by as much as 10% when compared to 2D FCN. 2D FCN produce noisy segmentations (row 1 and 2) because each axial slice is processed independently. Also, the misclassification between liver and kidney in presence of both renal and hepatic cysts is severe as compared to 3D FCN. Although 3D FCN in general resolve such misclassifications (row 1) because it learns from global 3D features, we show cases (row 2) where it fails. In such cases, we find that the proposed multi-task architectures achieve higher accuracy. One explanation could be that the encoder of multi-task architecture generates more rich features than single task architecture, because it is forced to learn an additional task of liver segmentation. Rich features thus make it easier to classify kidney from surrounding organs. The accuracy is also improved in cases where conventional 3D FCN misclassify spleen and kidney (row 3) or when the kidney is contrast enhanced (row 4). Conventional 3D FCN results in poor accuracy in case of high contrast kidneys because of lack of such cases in ADPK dataset. Obtaining better results with multi-task architecture without adding additional contrast enhanced ADPK in the dataset has interesting implications. Thus in summary, while the mean accuracy change from single-task to multi-task might not look significant (Table 1), for specific cases we find considerable improvement in accuracy. With respect to loss function; we find that simply bootstrapping cross entropy loss works as good as dice loss or even marginally better (Table 1). Results in Fig. 3 show both cases when bootstrap loss performs better (row 1) and vice versa (row 4). With respect to convergence speed, we find no difference between the two as shown in Fig. 4.

We evaluate the clinical usefulness of proposed method using a scatter plot (Fig. 5) which shows TKV error in percentage on entire dataset. The mean absolute error is 3.86% which is below the precision requirement of 5% for clinical applications. Although, for unique test cases or small kidneys, we find multiple cases with absolute error to be larger than 5%. Such cases can be reduced either by increasing the dataset size of ADPK or including additional tasks such as spleen or colon segmentation using multi-task approach.

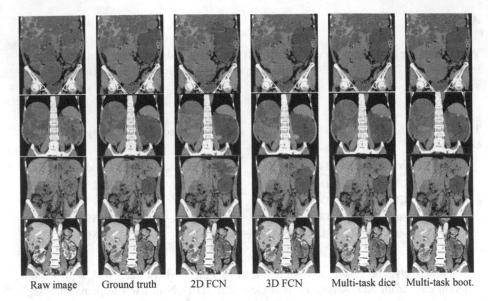

|Raw image|Ground truth|2D FCN|3D FCN|Multi-task dice|Multi-task boot.|

Fig. 3. Qualitative comparison of results. Rows represents coronal slice each taken from a different case in ADPK dataset. Columns represent results obtained from different experiments.

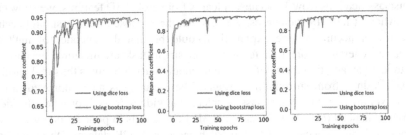

Fig. 4. Comparison of mean kidney dice coefficient on validation set A, B and C obtained using multi task dice (Red) and multi-task bootstrap (Green) methodology

5   Conclusion and Future Work

In this work, we propose a multi-task 3D FCN for ADPK segmentation and achieve a mean TKV error acceptable to be directly used in clinical applications. After analyzing both conventional single task 3D FCN approach and proposed multi-task 3D FCN approach we find that multi-task approach improves the segmentation accuracy especially for high contrast ADPK and cases where both renal and hepatic cysts are present. Higher accuracy achieved using multi-task architecture implies that segmentation performance can be improved without explicitly adding data corresponding to target segmentation anatomy. In the future, we would like to analyze the performance by adding additional tasks such as spleen, colon or even segmentation of unrelated anatomies like heart and lung. We also analyzed in this work that simply bootstrapping cross entropy loss works similar to dice loss to counter class imbalance issue. It would be interesting to analyze its performances for even severe inter and intra class imbalance tasks such as aorta segmentation from CT images.

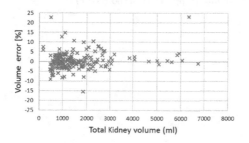

Fig. 5. Scattered plot showing percentage TKV error over the entire dataset

Acknowledgements. We acknowledge using Reedbush-L (SGI Rackable C2112-4GP3/C1102-GP8) HPC system in the Information Technology Center, The University of Tokyo for GPU computational resources used in this work.

References

1. Muto, S., Kawano, H., Isotani, S., Ide, H., Horie, S.: Novel semi-automated kidney volume measurements in autosomal dominant polycystic kidney disease. Clin. Exp. Nephrol. **22**(3), 583–590 (2017)
2. Gansevoort, R.T., Arici, M., Benzing, T.: Recommendations for the use of tolvaptan in autosomal dominant polycystic kidney disease: a position statement on behalf of the ERA-EDTA working groups on inherited kidney disorders and european renal best practice. Nephrol. Dial. Transpl. **31**(3), 337–348 (2016)
3. NIH homepage: https://ghr.nlm.nih.gov/condition/polycystic-kidney-disease#statistics. Accessed 03 Feb 2017
4. Sharma, K., Rupprecht, C., Caroli, A.: Automatic segmentation of kidneys using deep learning for total kidney volume quantification in autosomal dominant polycystic kidney disease. Sci. Rep. **7**(1), 2049 (2017)
5. Çiçek, Ö., Abdulkadir, A., Lienkamp, S.S., Brox, T., Ronneberger, O.: 3D U-Net: Learning Dense Volumetric Segmentation from Sparse Annotation. In: Ourselin, S., Joskowicz, L., Sabuncu, M.R., Unal, Gozde, Wells, W. (eds.) MICCAI 2016. LNCS, vol. 9901, pp. 424–432. Springer, Cham (2016). https://doi.org/10.1007/978-3-319-46723-8_49
6. Milletari, F., Navab, N., Ahmadi, S.A.: V-net: Fully convolutional neural networks for volumetric medical image segmentation. In: Fourth International Conference on 3D Vision (3DV), 2016, pp. 565–571. IEEE (2016)

7. Moeskops, P., et al.: Deep Learning for Multi-task Medical Image Segmentation in Multiple Modalities. In: Ourselin, S., Joskowicz, L., Sabuncu, M.R., Unal, G., Wells, W. (eds.) MICCAI 2016. LNCS, vol. 9901, pp. 478–486. Springer, Cham (2016). https://doi.org/10.1007/978-3-319-46723-8_55
8. Pohlen, T., Hermans, A., Mathias, M., Leibe, B.: Full-resolution residual networks for semantic segmentation in street scenes. In: Proceedings of the IEEE Conference on Computer Vision and Pattern Recognition, pp. 4151–4160 (2017)

Dynamic Routing on Deep Neural Network for Thoracic Disease Classification and Sensitive Area Localization

Yan Shen[✉] and Mingchen Gao

Department of Computer Science and Engineering, University at Buffalo,
Amherst, NY, USA
yshen22@buffalo.edu

Abstract. We present and evaluate a new deep neural network architecture for automatic thoracic disease detection on chest X-rays. Deep neural networks has shown great success in a plethora of vision recognition tasks such as image classification and object detection by stacking multiple layers of convolutional neural networks (CNN) in a feed forward manner. However the performance gain by going deeper has reached bottlenecks as a result of the trade-off between model complexity and discrimination power. We address this problem by utilizing recently developed routing-by-agreement mechanism in our architecture. A novel characteristic of our network structure is that it extends routing to two types of layer connections (1) connection between feature maps in dense layers, (2) connection between primary capsules and prediction capsules in final classification layer. We show that our networks achieves comparable results with much fewer layers in the measurement of AUC score. We further show the combined benefits of model interpretability by generating Gradient-weighted Class Activation Mapping (Grad-CAM) for localization. We demonstrate our results on the NIH chestX-ray14 dataset that consists of 112,120 images on 30,805 unique patients including 14 kinds of lung diseases.

1 Introduction

It is a relatively easy task for radiologists to read and diagnose chest X-ray images. However, teaching a computer to process hospital-scale of chest X-ray scans is extremely challenging. Chest X-rays is the most common imaging examinations in practice, with approximately 2 billion procedures per year [8]. The success of chest X-ray disease detection will lay the groundwork for more complex systems to provide consistent, trustable and interpretable second opinions on reading medical images of all kinds of modalities.

Deep Learning methods have been applied to disease classification, sensitive area localization and tissue segmentation [7]. The success of deep learning has made computer program an indispensable aid to physicians for disease analysis

© Springer Nature Switzerland AG 2018
Y. Shi et al. (Eds.): MLMI 2018, LNCS 11046, pp. 389–397, 2018.
https://doi.org/10.1007/978-3-030-00919-9_45

[11]. "ChestX-ray14" is so far the largest publicly available chest X-rays dataset [13]. Along with the collection of the dataset, baseline models were also tested on this dataset. The best is a 50 layers ResNet. There are many followed up works on this dataset, such as DenseNet based models [8,14] or attention guided CNN to integrate disease-specific region and global cues [3]. However most of the current work randomly split the data into training, validation and testing. It is likely to have images from the same patient appear in both training and testing set. Such experimental setting makes the direct comparisons of reported evaluation metrics problematic. Yao [15] uses a learnable Log-Sum-Exp pooling functions in their network for classification and use Log-Sum-Exp pooling function to generate salient maps at different resolutions to indicate regions of interest (ROI). We also follow the split suggestion by Wang [13,15] and does not use additional training data.

A highly correlated task with disease classification is to localize the sensitive area related to diseases. Weakly-supervised pathology localization has been used to generate heatmap based on class activation mappings (CAMs) [16]. RR Selvaraju [10] used Gradient-weighted Class Activation Mapping (Grad-CAM) as a more generalized form of CAMs without the need of global average pooling at last layer of feature maps. Zhe et al. proposed a unified approach to simultaneously perform disease identification and localization [6].

Current advancement in deep network's recognition power is typically achieved by going deeper with more layers and denser connections. One exception is Hinton's Capsule net [9] which shows promising potential by its novel structure. The network's connectivity adapts to the coherence of input feature vectors other than being optimized through back propagation. The activations in higher levels are achieved by routing-by-agreement iteration. Dilin et al. [12] views Capsule net as minimizing a clustering loss function with a KL divergence regularization iteratively. Capsule network has been extended to many applications, includes but not limited to pathology lung segmentation [5] and brain tumor type classification [1].

Inspired by Hinton's work, this paper proposes a new implementation of Capsule net on CNNs. Our model involves three key contributions.

- We introduce dense connectivities with dynamic routing into our network. Dense connectivity is achieved by a 1×1 convolutional layer that takes all of the previous feature maps as input. And we extend the routing-by-agreement mechanism to that 1×1 convolutional layer. This preserves DenseNet's nice property of facilitating training process while incorporates Capsule Net's routing mechanism to select more relevant feature maps in a bottom-up fashion. To the best of our knowledge, our paper is the first work that extends dynamic routing to convolutional layers.
- Our model is efficiently implemented using kernel trick. Feature maps need only to be calculated once per layer. The routing coefficient is set to be trainable only at the last iteration. Such implementation reduces the time for training and inference as its complexity is comparable to a single layer without routing iterations.

- Rather than generating heatmap before global average pooling layers or fully connected layer, we generate heatmap before an average pooling layer of strides 4 × 4 and a fully connected dynamic routing layer before prediction layer. Our generated heatmap preserves the benefit of model interpretability as CAM without sacrifice classification accuracy by introducing global average pooling.

2 Methods

In our networks, chest X-ray images are firstly pre-processed and then passed to a down-sampling block of Conv-Pool-Conv-Pool. The first convolutional layer is of size 7 and stride 2. And then the second pooling layer is using max-pooling of size 3 and stride 2. Following with the max-pooling layer, we use a convolutional layer of size 1 and stride 2. Finally we use average-pooling layer of size 2 and stride 2 before feeding to our dense layer.

We use dense blocks after down-sampling blocks. Our dense block follows the pattern in [4] except for the 1 × 1 convolutional layer. A dense layer consists of consecutive layers of composite functions which takes concatenated output produced in previous layers. Each composite function $H_l(\cdot)$ consists 6 consecutive operations: BN-ReLu-Conv(1 × 1)-BN-ReLu-Conv(3 × 3). In our network, dynamic routing is included between the connections of 1 × 1 convolution layer. A dynamic routing dense block is illustrated in Fig. 1.

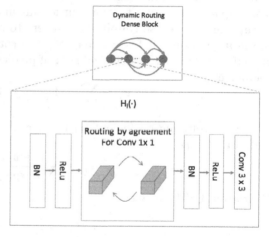

Fig. 1. Each dense block consists 8 layers of composite functions. 1 × 1 convolutional layer is updated using dynamic routing.

Subsequent to dense blocks, we use a larger size convolutional layer with size 9 and stride 1. Then we use a average pooling layer of size 4 and stride 4 before we use a fully connected capsule layer to class labels. In our fully connected capsule layer, we reshape the feature map to primary capsules by taking 8 consecutive feature maps of each pixel as one capsule. Then we route the fully connected layer between primary capsules and disease label capsule following the routing by agreement mechanism in [9]. Finally, we take the L_2 norm of each vectors in digit capsules as the digit of each disease label.

2.1 1×1 Convolutional Capsule Layer

In Capsule net, the coupling coefficient is updated iteratively as the agreements between input and output from the layer below. We extend the routing-by-agreement mechanism [9] to 1×1 convolutional layer. The output capsule vector and routing coefficient can be computed element-wisely. However this brute-force effort is computational exhaustive and not feasible. The convolutional kernels and coupling coefficient share the property of parameter sharing. We propose to use kernel trick to implement dynamic routing on feature maps efficiently. Recall that in 1×1 convolutional layer, every output of feature map $\mathbf{g}_j$ is the linear combination of input feature maps $\mathbf{f}_i$.

$$\mathbf{g}_j = \sum_i K_{i,j} \mathbf{f}_i, \tag{1}$$

where $K_{i,j}$ is the scalar element of convolutional kernel. Here we follow the dynamic routing and define the term $\hat{\mathbf{f}}_{j|i} = W_{i,j} \mathbf{f}_i$ as the "prediction vector" from input feature map $\mathbf{f}_i$ to output feature map $\mathbf{g}_j$. Similarly as the mechanism of capsule net, we use coupling coefficient to represent the agreements between the input and output feature map of 1×1 convolutional layer. Specifically, the output feature maps is weighted sum of prediction vectors weighted on coupling coefficient.

$$\mathbf{g}_j = \sum_i c_{i,j} \hat{\mathbf{f}}_{j|i} = \sum_i W_{i,j} c_{i,j} \mathbf{f}_i, \tag{2}$$

where the coupling coefficient term $c_{i,j}$ is updated by the following two steps:
Softmax Step:

$$c_{i,j} = \frac{\exp(b_{i,j})}{\sum_k \exp(b_{i,k})} \tag{3}$$

Evidence Update Step:

$$b_{i,j} \leftarrow b_{i,j} + \hat{\mathbf{f}}_{j|i} \cdot \text{squash}(\mathbf{g}_j) \tag{4}$$

Rather than getting the new couping coefficient by updating the whole feature map in every iteration. We can take the simplified step by applying kernel tricks.

$$\hat{\mathbf{f}}_{j|i} \cdot \text{squash}(\mathbf{g}_j) = \frac{|\mathbf{g}_j|}{1 + |\mathbf{g}_j|^2} \hat{\mathbf{f}}_{j|i} \cdot \mathbf{g}_j \tag{5}$$

The term $\hat{\mathbf{f}}_{j|i} \cdot \mathbf{g}_j$ can be computed as:

$$\hat{\mathbf{f}}_{j|i} \cdot \mathbf{g}_j = \sum_l \hat{\mathbf{f}}_{j|i} \cdot c_{i,j} \hat{\mathbf{f}}_{j|l}$$

$$= \sum_l W_{i,j} W_{l,j} c_{l,j} \mathbf{f}_l \cdot \mathbf{f}_i$$

And the norm of feature maps $|\mathbf{g}_j|$ can be computed as the weighted sum of $\hat{\mathbf{f}}_{j|i} \cdot \mathbf{g}_j$:

$$|\mathbf{g}_j|^2 = \mathbf{g}_j \cdot \mathbf{g}_j = \sum_{i=1} c_{i,j} \mathbf{g}_j \cdot \hat{\mathbf{f}}_{j|i} \tag{6}$$

So we only need vector product of input feature maps $\mathbf{f}_l \cdot \mathbf{f}_i$, convolutional kernel $W_{i,j}$ and routing coefficient $\mathbf{c}_{i,j}$ produced in last step to compute the term $\hat{\mathbf{f}}_{j|i} \cdot \mathrm{squash}(\mathbf{g}_j)$ to update routing coefficient. The inner product of input feature maps $\mathbf{f}_i \cdot \mathbf{f}_j$ only need to be computed once and are shared in every step of iteration.

3 Experiment Results

ChestX-ray14 dataset includes front view of chest X-ray images. Each one is annotated with multiple of 14 categories of lung diseases. We augment our training data by flipping the training images, randomly adjusting their brightness and contrast. To make our training and inferencing tractable, we resize the original chest X-ray image from original resolution 1024×1024 to 256×256. Those images are then standardized to zero mean and unit scale as the first step of our network. To validate the performance of our model, we follow the training and testing partition suggested by [13] with 86524 training/validation images and 25596 testing images.

Our neural network model is implemented using Tensorflow. Models are trained using Adam optimizer. The learning rate is set to $\alpha = 0.001$, $\beta_1 = 0.9$, $\beta_2 = 0.999$ and $\epsilon = 10^{-8}$ as our default parameters. Parameters are initialized using random normal initializations.

Curriculum learning is used in our training to stabilize our training process [2]. As sparse positive labels in training data favors negative prediction, we set a down-scaling parameter on negative labels to compensate for that. We firstly set $\lambda_+ = 1$ and $\lambda_- = 0.05$. And then we shifted to $\lambda_+ = \frac{|N|}{|P|+|N|}$ and $\lambda_- = \frac{|P|}{|P|+|N|}$ after 50 epochs. Our whole training takes around $400,000$ global steps from random initialization and converges in $150,000$ global steps. We use GTX-1080Ti to accelerate our training process. It takes about 30 h for our whole training process. We train our network only on chest X-ray dataset without any pre-training.

We explore the impact of dynamic routing on 1×1 convolutional capsules and the variations of network architectures on the performance of disease classifications. We replace the 1×1 convolutional capsule in our proposed model to standard 1×1 convolutional in our baseline. All the variations in network architectures are trained using the same settings to compare apple to apple.

Table 1. Compared to our baseline model, our proposed model achieves performance increase with replacing the 1×1 convolutional layer with our 1×1 capsule convolutional layer. The gain is brought by the increased generalization ability through routing-by-agreement between capsules. Our results also outperforms state-of-the-art algorithm in the literature.

Pathology	Wang et al. [13]	Yao et al. [15]	Our proposed	Our baseline
Atelectasis	0.7003	0.733	**0.766**	0.616
Cardiomegaly	0.8100	**0.856**	0.801	0.761
Effusion	0.7585	**0.806**	0.797	0.710
Infiltration	0.6614	0.673	**0.751**	0.611
Mass	0.6933	**0.777**	0.760	0.589
Nodule	0.6687	0.718	**0.741**	0.534
Pneumonia	0.6580	0.684	**0.778**	0.569
Pneumothorax	0.7993	**0.805**	0.800	0.662
Consolidation	0.7032	0.711	**0.787**	0.617
Edema	0.8052	0.806	**0.820**	0.744
Emphysema	0.8330	**0.842**	0.773	0.672
Fibrosis	**0.7859**	0.743	0.765	0.630
Pleural thickening	0.6835	0.724	**0.759**	0.611
Hernia	**0.8717**	0.775	0.748	0.441
Average	0.738	0.761	**0.775**	0.626

Finally, we generate Grad-CAM for as interpretation of our model's prediction. We investigate these regions that are considered important for our disease predictions and compare it with the bounding box that are provided by professional physicians. To define the important region of our generated Grad-CAM, we normalize our Grad-CAM from 0 to 1, and preserve those areas with an activation larger than 0.1 as the important region.

Classification Accuracy Many of the follow up works on this dataset split the dataset randomly rather follow the suggestion given in the original dataset [13]. We compare our models with the only two utilizing the official splits of training and testing data. Our model is demonstrated to be the state-of-the-art as shown in Table 1.

Convolutional capsule net achieves stable results in every category of pathology label predictions with much smaller number of layers and simpler network structures. Replacing our 1×1 convolutional capsules with standard 1×1 convolutional layer results in degraded accuracies in nearly all categories of pathology. In average, the standard standard 1×1 convolutional layer reduced accuracy by 15%. The increased accuracy reported in test dataset by our proposed model demonstrated the effectiveness of adopting capsule routing in convolutional layers.

Disease Localization We generate heap-map to visualize the area that is indicative of a suspect disease. We use the Grad-CAM to generate heat-map for disease area localization. We generate Grad-CAM M_c from primary capsules at the resolution of 32×32 before 4×4 average pooling layer. And then we up-sample it to the dimensions of input image and overlay it with the corresponding images. Figure 2 shows the heat-map generated by two chest x-ray images of patients diagnosed with Atelectasis. Qualitatively, the Grad-CAM of our model almost overlaps with the sensitive area of lung that are diagnosed with the corresponding pathology. Specifically in Fig. 2(a), the patient has Atelectasis in upper part of his left lung. The Grad-CAM of his chest X-ray image overlaps with his upper-left lung. Similarly in Fig. 2(b) generated Grad-CAM for patient with upper-right lung pathology is activated at upper-right lung. We find that the heat-map generated at primary capsule level is indicative to disease area even though it is generated at low resolution.

For a quantitative analysis, We compare our generated Grad-CAM with the hand annotated ground truth (GT) boxes included in ChestX-ray14. Although the total number of B-Box annotations (1600 images) is relatively small compared with the entire dataset, it is still reasonable to estimate on the interpretation of our model. To exam the accuracy of our computed Grad-CAM versus the GT B-Box, we use Intersection over the detected B-Box ratio (IoBB) for measurement. Table 2 illustrates the localization accuracy (Acc.) for each disease type, with $T(IoBB) \in \{0.1, 0.25, 0.5\}$.

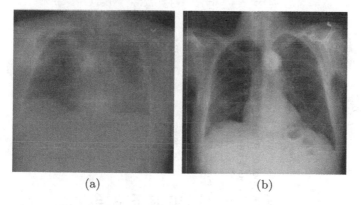

(a)   (b)

Fig. 2. Two Patients with lung Atelectasis. The dynamic routing dense model along with Grad-CAM identifies the left or right upper lung Atelectasis, respectively and correctly classifies the pathology.

Table 2. Pathology localization accuracy for 8 disease classes. Because our primary capsule only have a resolution of 8×8, we use the layer before 4×4 average pooling that have a resolution of 32×32. Our generated Grad-CAM is like neuralization on CAM and Grad-CAM that trades-off on model interpretation and classification

T(IoBB)	Atelectasis	Cardiomegaly	Effusion	Infiltration	Mass	Nodule	Pneumonia	Pneumothorax
T(IoBB) = 0.1								
Acc.	0.6977	0.8333	0.6234	0.635	0.4324	0.1234	0.6973	0.4687
T(IoBB) = 0.25								
Acc.	0.4534	0.8277	0.4840	0.5734	0.3866	0.0023	0.5342	0.3512
T(IoBB) = 0.5								
Acc.	0.2198	0.5231	0.2473	0.2412	0.1854	0.0019	0.3693	0.0716

4   Conclusion

In this work, we handle the disease detection problem by using dynamic routing between 1×1 convolutional layers in dense block. We further test our network's detection accuracy and model interpretability in our experiment. For future work, we plan to improve disease localization by integrating location information provided in the dataset using semi-supervised learning.

References

1. Afshar, P., Mohammadi, A., Plataniotis, K.N.: Brain tumor type classification via capsule networks. arXiv preprint arXiv:1802.10200 (2018)
2. Bengio, Y., Louradour, J., Collobert, R., Weston, J.: Curriculum learning. In ICML, pp. 41–48. ACM (2009)
3. Guan, Q., Huang, Y., Zhong, Z., Zheng, Z., Zheng, L., Yang, Y., et al.: Diagnose like a radiologist: Attention guided convolutional neural network for thorax disease classification. arXiv preprint arXiv:1801.09927 (2018)
4. Huang, G., Liu, Z., van der Maaten, L., Weinberger, K.Q.: Densely connected convolutional networks. In: CVPR (2017)
5. LaLonde, R., Bagci, U.: Capsules for object segmentation. arXiv preprint arXiv:1804.04241 (2018)
6. Li, Z., et al.: Thoracic disease identification and localization with limited supervision. In: CVPR (2017)
7. Litjens, G., et al.: A survey on deep learning in medical image analysis. Med. Image Anal. **42**, 60–88 (2017)
8. Rajpurkar, P., et al.: Chexnet: radiologist-level pneumonia detection on chest x-rays with deep learning. arXiv preprint arXiv:1711.05225 (2017)
9. Sabour, S., Frosst, N., Hinton, G.E.: Dynamic routing between capsules. In: NIPS, pp. 3859–3869 (2017)
10. Selvaraju, R.R., Cogswell, M., Das, A., Vedantam, R., Parikh, D., Batra, D., et al.: Grad-cam: visual explanations from deep networks via gradient-based localization. In: CVPR, pp. 618–626 (2017)
11. Shin, H.-C., et al.: Deep convolutional neural networks for computer-aided detection: Cnn architectures, dataset characteristics and transfer learning. TMI **35**(5), 1285–1298 (2016)
12. Wang, D., Liu, Q.: An optimization view on dynamic routing between capsules. In: ICLR workshop (2018)
13. Wang, X., Peng, Y., Lu, L., Lu, Z., Bagheri, M., Summers, R.M., et al.: Chestx-ray8: hospital-scale chest x-ray database and benchmarks on weakly-supervised classification and localization of common thorax diseases. In: CVPR, pp. 3462–3471. IEEE (2017)
14. Yao, L., Poblenz, E., Dagunts, D., Covington, B., Bernard, D., Lyman, K., et al.: Learning to diagnose from scratch by exploiting dependencies among labels. arXiv preprint arXiv:1710.10501 (2017)
15. Yao, L., Prosky, J., Poblenz, E., Covington, B., Lyman, K.: Weakly supervised medical diagnosis and localization from multiple resolutions. arXiv preprint arXiv:1803.07703 (2018)
16. Zhou, B., Khosla, A., Lapedriza, A., Oliva, A., Torralba, A.: Learning deep features for discriminative localization. In: CVPR, pp. 2921–2929. IEEE (2016)

Deep Learning for Fast and Spatially-Constrained Tissue Quantification from Highly-Undersampled Data in Magnetic Resonance Fingerprinting (MRF)

Zhenghan Fang[1], Yong Chen[1], Mingxia Liu[1], Yiqiang Zhan[2], Weili Lin[1], and Dinggang Shen[1(✉)]

[1] Department of Radiology and BRIC, University of North Carolina at Chapel Hill, Chapel Hill, NC 27599, USA
zhenghan@ad.unc.edu, dgshen@med.unc.edu
[2] Institute for Medical Imaging Technology, School of Biomedical Engineering, Shanghai Jiao Tong University, Shanghai 200240, China

Abstract. Magnetic resonance fingerprinting (MRF) is a novel quantitative imaging technique that allows simultaneous measurements of multiple important tissue properties in human body, e.g., T1 and T2 relaxation times. While MRF has demonstrated better scan efficiency as compared to conventional quantitative imaging techniques, further acceleration is desired, especially for certain subjects such as infants and young children. However, the conventional MRF framework only uses a simple template matching algorithm to quantify tissue properties, without considering the underlying spatial association among pixels in MRF signals. In this work, we aim to accelerate MRF acquisition by developing a new post-processing method that allows accurate quantification of tissue properties with *fewer* sampling data. Moreover, to improve the accuracy in quantification, the MRF signals from multiple surrounding pixels are used together to better estimate tissue properties at the central target pixel, which was simply done with the signal only from the target pixel in the original template matching method. In particular, a deep learning model, i.e., U-Net, is used to learn the mapping from the MRF signal evolutions to the tissue property map. To further reduce the network size of U-Net, principal component analysis (PCA) is used to reduce the dimensionality of the input signals. Based on *in vivo* brain data, our method can achieve accurate quantification for both T1 and T2 by using only 25% time points, which are *four times* of acceleration in data acquisition compared to the original template matching method.

Keywords: Magnetic resonance fingerprinting · Relaxation times
Deep learning

1 Introduction

Quantitative imaging, i.e., quantification of tissue properties in human body, is desired in both clinics and research. The quantified tissue properties allow physicians to better distinguish between healthy and pathological tissues [1] with certain quantitative

The original version of this chapter was revised: an Acknowledgements section has been added. The correction to this chapter is available at https://doi.org/10.1007/978-3-030-00919-9_47

metrics, thus making it easier to objectively compare different examinations in longitudinal studies [2]. Also, these quantitative measurements could be more representative of the underlying changes at the cellular level [3, 4], compared to qualitative results obtained from standard MR imaging data. [5]

One of the major barriers of translating conventional quantitative imaging techniques for clinical use is the prohibitively long data acquisition time. Recently, a new framework for MR image acquisition and post-processing, termed as Magnetic Resonance Fingerprinting (MRF) [6], has been introduced, which can significantly reduce the acquisition time needed for quantitative measurement. The MRF framework first acquires a series of highly-undersampled MR images with different contrast weightings using pseudo-randomized acquisition parameters, such as repetition times and flip angles. Note that different tissues or materials have unique signal evolutions that depend on multiple tissue properties. Then, the signal evolution from each pixel is matched to a precomputed dictionary, containing the signal evolutions of a wide range of tissue types. The entry with the best matching signal evolution in the dictionary is selected, with its tissue properties finally assigned for this pixel. The simultaneous measurement of multiple tissue properties and high undersampling rate in the acquisition enable fast quantitative imaging using MRF.

While MRF has demonstrated higher scan efficiency as compared to conventional quantitative imaging techniques, further acceleration is needed as the current scan time is still too long for certain subjects such as infants and young children. In the MRF framework, the acquisition time is approximately proportional to the number of time points used in the imaging sequence, i.e., the number of acquired images with different contrast weightings. In this study, we propose to reduce the acquisition time by reducing the number of time points acquired in each scan. However, the reduction of time points will result in a shorter signal evolution and therefore the loss of useful information at each pixel, which influences the accuracy of tissue quantification.

To compensate for the loss of information at each pixel and improve the quantification accuracy, we propose to use additional information from the space domain, i.e., signal evolutions at neighboring pixels, to assist the estimation at each target pixel. We believe that spatial context information is critical for the following two reasons. *First*, the tissue properties at different pixels are not independent, but actually correlated. For example, the adjacent pixels of one tissue are likely to have similar tissue properties. Therefore, neighboring pixels could be used together as spatial constraint to regulate the estimation and correct errors at the central target pixel. *Second*, the undersampling in k-space in MRF acquisition results in aliasing in the image space, due to distribution of the target pixel signal to neighboring pixels. Therefore, using spatial information may help retrieve the scattered signals and finally provide a better quantification with MRF.

To achieve the aforementioned spatially-constrained quantification, we resort to a deep learning model, i.e., U-Net [7], to learn the mapping from the MRF signals of a cross-section slice to its tissue property map. Because of using the convolution and down- and up-sampling operations in the U-Net, quantitative tissue properties from one pixel in the output space are spatially correlated with signal evolutions from multiple neighboring pixels in the input space. In addition, a principal component analysis (PCA) is further performed to reduce the dimensionality of the MRF signals before feeding them into the U-Net, thus significantly reducing network size as well as facilitating network training and finally improving accuracy in tissue quantification.

Note that deep learning has been used for MRF post-processing in previous studies. For example, [8] used a neural network to map the signal evolution at each pixel to the underlying tissue properties. For the same mapping, [9] used a convolutional neural network, where each signal evolution was treated as a time sequence and the convolution was done in time domain. The results of these studies demonstrated potential of deep learning methods for tissue quantification in MRF. However, both studies focused only on improving the quantification speed, instead of accelerating MRF scanning. In addition, these previous studies used *either* fully-sampled MRF images *or* phantom data for method validation. The performance using the actual highly-undersampled *in vivo* data as proposed in the MRF framework needs to be evaluated.

2   Materials and Method

In our spatially-constrained tissue quantification method, the MRF images are fed into a U-Net to first extract spatial features and then estimate the tissue property map. One network is trained for each tissue property under estimation, i.e., T1 or T2. To deal with the large quantitative range of tissue properties in human body, we develop a relative difference based loss function to balance the contributions of tissues with different property ranges. Also, to address the across-subject variation and high-dimensionality of MRF signals, we propose two data pre-processing strategies, i.e., (1) energy-based normalization, and (2) PCA-based compression. In the following, we first introduce the data acquisition and pre-processing methods in Sect. 2.1, and then present our proposed deep learning based method in Sect. 2.2.

2.1   Data Acquisition and Pre-processing

Data Acquisition. We acquired MRF data of cross-section slices of human brains on a Siemens 3T Prisma scanner using a 32-channel head coil. Highly-undersampled 2D MR images were acquired using fast imaging with steady state precession (FISP) sequence. For each slice, 2,304 time points were acquired and each time point consists of data from only one spiral readout (reduction factor = 48). Other imaging parameters included: field of view (FOV): 30 cm; matrix size: 256×256; slice thickness: 5 mm; flip angle: $5°–12°$.

The MRF dictionary was simulated with 13,123 combinations of T1 (60–5000 ms) and T2 (10–500 ms). The reference tissue property maps were obtained by dictionary matching from all 2,304 time points. These maps are considered as "ground truth" in this work.

Energy-based Data Normalization. Since the magnitude of MRF signals varies largely across different subjects, it is critical to normalize these signals to a common magnitude range in MRF-based learning framework. In this work, we propose to normalize the energy (i.e., sum of squared magnitude) of the acquired signal evolution at each pixel to 1.

PCA-based Compression. MRF implementation typically acquires a large number of images with different contrast weightings for one subject, i.e., 2,304 in total and 576 after undersampling. In this case, it is unreasonable to feed such high-dimensional data directly into U-Net, as it results in a prohibitively large network size, which is challenging for efficient training and good generalization. Inspired by a previous work [10], we propose to perform PCA for dimensionality reduction of the signal evolutions after normalization. Specifically, the bases of the principal component subspace are obtained from signal evolutions in the dictionary. The k largest eigenvalues are retained with a threshold energy E (i.e., $E = 99.9\%$ and $k = 17$ in our study). As a result, the input channels of U-Net are compressed to $2k$, with each channel representing the real or imaginary part of the coefficient along one basis.

2.2 Proposed U-Net Model

In conventional template matching method, only the signal evolution from a particular local pixel is used to estimate tissue properties at the corresponding pixel in the tissue property map, without considering the global context information (e.g., spatial association among pixels) of the input MRF images. Actually, for each pixel, signals from its neighboring pixels may also provide important *spatial constraints* for estimating the tissue properties. Therefore, in this work, we resort to U-Net to capture both the local and global information of MRF images, with the architecture shown in Fig. 1.

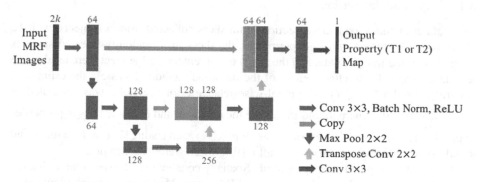

Fig. 1. U-net architecture. Each blue block represents a multi-channel feature map, and gray blocks represent copied feature maps. The number of channels is denoted at the top or bottom of each block. The arrows denote different operations.

As shown in Fig. 1, this network consists of an encoder sub-network (i.e., left part of Fig. 1) that extracts multi-scale spatial features from the input MRF images, and a successive decoder sub-network (i.e., right part of Fig. 1) that uses the extracted features to generate the output tissue property (T1 or T2) map. During alternate feature extraction (3×3 convolution followed by ReLU activation) and down-sampling (2×2 max pooling) operations in the encoder sub-network, the information from distributed signals due to aliasing in MRF images is retrieved and summarized. Also, the spatial constraints among different pixels are now implicitly incorporated into the extracted feature maps. Then, the decoder sub-network expands (with the transpose convolution 2×2) the down-sampled feature maps and combines feature maps at different scales by copying and concatenating, to fuse global context knowledge with complementary local details, for accurate and spatially-consistent estimation of the tissue property map.

It is worth noting that T1 and T2 measures in human body have very large quantitative ranges. As a result, the loss function based on the conventional absolute difference between network estimation and ground-truth will be dominated by the tissues with high T1 or T2 values. To address this issue, we propose to use the *relative difference*, rather than absolute difference, in our loss function, as defined below:

$$L = \sum_{x \in \Omega} \left| \frac{\theta_x - \widehat{\theta}_x}{\theta_x} \right| \tag{1}$$

where Ω is the set of all pixels inside the brain region of a training slice, $\widehat{\theta}_x$ is the network output at pixel x, and θ_x is the corresponding ground-truth property. With Eq. (1), the loss function is balanced over tissues with different property ranges.

3 Experiments

3.1 Experimental Settings

Our dataset includes axial cross-section brain slices collected from 5 subjects, with 12 slices for each subject. In our experiments, the slices of 4 randomly selected subjects were used as the training data, and the slices of the remaining 1 subject were used as the testing data to validate effectiveness of the proposed method. To assess the estimation accuracy, similar to Eq. (1), the pixel-wise relative error at pixel x was computed as $e_x = \left| \theta_x - \widehat{\theta}_x \right| / \theta_x$, where θ_x and $\widehat{\theta}_x$ denote the reference and estimated tissue properties at pixel x. The average relative error over all pixels in each testing slice and the mean and standard deviation of the errors over all testing slices were also computed.

We first compared our proposed Spatially-constrained Tissue Quantification method (denoted as **STQ**) with the standard **D**ictionary **M**atching approach (denoted as **DM**). It is worth noting that there are three components in our method, including (1) energy-based data normalization, (2) relative difference based loss in Eq. (1), and (3) PCA-based compression. To evaluate the influence of each component, we further compared our proposed STQ method with its three variants: (1) **STQ** without data normalization (denoted as **STQ_N**), where the acquired MRF signals were directly used for the following PCA-based compression without energy normalization; (2) **STQ** using conventional absolute difference as loss function (denoted as **STQ_A**); and 3) **STQ** without using PCA-based compression (denoted as **STQ_P**), where the high-dimensional MRF signals were directly fed into U-Net without dimensionality reduction. For fair comparison, all these five competing methods were used to estimate tissue properties from the first 576 time points among all 2,304 time points (i.e., with the undersampling rate of 25%, or reducing the MRF acquisition time by 4 times).

3.2   Results

Comparison with Dictionary Matching. The tissue property maps of a testing slice obtained by DM and STQ, along with their error maps, are shown in Fig. 2. The estimation errors over the testing set achieved by DM are 19.4% (T1) and 12.3% (T2), and 5.6% (T1) and 8.8% (T2) by STQ, as shown in Table 1. We can see that our STQ method achieves 71.1% (T1) and 28.5% (T2) reductions in estimation errors compared

Table 1. The means and standard deviations of T1 and T2 estimation errors achieved by DM, STQ (our proposed method) and three variants of STQ (unit: %).

	DM	STQ	STQ_N	STQ_A	STQ_P
T1	19.4 ± 8.8	$\mathbf{5.6 \pm 1.8}$	7.7 ± 1.9	7.9 ± 3.7	6.9 ± 2.0
T2	12.3 ± 3.0	$\mathbf{8.8 \pm 1.9}$	10.8 ± 1.7	10.6 ± 3.2	9.0 ± 2.3

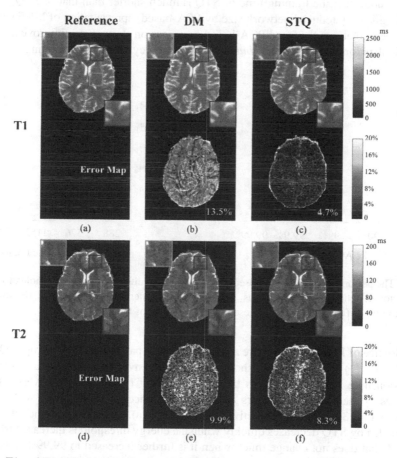

Fig. 2. T1 and T2 estimation results for a testing slice obtained by DM and STQ (our proposed method). (a) Reference T1 map. (b), (c) Estimated T1 maps and their corresponding relative error maps. (d) Reference T2 map. (e), (f) Estimated T2 maps and their corresponding relative error maps. For each error map, the mean relative error over brain area is shown at the lower-right corner.

to DM. Moreover, as shown by the visual results in Fig. 2, the quantitative maps of STQ have much less noise than those of DM, especially for T2 estimation, suggesting that the spatial constraint from neighboring pixels can help correct estimation errors and achieve more spatially-consistent quantification results. It is worth noting that the spatial resolution is not deteriorated by the denoising effect of STQ, i.e., the boundaries between different tissues are well-preserved (see the blue zoom-in boxes in Fig. 2). This advantage of our method is particularly important for the subsequent statistical analysis procedures such as segmentation of lesions.

Comparison with Three STQ Variants. We further compare our proposed STQ method with its three variants, with numerical results shown in Table 1. We can observe that our STQ method obtains the best results for both T1 and T2 estimations, compared with its three variants (i.e., STQ_N, STQ_A and STQ_P). These results clearly demonstrate the merits of our three proposed strategies, i.e., energy-based data normalization, relative difference based loss function, and PCA-based compression. It is worth noting that the training time of STQ is much shorter than that of STQ_P, due to the significantly reduced network size by PCA-based representation of MRF signals. This suggests that our proposed PCA-based compression strategy can improve *not only* the generalization of the network *but also* the efficiency of network training.

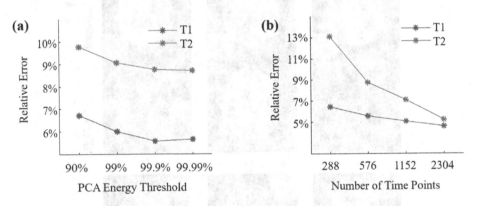

Fig. 3. The performance of the proposed method using (a) different energy thresholds for PCA eigenvector selection (with the x-axis representing the energy threshold), and (b) different acquisition times (with the x-axis representing the number of time points).

Influence of Parameters. There are two important parameters in our proposed STQ method, i.e., (1) the energy threshold for PCA eigenvector selection, and (2) data acquisition time (corresponding to the undersampling rate). Now we investigate the influences of these two parameters on the performance of our method, with results reported in Fig. 3(a) and (b), respectively. From Fig. 3(a), we can see that the estimation error yielded by STQ decreases quickly when the energy threshold is increased from 90 to 99.9%, but does not change much when it is further increased to 99.99%. Also, we change the acquisition time by extracting tissue properties from different numbers of time points, i.e., 288 (12.5%), 576 (25%), 1152 (50%), 2304 (100%). As shown in Fig. 3(b), there is a trade-off between acquisition time and quantification accuracy, and

STQ can achieve good estimation accuracy using 100%, 50% and 25% acquisition time. When the acquisition time is further reduced to 12.5%, the estimation error of STQ for T1 is still acceptable, but becomes much worse for T2 (i.e., relative error > 13%).

4   Conclusion

In this study, we have proposed a new MRF post-processing method for accurate tissue quantification from highly-undersampled data. Unlike the conventional method that performs estimation for each pixel separately, our method uses the signals at multiple pixels around the target pixel to jointly estimate its tissue property, resulting in more accurate and spatially-consistent quantification results. A deep learning model, i.e., U-Net, is used to learn the mapping from MRF signals to the desired tissue property map. The experimental results from *in vivo* brain data show that our method achieves good accuracy in T1 and T2 quantification using only 25% of time points (i.e., four times of reduction in acquisition time), and 71.1% (T1) and 28.5% (T2) reductions in estimation errors compared to the conventional dictionary matching method.

Acknowledgement. This work was supported in part by NIH grant **EB006733**.

References

1. Larsson, H.B.W., et al.: Assessment of demyelination, edema, and gliosis by in vivo determination of T1 and T2 in the brain of patients with acute attack of multiple sclerosis. Magn. Reson. Med. **11**(3), 337–348 (1989)
2. Usman, A.A., et al.: Cardiac magnetic resonance T2 mapping in the monitoring and follow-up of acute cardiac transplant rejection clinical perspective: a pilot study. Circ. Cardiovasc. Imaging **5**(6), 782–790 (2012)
3. Payne, A.R., et al.: Bright-blood T2-weighted MRI has high diagnostic accuracy for myocardial hemorrhage in myocardial infarction clinical perspective: a preclinical validation study in swine. Circ. Cardiovasc. Imaging **4**(6), 738–745 (2011)
4. Van Heeswijk, R.B., et al.: Free-breathing 3T magnetic resonance T2-mapping of the heart. JACC: Cardiovasc. Imaging **5**(12), 1231–1239 (2012)
5. Coppo, S., et al.: Overview of magnetic resonance fingerprinting. In: MAGNETOM Flash, 65 (2016)
6. Ma, D., et al.: Magnetic resonance fingerprinting. Nature **495**, 187–192 (2013)
7. Ronneberger, O., et al.: U-net: convolutional networks for biomedical image segmentation. In: International Conference on Medical Image Computing and Computer-Assisted Intervention. Springer, Cham (2015)
8. Cohen, O., et al.: Deep learning for rapid sparse MR fingerprinting reconstruction. arXiv preprint arXiv:1710.05267 (2017)
9. Hoppe, E., et al.: Deep learning for magnetic resonance fingerprinting: a new approach for predicting quantitative parameter values from time series. Stud. Health Technol. Inf. **243**, 202–206 (2017)
10. Mcgivney, D.F., et al.: SVD compression for magnetic resonance fingerprinting in the time domain. IEEE Trans. Med. Imaging **33**(12), 2311 (2014)

Correction to: Deep Learning for Fast and Spatially-Constrained Tissue Quantification from Highly-Undersampled Data in Magnetic Resonance Fingerprinting (MRF)

Zhenghan Fang, Yong Chen, Mingxia Liu, Yiqiang Zhan,
Weili Lin, and Dinggang Shen

Correction to:
Chapter "Deep Learning for Fast and Spatially-Constrained
Tissue Quantification from Highly-Undersampled Data
in Magnetic Resonance Fingerprinting (MRF)"
in: Y. Shi et al. (Eds.): *Machine Learning in Medical Imaging*,
LNCS 11046, https://doi.org/10.1007/978-3-030-00919-9_46

In the originally published version of this chapter, the Acknowledgements section was missing. This has been corrected and an Acknowledgements section has been added.

The updated version of this chapter can be found at
https://doi.org/10.1007/978-3-030-00919-9_46

Author Index

Printed in the United States
By Bookmasters